Anxiety and Depression
in Children and Adolescents

Thomas J. Huberty

Anxiety and Depression in Children and Adolescents

Assessment, Intervention, and Prevention

Springer

Thomas J. Huberty
Department of Counseling and Educational Psychology
School Psychology Program
Indiana University
Bloomington, IN, USA

ISBN 978-1-4614-3108-4   e-ISBN 978-1-4614-3110-7
DOI 10.1007/978-1-4614-3110-7
Springer New York Dordrecht Heidelberg London

Library of Congress Control Number: 2012932615

Printed on acid-free paper

Springer is part of Springer Science+Business Media (www.springer.com)

To Marsha, my life partner, soul mate, and best friend for her love, patience, support, and encouragement

To Christopher, who reaffirms my faith and hope in our children and youth

In memory of my mother

Preface

Anxiety and depression are two of the most prevalent mental health problems of childhood and adolescence, affecting up to as many as one-third of children and youth over their lifetimes, but also are among the most under-identified or misdiagnosed syndromes and disorders. They are also highly comorbid with each other and other disorders and are difficult to differentiate for clinical and research purposes. They present challenges in assessment, intervention, and consultation in clinical, community, and school settings. Because the conditions are so prevalent, complex, and comorbid, this book was conceptualized as an attempt to address the complexity from a combination of considering relevant research and applying that information to practice.

The book is based on principles and research in developmental psychopathology as the organizing theme, reflected in Part I that focuses on foundations with considerations for assessment and intervention. The first chapter describes major principles, concepts, and research in developmental psychopathology, with emphasis on protective and risk factors, vulnerability, and resilience. Historically, development has been conceptualized in five domains or contexts: (a) genetic factors, (b) biological factors, (c) cultural factors, (d) social factors, and (e) family factors. In this book, a sixth contextual factor has been added: *schools,* because children spend approximately one-fourth of their waking hours in school. Moreover, many of the emotional and behavioral problems of children and youth are related to school functioning and as many as half of mental health referrals originate from academic-related issues. Schools not only teach literacy skills, but are also major contributors to the development of social skills and competence, arguably making schooling the most important influence on children apart from the family. Thus, the chapter is organized around six contexts: genetic, biological, cultural, social, family, and school.

In Chap. 2, the developmental psychopathology and contextual themes are applied to anxiety and anxiety disorders, with emphasis on understanding the normal developmental aspects of anxiety. Unlike many disorders, anxiety is a normal developmental process that not only occurs in all people on almost a daily basis, but can be adaptive. When anxiety becomes so severe that it impairs personal, social, occupational, or academic functioning, interventions may be needed. The chapter summarizes the research with regard to the six contexts and concludes with implications for clinical practice.

Chapter 3 follows a similar format, recognizing that depression and mood disorders do not have the normal developmental progression as does anxiety. The third chapter follows the organization of Chap. 2 with regard to the six contexts and concludes with a discussion of clinical implications.

Chapter 4 addresses the important concept of emotion regulation, an area that has received increased research and practice attention in the last decade. Emotion regulation refers to the ability of a child to learn how to manage emotions and learn appropriate ways of expression. Some regulation processes are based on genetic and biological factors, but they are highly influenced by environmental factors, particularly parents, teachers, and peers who have strong influences on the development of regulation skills.

Part II contains two chapters that address how to conduct differential diagnosis of anxiety and depression, with emphasis on DSM-IV criteria. In Chap. 5, the primary anxiety disorders are discussed: Separation Anxiety Disorder, Generalized Anxiety Disorder, Obsessive-Compulsive Disorder, Social Phobia (Social Anxiety Disorder), Specific Phobia, Posttraumatic Stress Disorder, and Panic Disorder. Prevalence and epidemiology data are presented, along with primary symptoms and secondary features, comorbid disorders, differential diagnosis considerations, and typical assessment profiles. Chapter 6 follows the same format with discussion of Major Depressive Disorder, Dysthymia, and Bipolar Disorder. Both chapters conclude with discussion of a developmental psychopathology perspective on the anxiety and depressive disorders, respectively.

Part III focuses on assessment of anxiety and depressive disorders, with Chap. 7 presenting a summary of clinical assessment measures that are useful with internalizing disorders. This chapter emphasizes general principles of clinical interviewing, observation, and standardized rating scales and multidimensional measures. In Chaps. 8 and 9, more detailed description of the assessment of anxiety and depression are presented, including measures specific to each condition and how they are used with other assessment procedures. At the end of each chapter, a case study is provided that includes results from a psychological assessment.

Part IV contains Chaps. 10–13 that discuss interventions and prevention of anxiety and depression. Chapter 10 presents cognitive–behavioral therapy (CBT) as the primary direct intervention method for anxiety, as well as exposure, systematic desensitization, manualized CBT programs, and pharmacotherapy. Suggestions for conducting clinical and sample interview dialogues are presented. In Chap. 11, a similar format is followed for interventions for depression and mood disorders, with discussion of three primary therapeutic interventions: CBT, Interpersonal Psychotherapy, and Positive Psychotherapy. Discussion of treatment of the anxious-depressed syndrome that has features of both anxiety and depression is presented. Content about the relative effectiveness of CBT and medications is provided, as well. Discussion of intervening with suicidal children and adolescents is presented. Finally, the case example introduced in Chap. 9 is revisited with attention to developing interventions based on the assessment data.

Part IV also includes Chap. 12, which addresses school-based interventions for anxiety and depression. Emphasis is placed on screening for anxiety and depression and using a three-tier, problem-solving approach to interventions that can be done is schools. Primary topics include providing direct, indirect/consultative, and systems interventions in schools that are feasible and acceptable to school personnel, students, and parents.

The last chapter in Part IV addresses approaches toward prevention of anxiety and depression. Many of the mental health prevention programs for children and youth, including anxiety and depression, have been implemented in school settings, consistent with the perspective that schools provide the best opportunity to reach large numbers of youth. Community-based prevention programs also exist; therefore, discussion includes general principles for developing effective prevention programs. Descriptions of evidence-based prevention programs for anxiety and depression at the universal, selected, and indicated levels are presented.

Part V contains one chapter that addresses legal issues in educating anxious and depressed students in schools. Children and youth with anxiety and depression often are not identified, but may need help to progress in school. The *Individuals with Disabilities Education Act* (IDEA) and *Section 504 of the Rehabilitation Act of 1973* (Section 504) are the primary avenues for providing special education services and accommodations for students who have disabilities. The chapter is organized primarily around the IDEA and its definition of Emotional Disturbance and how children and adolescents who are depressed or anxious may or may not be served in special education. Issues regarding eligibility, evaluations, and procedural issues are discussed within the context of illustrative court cases and the author's extensive experience as an administrative law judge/independent hearing officer for due process hearings under the IDEA and Section 504.

In closing, the author hopes that the reader finds the book to be a relatively comprehensive treatment of anxiety and depression in children and adolescents, and that it will be informative with regard to current research, how research is linked with practice, and how the practitioner can apply research in everyday practice. Hopefully, the practitioner will gain valuable information that can be used to provide services to anxious and depressed children and adolescents using evidence-based practices from a developmental psychopathology perspective. The book may be useful for graduate students in clinical, counseling, and school psychology and related disciplines who are interested in anxiety and depression and how to use evidence-based concepts and literature in their work. Ultimately, our goal should be to help children and youth become psychologically healthy and happy adults. They deserve no less than our best efforts.

Bloomington, IN, USA   Thomas J. Huberty

Acknowledgments

The author wishes to acknowledge the support and encouragement of Judy Jones, Senior Editor at Springer, in the development of this book. She has been exceptionally helpful, insightful, and supportive in the development and production of this work, which is sincerely appreciated. Appreciation is also given to Garth Haller at Springer for his help in the production of the book.

Appreciation is extended to Michael Axelrod, Ph.D., for reviewing some of the chapters and providing valuable feedback.

Appreciation is also given to Kevin McDowell, J.D., Deputy Attorney General for the State of Indiana for his careful and insightful review and suggestions for Chap. 14, *Legal Issues in Educating Anxious and Depressed Students,* as well as for his friendship and mentoring in special education law over many years.

The author also expresses his gratitude to former and current graduate students at Indiana University, who have provided inspiration in the development of this book.

Contents

Part IV   Intervention and Prevention

Part VI   Appendices

Part I
Foundations

Chapter 1
Foundations of Developmental Psychopathology

Historical Context of Child and Adolescent Psychopathology

Research and interest in child psychopathology have burgeoned in the last two decades, resulting in a research base has led to greater understanding of the development and treatment of childhood disorders (Achenbach, 1982; Lewis, 2000; Sroufe, 1997). Views of childhood psychological problems have changed over time from early Greek and Roman perspectives when disorders were viewed as being due to organic imbalances or other inherent problems. Children with psychological or physical disabilities were viewed as burdens on society and often were scorned, abandoned, or put to death. Other conceptualizations about children with mental and psychological problems viewed them as being inherently evil or possessed by demons. Until the mid-1800s, it was not uncommon for children with disabilities to be kept in cages and cellars (Silk, Nath, Siegel, & Kendall, 2000), and they did not receive help or education. Fortunately, attitudes toward children with psychological and developmental problems have changed significantly, and they are more likely to be given help and to be protected under various federal and state laws that govern neglect and abuse, mental health services, public education, and others.

Nevertheless, views of child mental health disorders early in the twentieth century were comparable to adult disorders, and there was little published research on child psychopathology except for "mental defectives." There were no significant, integrated theories of child psychopathology, and it was assumed that the problems originated within the child, with little attention given to other factors, such as family, environment, or education. These perspectives continued relatively unchanged until the late 1970s and early 1980s when researchers began conducting studies about the nature of child psychopathology (Achenbach, 1982), development of psychopathology over the lifespan (Ingram & Price, 2001), empirically supported treatments (Lonigan, Elbert, & Johnson, 1998), and prevention (Institute of Medicine, 1994). Consequently, recognition and acceptance that children's psychological disorders differ in important fundamental developmental ways from adults have

T.J. Huberty, *Anxiety and Depression in Children and Adolescents:*
Assessment, Intervention, and Prevention, DOI 10.1007/978-1-4614-3110-7_1,
© Springer Science+Business Media, LLC 2012

emerged. Children are not "mini" adults who vary quantitatively from adults in the number of disorders or symptoms they manifest, but also differ in many qualitative developmental perspectives that are critical to successful outcomes and intervention efforts. These new perspectives and emphases have resulted in a substantial research base, advances in theories and models of child psychopathology, and a recognized developmental psychopathology framework.

The Emergence of Developmental Psychopathology

Developmental psychopathology has been defined as "...*the study and prediction of maladaptive behaviors and processes over time*" (Lewis, 2000, p. 3). Kerig and Wenar (2005) describe developmental psychopathology as "normal development gone awry." As such, developmental psychopathology is concerned with changes over the lifespan of the child and adult and the factors that contribute to these changes. This perspective represents a broad and integrative framework that incorporates and utilizes input from a variety of disciplines, including psychology, psychiatry, medicine, neurology, and others (Cichetti & Sroufe, 2000). The result of this integration has been the development of research that has had significant impact on understanding of childhood psychopathology and continues to influence clinical practice. In particular, developmental psychopathology has an important role in understanding, treating, and preventing anxiety and depression, which will be presented throughout this book.

Developmental psychopathology has as its cornerstone the consideration of how emotional and behavioral problems develop and change over time and seeks to determine the factors that contribute to change or stability. Thus, developmental psychopathology emphasizes how emotional and behavioral problems of children and youth emerge, develop, and change over time. These changes can range from the presence of no symptoms at one point in time to those that appear at another point in time. Differences in manifestations of symptoms at different points in time have significant implications for understanding, assessing, and treating childhood emotional and behavioral problems. For example, if a child remains symptom-free across time, there are implications for understanding resilience and how he might show typical development despite the presence of risk factors. Similarly, if a child shows problem at one point in time and later appears symptom-free, there may be implications for the effects of treatment. The table below shows the four types of patterns of change over time, their descriptions, and possible explanatory factors for each.

A major challenge for clinicians working with children is how to distinguish typical developmental variations of behavior from those that indicate psychopathology. This issue is important because failure to do so can have at least one of two consequences: (a) typical developmental variations may be erroneously considered to be pathological, or (b) significant pathological patterns may be seen as typical behaviors that the child will "grow out of." Either of these errors, often referred to as Type I or Type II errors, respectively, can lead to inappropriate intervention or no intervention when it is warranted. In general, the behaviors that children exhibit as manifestations of problems (i.e. "symptoms") vary in intensity, frequency, or duration of typical behaviors. For example, preschool children often are impulsive or active, which is considered typical for that age. When these behaviors are extreme or occur at school, they may be considered problematic and indicative of problems. The primary indicator of whether variations in typical behaviors constitute pathology is if they are expected based on the child's developmental level (not merely age) and if they cause impairment in personal, social, or academic functioning. It can be misleading to focus on isolated behaviors, particularly if they are variations of typical behaviors that are often seen in children at one time or another (Achenbach, 1993). Thus, it is necessary to look at patterns or clusters of symptoms over sufficient periods of time to conclude whether psychopathology exists.

When attempting to confirm the presence of anxiety or depression in children or youth, however, identifying symptoms can be challenging, because the associated behaviors often are not disruptive or at a high level of intensity, frequency, or duration that cause concern in adults. To a considerable extent, determination of psychopathology is influenced by the point in time that the child is observed and who is the observer. It is not uncommon for adults to differ in their perspectives on the presence or severity of emotional and behavioral problems. For example, in their often-cited study of multiple informants of child behavior problems, Achenbach, McConaughey, and Howell (1987) found low correspondence of ratings among parent, teacher, and child self-reports.

Various approaches to understanding childhood problems have included illness, diagnosis, and symptoms, which have had various effects on how childhood psychopathology has been conceptualized (Richters & Cichetti, 1993). A consequence of the traditional, diagnostic approach has been the view that the source of children's problems lies within the child, with relatively little attention to other factors, such as environment and parenting practices. The emergence of the field of developmental psychopathology has shifted emphasis toward looking at multiple factors, which has had a positive effect on clinical assessment, intervention, and prevention research and practice.

Core Concepts in Developmental Psychopathology

Developmental psychopathology is a dynamic, interactive approach that requires the clinician to consider multiple concepts simultaneously when identifying, assessing, and treating children who present with emotional and behavioral symptoms that suggest impairment in personal, social, or academic functioning. Depending upon the nature of the symptoms, the contributing factors, child characteristics, environmental influences, genetics, and other factors, these core concepts are important in conceptualizing child psychopathology at the group and individual levels, as well as in intervention and prevention efforts.

Developmental Continuity

In general, the cognitive, social, physical, linguistic, academic, and emotional/behavioral skills of children will progress qualitatively and quantitatively in a rather uniform fashion within a broad range of "normal." Behaviors that deviate from these expected patterns are considered "symptoms" of a problem only if they are developmentally inappropriate in frequency, intensity, or duration and impair functioning. When development proceeds in a predictable and orderly fashion with only occasional deviations that are not indicative of problems, *developmental continuity* is present.

When considering disordered behavior from a developmental psychopathology perspective, we are interested in the degree of continuity or discontinuity over time. Some behaviors show relative continuity over time, such as moderate to severe shyness. Although significant shyness may improve over time, the behaviors are likely to persist at less severe levels over childhood and adolescence. Conversely, oppositional behavior commonly seen in preschoolers tends to dissipate with time as children participate in school and develop social and emotion regulation skills. As will be discussed later, anxiety symptoms tend to remain rather stable over time, beginning in childhood and developing into anxiety disorders that become chronic into adulthood (Achenbach, Howell, McConaughey, & Stanger, 1995). Developmental disorders, such as an autism or mental retardation, tend to show a higher degree of continuity, and the course of the development tends to be more predictable than nondevelopmental disorders. In both of these cases, significant impairment in cognitive, linguistic, social, adaptive, and behavioral development occurs, although there tends to be relative continuity of the behaviors over time. Therefore, the continuity of disorders from childhood through adulthood varies depending on the nature of the disorder and contributory or maintenance factors, such as parenting or socioeconomic status. In general, externalizing patterns tend to be more stable over time than do internalizing patterns, but much depends on the specific nature of the problem, assessment methods, and other factors (Mash & Dozois, 2003). In general, research supports the position that childhood disorders tend to have relative continuity with some, but not all, adult disorders over time and into adulthood. While anxiety and depression tend to have chronic courses that may persist into adulthood, disorders such as encopresis and enuresis are primarily childhood disorders (Mash & Dozois).

Another factor contributing to continuity or discontinuity is the *pervasiveness* of a disorder. For example, moderate to severe developmental disorders tend to have pervasive effects across social, personal, and academic spheres. Conversely, children who have average cognitive ability but have a reading disorder may do quite well in other subject areas and in social and recreational interests. Therefore, less pervasive patterns tend to be associated with more developmental continuity and less impairment in overall functioning. In summary, the progression of psychological disorders of children over time and into adulthood is characterized by both continuous and discontinuous patterns that are mediated by a complex number and interaction of variables operating at different times and degrees in direct and indirect ways.

Developmental Pathways

A central concept in developmental psychopathology is *developmental pathway*, which refers to the direction or pathway of childhood disorders. Table 1.1 describes the four types of pathways or trajectories that can be shown in childhood at two points in time. Of course, more times could be included in research or clinical practice, any of which could change. For example, a child might appear to be doing well at preschool and early childhood (Time I), but a problem could develop at a later time, such as severe depression (Time II) that would cause clinicians to consider what happened between Time I and Time II that contributed to the development of the disorders. Thus, developmental trajectories or pathways are not necessarily fixed and, in fact, are subject to change over time, particularly for nondevelopmental disorders that are highly influenced by environmental circumstances, such as traumatic events or the emergence of medical problems that have accompanying psychological correlates, for example, diabetes or seizure disorders. To fully understand how individual pathways develop in children, it is best to try to trace the child's development prior to the onset of problems, which facilitates understanding the heterogeneity of disorders (Sroufe, 1997). Typically, clinical research has focused on identifying variables associated with the development of psychopathology, such as child characteristics and environmental contributors. An alternative is to take a person-centered approach to developmental pathway research, which focuses on identifying rather homogenous subgroups in order to more precisely identify factors that contribute to and maintain psychopathology and how changes occur over time (Cichetti & Rogosch, 1996).

There is a multitude of possible developmental pathways that children can take and which are affected by an almost infinite number and combination of variables. There are some developmental pathways that are well established in research and clinical practice and serve as examples of how patterns evolve and become predictable over time. For example, early-onset conduct disorder occurs most often in boys and tends to be predictive of antisocial behavior and substance abuse at adolescence and early adulthood (Hinshaw & Lee, 2003). Children who show extreme shyness and withdrawal are more likely to develop anxiety disorders (Kagan, Reznick, & Snidman, 1987), increasing their chances of developing a depressive disorder. By understanding developmental pathways, clinicians are better able to inform parents of potential outcomes of emotional and behavioral problems and to help develop efforts to alter maladaptive trajectories and prevent or reduce negative long-term outcomes.

Table 1.1 Patterns of development of psychopathology

Pattern	Time 1	Time 2	Description	Explanatory factors
I	Symptoms absent	Symptoms absent	At Time 1 and Time 2, there are no symptoms of problems that deviate significantly from typical developmental expectations	Child continues to develop typically; genetic predispositions remain dormant; environment remains positive, stable, and supportive and promotes resilience; if primary prevention approaches are implemented, they likely are effective
II	Symptoms absent	Symptoms present	At Time 1, there are no problems that deviate significantly from typical developmental expectations. At Time 2, symptoms onset after a period of apparent typical development	Genetic predispositions to psychopathology begin to emerge; previously undetected patterns are identified; child's development begins to deviate from typical in one or more areas; child is unable to continue to learn developmentally appropriate coping skills; environment becomes unstable and unsupportive and does not promote resilience; ineffective primary prevention efforts; new risk factors introduced that are not managed effectively; decline in parenting behavior
III	Symptoms present	Symptoms absent	Symptoms are present at Time 1 that deviate significantly from typical developmental expectations. At Time 2, child's behavior is within range of typical developmental expectations	Initial developmental problems are resolved; environment becomes stable and supportive; improved parenting behaviors; effective interventions
IV	Symptoms present	Symptoms present	Symptoms are present at Time 1 that deviate significantly from typical developmental expectations. At Time 2, the same symptoms exist or other ones have emerged in addition to the original patterns or different symptoms have emerged	Developmental problems persist; unstable and unsupportive environment remains so or worsens; continued parenting problems; lack of interventions; ineffective interventions

Equifinality and Multifinality

Important to understanding the concept of developmental pathways are the concepts of *equifinality* and *multifinality*. Clinicians and researchers alike have often observed that children with diverse backgrounds and circumstances can demonstrate similar developmental outcomes (equifinality). The fact that similar outcomes result from diverse circumstances indicates that the contributory factors vary in complexity, onset, number, and interactions. Conversely, a single risk factor may have a number of implications, depending on variables operating within the child and the environment (multifinalilty) (Cichetti & Rogosch, 1996). Of similar interest is that some children who live in stressful and high-risk environments nevertheless have positive developmental outcomes, presumably due to a combination of inherent strengths and positive, supportive environments.

Risk and Protective Factors

In developmental psychopathology, the roles of risk and protective factors are central to understanding developmental pathways, outcomes, equifinality, and multifinality. Risk factors are those variables that, depending on the individual child and circumstances, increase the probability of negative pathways and outcomes. Conversely, protective factors are those variables that serve to prevent or minimize negative outcomes in children who are exposed to stressful or risk-producing situations. Understanding risk and protective factors is not merely a matter of a large number of them increasing the chances of negative outcomes compared to a small number of factors. Although it is true that a greater number of risk factors increase the chances of negative outcomes, the issue is not that simple. A seemingly singular event may set a series of consequences in motion that create conditions for other risk factors to emerge. For example, a child born into poverty faces a large number of risk factors that co-occur and increase the probability of negative outcomes, such as parenting, less adequate education, and nutrition. Over time, risk factors that by themselves may not cause negative outcomes, the cumulative effects may, at some point in development, "trigger" the onset of emotional and behavioral problems. Risk and protective factors exist in a range of circumstances and contexts and are summarized in Table 1.2.

Categorical Classification vs. Developmental Psychopathology

As most psychologists in the USA are aware, the *Diagnostic and Statistical Manual of Mental Disorders-Fourth Edition* (DSM-IV; American Psychiatric Association, 2000) is the primary reference and classification systems for mental disorders. In other countries, the International Classification of Diseases-10 (ICD-10; World Health Organization, 1993) that includes both medical and psychological/psychiatric

Table 1.2 Partial list of risk factors

Context	Risk factors	Vulnerabilities	Protective factors
Genetic	• Genetic disorders or predispositions • Heredity factors	• Problems associated with genetic or hereditary disorders, e.g. language and self-help skill deficits	• Absence of genetic or hereditary disorders • Minimal influence of genetic or hereditary disorders • Lack of stressors that might "trigger" predispositions
Biological	• Prenatal infections or injury • Neuropsychological deficits/brain damage • Poor maternal care and nutrition • In utero exposure to toxins • Maternal substance abuse	• Difficult temperament • Problems associated with neurological and biological problems, e.g. cortical dysfunction, adaptive skill deficits	• Easy temperament • Absence of or minimal effects of biological or neurological problems
Personal/individual	• Low intelligence • Poor emotional regulation • Low self-efficacy • Low self-esteem • Impulse control problems • Extreme shyness	• Gender • Poor planning ability • Emotional regulation problems • Sociability and social skills deficits • Impulse control • Attention problems • Executive functioning problems	• Gender • Average or above intelligence • Good social acumen and skills • Good emotional regulation skills appropriate for developmental level and situation • Absence of impulse control and attention problems

Family	• Poor parenting practices • Inadequate supervision • Insecure attachment • Parental psychopathology • Parental conflict • Unstable home environment	• Parent–child conflicts • Presence of a developmental, medical, or physical disability • Inadequate coping strategies based on current developmental capacity	• Cohesive family functioning • Good parenting practices • Absence of parental psychopathology • Good coping skills • Able to accept developmentally appropriate personal responsibility
Social	• Antisocial friends • Limited friendships • Limited access to positive social interactions • Poor social models • Socially marginalized	• Social skill deficits • Performance skill deficits • Fluency skill deficits • Social information-processing deficits	• Able to make friends and engage in age-appropriate reciprocal relationships • Absence of or minimal social, performance, and fluency deficits • Good social problem-solving skills • Positive role models
Cultural	• Poverty • Racism • Prejudice • Being a member of a minority cultural or ethnic group within a larger cultural context • Unstable, chaotic, or violent community environment	• Personal characteristics, including disabilities, that are not compatible with the larger social context • Degree of cultural assimilation of child	• Personal characteristics compatible with cultural context • Child is well assimilated into the culture • Positive socioeconomic status • Stable, supportive environment

(continued)

Table 1.2 (continued)

Context	Risk factors	Vulnerabilities	Protective factors
Educational/academic	• Poor school environment • Inadequate instruction • Lack of support for mental health and social development in the school setting • "Mismatch" between child's needs and characteristics and the instructional environment • Disproportional instructional or disciplinary practices • Bullying and relational aggression • Limited family involvement in child's education	• Learning disorders • Difficulties adjusting to demands of school setting • Attention problems • Impulse control problems • Developmental delays	• Positive instructional, mental health, and social school environment • Absence of learning disorders and developmental delays • Individualized instruction adapted to the child's needs • Cultural, racial, and ethnic equity with regard to instruction and discipline • School recognizes and effectively addresses bullying and relational aggression • Active family involvement in child's education

Vulnerabilities and protective factors in developmental psychopathology by contextual influences
Adapted from (Kerig & Wenar, 2005)

disorders is commonly used. Both of these systems are categorical in nature and present a nomenclature to identify clusters of symptoms that lead to a specific diagnosis. The DSM-IV is designed to be a *mutually exclusive* approach, i.e. with accurate diagnosis, the person's behavioral can be classified into specific categories. It is possible to have multiple diagnoses although there may be behaviors common to multiple diagnoses, such as inattention or irritability. For multiple diagnoses to be given, however, some behaviors or patterns must be sufficiently distinct that cannot be explained by a primary or single diagnosis.

The DSM-IV is a *polythetic* approach, because a child does not have to meet all criteria or the same criteria as another child to be given the same diagnosis. For example, if a child must meet six of eight criteria, a child who meets the first six and one who meets the last six criteria may be given the same diagnosis, but have very different treatment needs. While useful from a descriptive and administrative perspective, the implications for treatment by DSM-IV categories may be limited, because the categories do not provide sufficient guidance for establishing intervention goals and plans for individual children. In addition to these limitations, the DSM-IV has been criticized on other points as well. Although it is much improved over its predecessors, especially with the multiaxial system, it does not adequately consider developmental variations, cultural factors, or the role of contributing factors, such as socioeconomic status or parenting variables, all of which are known to be related to the development and maintenance of psychopathology.

Historically, the approach to child psychopathology has mirrored adult psychopathology with an emphasis on the medical model where problematic behaviors are seen as symptoms of a disorder that are diagnosed and classified. The DSM-IV and its previous versions are the primary examples of this categorical approach. Both adult and child disorders are included in the DSM-IV, with the intent to classify behaviors into mutually exclusive categories. Although the DSM-IV has significant clinical utility, it has been criticized for the static nature of the categories compared to ongoing dynamic nature of children's development. As an alternative to this approach, there has been increased research and practice of child psychopathology from a developmental perspective, particularly with regard to differentiating typical developmental anxiety and mood variations from those that indicate an impairing condition requiring professional help. The developmental approach to psychopathology considers how childhood emotional and behavioral problems emerge, develop, and change over time. Lewis (1990) has defined developmental psychopathology as "…the study and prediction of maladaptive behaviors and processes over time" (p. 3). Therefore, this book describes assessment and intervention for anxiety and depression in children primarily from a developmental perspective.

The Contexts of Developmental Psychopathology

Historically, views of child development have focused on a person–environment perspective and the interaction between them. Despite this recognition, the child often has been seen as the primary source of disordered behavior, suggesting that the focus of treatment should be on alleviating or reducing individual symptomatology. Most psychologists and mental health professionals would agree that children do not develop in a vacuum and that their social, emotional, personal, and academic development is affected by several interacting factors or contexts. These contexts most often are represented by genetic, biological, social, cultural, and familial factors. An often overlooked or minimized context, however, is an academic perspective. Apart from family, children spend more time in school and around many same-age peers than at any other time. Indeed, during a typical school year, children spend approximately one-third of their waking hours per week at school where they learn academic and social behaviors. This is a significant developmental context, especially when one considers that a large number of referrals to mental health professionals are related to school-related problems. These contexts will be discussed throughout the book as important considerations in working with children and adolescents who have anxiety or depression. In considering these contexts, it is important to remember that they do not operate as singular entities, but often have interactive and cumulative effects. For example, a child with a genetically based developmental disorder is much more likely than his typical peers to have social and academic problems.

The contributions of culture to developmental outcomes of children are multiple and complex, including racial, ethnic, socioeconomic, and religious factors. In an important conceptualization about the context of culture, Messick (1983) suggested that child psychopathology must consider three contexts: (a) the child as context, i.e. the child presents specific traits and predispositions that impact the individual developmental course; (b) the child of context, i.e. that his or her background consists of family, school, community, and cultural variables that impact development; and (c) the child in context, i.e. the child is rapidly changing and that behaviors seen as one point in time may be quite different than those seen at other times. The interactions of the child within multiple cultural contexts must be considered simultaneously, and attempts to do otherwise will result in an incomplete and erroneous understanding of child psychopathology.

The Genetic Context

There is no doubt that genetic factors play a role in human development, although the nature of their contributions to the development of psychopathology is not completely clear. The effect of a genetic context can occur in one of two ways: (a) as identified genetic or hereditary influences with reasonably predictable development trajectories (e.g. Down syndrome, autism spectrum disorders) or (b) as genetic or hereditary dispositions that may emerge spontaneously at some point or may be "triggered" by environmental factors. Genetic influences can be pervasive or specific in their effects. Apart from known developmental disorders, however, genetic and hereditary effects tend to account for about one-third of the variance in the development of psychological disorders. Even if there is a genetic tendency, often it is manifested as a trend toward general patterns of symptoms, rather than for specific disorders (e.g. Eley, 2001). Some children may have family genetic histories and demonstrate some characteristics of a genetic problem, but the effects may be minimal to nonexistent, depending on environmental contexts and circumstances.

An important topic in psychological research is the contribution of genetic factors to the development of psychopathology vs. the contribution of nongenetic factors, such as family and environmental variables. There is substantial evidence that genetics contributes to many forms of psychopathology, including anxiety and depression. However, it is often difficult to determine which factors are genetic and how much they contribute to the development of psychopathology. Pennington (2002, p. 44) proposes four questions to consider when determining the contribution of genetics to a trait or phenotype:

1. Is the trait familial?
2. If so, is the familiality due in part to genetic influences? In other words, is the trait heritable?
3. If so, what is the mechanism of genetic transmission?
4. What is the actual location of the gene or genes involved?

Pennington (2002) notes that these questions do not apply if a trait having a genetic basis is not familial. If a trait is not familial, then it is not heritable. An example of this circumstance is children with trisomy 21 and mosaic trisomy 21 where some or all of the cells have 47 chromosomes and there is an extra chromosome 21. The syndrome is genetic, but is not heritable because it is not familial. Some psychiatric disorders do have heritable, familial bases, including ADHD, schizophrenia, bipolar disorder, major depression, autism, and dyslexia. Although familiality does not necessarily prove that a trait has a genetic basis due to the fact that it could be mediated by environmental circumstances, twin and molecular studies have demonstrated that genetics contributes substantially to the familiality of these disorders (Pennington).

The Biological Context

The biological context has implications for psychopathology when physical abnormalities, neurological conditions, or inborn characteristics contribute to maladaptive pathways. Obvious conditions include neurological damage, neuropsychological deficits, or seizure disorders. Much research has focused on specific neurological structures in behavior and psychopathology, such as structures in the limbic system (e.g. amygdala) and cortical areas, such as the prefrontal cortex. The hypothalamic–pituitary–adrenal axis regulates human stress reactions and has been implicated as a factor in the development and maintenance of some forms of psychopathology, including anxiety and depression (Meyer, Chrousos, & Gold, 2001).

One of the most studied biological contributors to development and psychopathology is a child's temperament. Research has established the important role of temperament in behavior and how it tends to be stable over time and to be predictive of developmental pathways. As a relatively stable personality pattern, temperament can be seen as a vulnerability construct where it can predispose a child to develop certain forms of psychopathology (Tackett & Kruger, 2005). This concept suggests that personality and psychopathology are on a continuum and are related dimensionally to each other (Tackett & Kruger). Behavioral inhibition is an example of a personality/temperament variable that is associated with psychopathology, such as anxiety and depression. Having an inhibited temperament is biologically based and places children at greater risk of developing an anxiety or mood disorder. Even if a child is not considered to be behaviorally inhibited but shows a high level of withdrawal, there is a greater risk for the development of internalizing problems in middle childhood (Young Mun, Fitzgerald, Von Eye, Puttler, & Zucker, 2001). Children with inhibited temperaments are more likely to be socially anxious and withdrawn, be subject to parental overprotection, and to have impaired coping skills. Despite the consistent findings that temperament often presents as a risk factor for psychopathology, the relationship between them should not be seen from a fatalistic or immutable perspective. Although temperamental characteristics tend to be predictive of certain developmental trajectories, they do not represent a *fait accompli*, i.e. many factors contribute to outcomes, including socioeconomic status, parental psychopathology, and culture. Behaviors associated with temperament can be affected by many variables, including parenting and social support, and can be changed through exposure to environmental events, including psychotherapy.

The Cultural Context

The cultural context, which includes ethnic, racial, socioeconomic, and religious factors, plays a central role in what behaviors are expected by society, family, and others and also dictates to a significant extent how feelings, distress, and emotions are expressed. For example, shyness and oversensitivity have been found to be seen as sources of social difficulties in Western culture, but associated with leadership qualities and school success in Chinese children (Chen, Rubin, & Li, 1995). Conceptions of psychopathology vary across cultures, affecting how normalcy is viewed and how diagnostic criteria are applied. Patterns of behaviors and symptoms vary across and within cultures (Hoagwood & Jensen, 1997), and different terminologies of conceptions of disorders tend to be culturally specific (López & Guarnaccia, 2000).

Moreover, assessment of psychopathology across cultures is complicated by the fact that the majority of standardized instruments have been developed on European American children and translated into other languages and then used in cross-cultural research. Whether those instruments accurately reflect psychopathology in those cultures is unclear, and more research is needed. A study by Ivanova, Achenbach, Dumenci et al. (2007) using the Child Behavior Checklist (CBCL; Achenbach & Rescorla, 2001) found that the dimensions measured by the CBCL appear to have cross-cultural correspondence. Therefore, clinicians must consider the cultural context of child psychopathology, including how their own cultural values and views may or may not be consistent with that of their clients and may affect delivery of services.

The Social Context

There is little doubt or dispute that social factors exert a significant effect on the development of both typical and atypical psychological development. Although temperament and personality traits play an important role in development and as risk factors for psychopathology, socialization also exerts a powerful influence on how children adapt to stressors they encounter. Socialization and life experiences modify personality traits and influence how they are expressed. Cohen (1999) found that, although temperament is important in a child's behavior and adaptation, teachers, parents, and others are highly influential in helping a child to develop coping strategies, impulse control, self-regulation, and social skills. Conversely, negative relationships with others are associated with greater risk for psychopathology, such as parents who have dysfunctional attachment styles with their children (Sroufe, Carlson, Levy, & Egeland, 1999). If a child experiences significant stressors and adversity, the socialization process does not progress normally beyond the family, leading to increased risk for psychopathology (Cohen; Johnson, Cohen, Kasen, Smailes, & Brook, 2001). Even if negative personality traits do emerge during childhood, they tend to diminish from late childhood or early adolescence through late adolescence into early adulthood, partly due to socialization experiences (Stein, Newcomb, & Bentler, 1986).

In the extreme, the social environment can present such aversive conditions that interpersonal competence is inhibited or directly interferes with development. Garbarino (1997) refers to such environments as "socially toxic" to children and that "...the social context in which they grow up has become poisonous to their development" (p. 141). Garbarino suggests that these "toxins" include family dysfunction that creates conditions for the development of psychopathology. These family dysfunctions can lead to impaired attachment, ineffective parenting behaviors, and poor parent–child communication. Over time, the risk for disorders increases, including anxiety and depression.

The Family Context

An excellent example of context is the role of the family in a child's personal, social, and academic development. There are multiple family contextual variables that can contribute to the development of typical or atypical development. Family stressors including marital discord, financial limitations, single-parent families, parenting practices, and parental psychopathology are but some of the risk factors that can contribute to the development of behavioral problems and exacerbate current difficulties or increase the probability of their emergence. For example, research has shown that mothers of anxious children tend to engage in overprotective behavior, therefore reinforcing anxiety and depression patterns (Ingram, Miranda, & Segal, 1998).

An area of research with regard to parenting styles has focused on parents who engage in overcontrolling and overprotective behaviors. Baumrind (1991) found that parents who exhibit overcontrol are more likely to have children who develop anxiety and depression and vulnerability to other childhood disorders. Chorpita and Barlow (1998) suggested that these parental behaviors may impede the development of children's sense of controllability and predictability over events by limiting their opportunities to experience anxiety-producing situations. They also reinforce a child for choosing avoidant behaviors when encountering stress. Consequently, the child does not learn coping skills, which tends to reinforce a cycle of anxiety, avoidance, and withdrawal.

The School Context

An often overlooked or minimized context is the role of education in children's development. Over 90% of US children attend public schools, which vary in their quality, available resources, and support for mental health. All states in the USA have compulsory attendance laws, usually at least until the age of 16. Approximately 25–30% of high school students fail to graduate (Greene & Winters, 2005), increasing the likelihood of social and mental health problems into adulthood. Up to 30% of children in public schools have recognized learning or behavioral problems or are at risk for developing them over their time in school. Approximately 5% of public school children have learning disabilities, and about half of those have a reading disability (Lyon, 1996). Children with learning disabilities also are at higher risk of developing social or emotional problems, including conduct disorder and ADHD (Frick et al., 1991), although whether one disorder causes the other is not fully understood. There may be a common set of factors that predispose some children to developing both learning and behavioral problems. In fact, many, if not most, referrals to community mental health professionals include concerns about problems at school, most often for attention and behavioral issues. Children spend up to 40 hours per week in school, where they must develop learning and social/emotional skills. For those who have difficulty in either of these spheres, there is increased probability of developing one or more forms of psychopathology over time, including anxiety, depression, conduct problems, and substance abuse.

Risk and Protective Factors from a Contextual Perspective

Compared to the rather static perspective of the medical model of psychopathology, developmental psychopathology focuses on factors that create risk for problems and those that appear to be protective. By conceptualizing risk and protective factors, we are interested in the likelihood of problems developing and changing over time. Risk factors predispose children to a higher probability of developing problems, but whether such problems occur depends on the dynamic nature of development and the various contextual factors that may or may not occur for the effects of risk factors to be realized. For example, a child who lives in an environment where he has experienced abuse would be considered to be at higher risk of developing emotional problems if he remains in that environment. Conversely, a child who has experienced abuse but who is placed in a supportive environment is more likely to follow an adaptive developmental trajectory and may not show significant negative effects.

Risk and protective factors may appear to be the opposite of each other, i.e. the presence of a risk factor indicates that it is not protective. However, the relationship between them is not that simple, because the role of each depends on the various contexts and the nature of developmental pathways. Lower intelligence is a risk factor for both learning and behavioral problems, while higher intelligence reduces the risk of the development of such patterns.

From a gender perspective, being a boy or girl can be a risk or a protective factor. Girls are two to three times more likely to develop anxiety disorders over their lifespan, as compared to boys (e.g. Lewinshohn, Gotlib, Lewinsohn, Seeley, & Allen, 1998). The possible reasons for this developmental pathway difference are complicated but likely involve genetic, biological, social, and family contexts. Conversely, boys are at a 3:1 to 6:1 greater likelihood of developing conduct disorder (APA, 2000) and are more likely to be physically aggressive and overtly antisocial than are girls. The role of risk and protective factors is complex and operates both within and across contexts, creating challenges to researchers to define and operationalize them and to clinicians who are involved in intervention and prevention.

Resilience

Resilience is a central concept in developmental psychopathology and refers to the degree to which a child can cope with or adapt to adverse circumstances (Luthar, Cichetti, & Becker, 2000). The existence of risk factors and adverse circumstances does not necessarily dictate that a child will proceed on a negative developmental trajectory. The presence and degree of impact of contextual factors that might portend a negative trajectory frequently are mediated by a wide range of interacting variables that can emerge and change over time. Defining and operationalizing resilience remains unclear. It can be an elusive concept because its demonstration depends on the presence of adverse circumstances. If a child has negative experiences and copes well, it might be said that he is "resilient." On the other hand, a child may have resilient qualities that are not shown in the absence of environmental stressors. Thus, a child might have a predisposition to being resilient or nonresilient, but the role of the environment, child characteristics, and late-appearing genetic factors will affect how "resilient" a child might be.

Despite the lack of clarity, the conceptualization of resilience offered by Werner (1995) is useful and generally describes it as children who (a) are able to have positive outcomes or avoid negative despite the presence of significant risk factors, (b) manage to function well while under stress, or (c) recover well from traumatic events. Children may be quite resilient in some areas, but less so in other areas, depending on variables such as child characteristics, situational demands, severity of stressors, and risk and protective factors that interact and change over time.

Vulnerability

A key concept in developmental psychopathology is *vulnerability*, which refers to the degree to which a child may be susceptible or "vulnerable" to the impact of risk factors across and within developmental contexts. Vulnerability is seen as a continuum from low to high and is mediated by the dynamic interplay of risk and protective factors. The degree to which vulnerability is shown depends to a large degree on the severity of stressors and the resilience of the child. Moreover, a child may be more vulnerable to some stressors than others. For example, a child with a high level of intelligence but who has social skills difficulties may not be highly vulnerable to learning problems at school, but have much difficulty in interpersonal relationships. Thus, the thresholds for vulnerability vary according to an interaction of child characteristics, contextual variables, and the type and degree of perceived stressors. It should be noted that what a stressor is for one child may not be a stressor or be as stressful for another child.

Diathesis–Stress Models of Vulnerability

A useful concept in developmental psychopathology and vulnerability is *diathesis–stress*. *Diathesis* originally referred to the medical concept that people have a predisposition to illness that is based in endogenous biological or constitutional factors (Ingram & Price, 2001). The concept has been expanded in developmental psychopathology to discuss how a child might show predispositions to a disorder that are the result of genetic, biological, psychological, or other vulnerabilities. Diathesis and vulnerability have been conceptualized as being interchangeable terms and are related to the presence of stress (Ingram & Luxton, 2005). Whether a diathesis or vulnerability is manifested, however, depends greatly on the presence and significance of stressors. If a stressor is perceived, then the degree of difficulty adapting to it is an index of vulnerability, as well as an indicator of resilience capacity. Children with multiple risk factors or disabilities are likely to have greater diatheses and have more difficulty coping with stress. An intervention or prevention implication of the diathesis–stress model is to reduce the impact of various stressors, which may reduce the severity or prevent the emergence of a disorder in children who are predisposed to developing a disorder.

Resilience, Risk, and Vulnerability

Resilience, risk, and vulnerability are interrelated concepts, but are distinct from each other. However, vulnerability differs from risk in that risk refers more to the increased probability of a disorder, whereas vulnerability is an endogenous factor that may be considered a trait (Ingram & Price, 2001). Vulnerability can increase through continued stress or reduced through changes in circumstances, intervention, or prevention. Thus, risk and vulnerability are related, in that children who are considered highly vulnerable to psychopathology are more likely to be affected by risk factors and stressors than are those considered to be less vulnerable, i.e. a high level of vulnerability increases the probability that a factor increases the risk for problems.

Models of vulnerability and stress typically incorporate vulnerability, resilience, and stress as factors in the likelihood of onset of a disorder. Children with high vulnerability are seen as having less resilience and are at greater risk of developing a disorder, with the severity of a disorder being related to the severity of one or more stressors. If a child with high vulnerability is exposed to severe stress, the likelihood of a disorder increases. Conversely, a child might have significant generic, biological, psychological, or other vulnerabilities, but is less likely to develop a disorder if stressors are not significant. Therefore, each child has a different threshold for the development of a disorder, based upon the degree of vulnerability, resilience, risk factors, and stress.

Ingram and Price (2001) view vulnerability and resilience on a single continuum with implications for the effects of risk factors and stressors. Children with high resilience (i.e. low vulnerability) are not immune to experiencing psychopathology, but are less likely than less resilient or more vulnerable children to develop a disorder. This conceptualization suggests that vulnerability interacts with stressors to increase the threshold for development of psychopathology. If vulnerability is a trait, then it may not be directly alterable, but can be affected indirectly by reducing the effects of stressors through intervention and prevention, thus increasing resilience.

Figure 1.1 is a variation of the model presented by Ingram and Price (2001), which proposes that vulnerability and resilience are on a continuum that is associated with the threshold for the development of a disorder. If a child is at risk for developing a problem due to vulnerability, but there are no stressors to trigger it, no problems will be shown. Conversely, if a child has low vulnerability and is able to show resilience to stressful events, the likelihood of a disorder developing is reduced. The model presented in Fig. 1.1 suggests that vulnerability and resilience are separate, but inversely related constructs, i.e. as vulnerability increases, resilience decreases and vice versa. Whether high or low vulnerability and resilience will be shown is dependent on risk factors and the severity of the stressors experienced by the child. The solid line represents the maximum likelihood that a disorder will develop in combination with the degree of vulnerability, resilience, and the severity of stressors. The multiple dashed lines represent the concept that the likelihood of

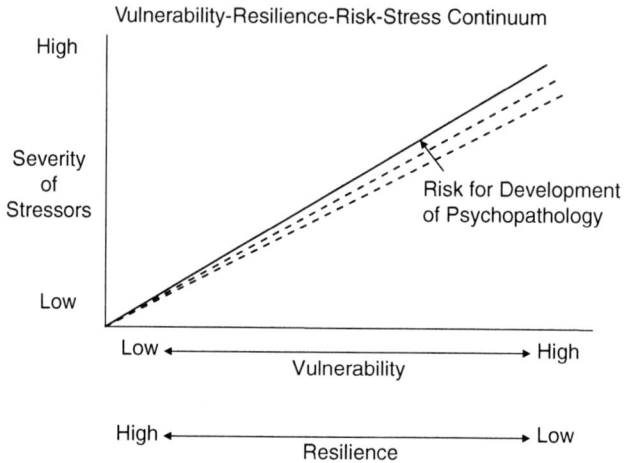

Fig. 1.1 Vulnerability–resilience–risk–stress continuum

development of a disorder is not fixed, but depends on the complex interplay among stressors, vulnerability, and resilience. For example, a child who has been raised in a highly stressful environment might be considered to have greater vulnerability and lower resilience to stress. However, if the child is placed in a safe, supportive, and caring environment where stressors are lessened, psychological or environmental vulnerability may be reduced and resilience enhanced, resulting in a lower likelihood of the onset of a disorder. As well as representing likelihood of the onset of a disorder, the lines may also help to account for the fact that many children have subsyndromal symptoms of disorders, but may not meet criteria for a disorder (e.g. Costello, Mustillo, Erkanli, Keeler, & Angold, 2003). As stressors, risk factors, and vulnerabilities change, the likelihood of subsyndromal patterns becoming diagnosable disorders also may be affected.

Diagnosis and Classification in a Developmental Psychopathology Perspective

The historical and predominant approach to conceptualizing psychopathology has been from a medical model with emphasis on identifying clusters of behaviors that characterize or describe a condition and formulating a specific diagnosis. The prominent example of this approach is the DSM-IV and its predecessors that emphasize diagnostic criteria and identifying one disorder from among many possibilities. These categories are presumed to improve communication among professionals and to offer guidelines for psychological and psychiatric treatment. The categorical approach assumes that when a child or adult meets sufficient criteria that indicate impairment, a DSM-IV disorder label can be applied.

The alternative approach to categorical classification is a dimensional approach, where symptoms are viewed as being on a continuum of severity. Often, however, dimensional approaches use a quasicategorical approach by establishing "clinical cutoffs" to indicate the presence of a disorder. For example, specific tests may suggest that scores at one or two standard deviations above the mean are suggestive of a disorder, although implicitly based on a dimensional concept. This approach is not without merit, however, because it helps to avoid "overpathologizing" of a range of typical behavior and creating diagnostic errors.

Achenbach (1982), Achenbach and Rescorla (2001), and others have described child and adolescent psychopathology from a dimensional perspective. Numerous studies have confirmed that, in general, children's behaviors cluster into internalizing and externalizing patterns, with some that do not clearly fit within either dimension. Internalizing patterns often are considered "overcontrolled" and as "emotional" problems. The primary internalizing patterns are anxiety and depression, although there is some debate whether they can be clinically separated, due to their high comorbidity. Typical symptoms of internalizing problems include anxiety, mood problems, withdrawal, somatic complaints, and sleeping difficulties. Externalizing patterns are described as "undercontrolled" and "behavior" problems and include disorders such as ADHD and conduct disorder. Typical behaviors include aggression, distractibility, and impulse control deficits (e.g. Achenbach & Rescorla).

It is possible that some disorders are better described in categorical terms and others in dimensional terms, although there is little agreement as to which ones best fit each approach (Mash & Dozois, 2003). Werry (2001) suggests that certain childhood disorders such as ADHD, anxiety, and depression may best be described on a dimensional basis as being personality problems. It may also be that disorders considered personality or trait problems may be best considered as dimensions for purposes of intervention, because the treatment goals often are reduction of rather than elimination of symptoms. This approach is particularly relevant for this book, which will address childhood anxiety and depression from both dimensional and categorical perspectives with regard to assessment and intervention.

Behaviors, Signs, Symptoms, Syndromes, and Disorders

Whether emphasizing a categorical or dimensional approach to classification of psychopathology, the common elements between them are to identify patterns, formulate a diagnostic picture, and develop recommendations. Diagnosis begins with examining patterns of behavior through formal or informal assessment that precipitate referral of a child for psychological or developmental problems. For the most part, behaviors of concern are not atypical of all children, but vary in frequency, intensity, or duration and are not developmentally appropriate. Atypical behaviors or patterns can occur, but are relatively rare, such as hallucinations, tics, and delusions. When behaviors appear to be indicative of a problem, they are considered *signs* that a problem is present that needs further investigation. When the clinician concludes that these signs are indicative of a problem, they are considered *symptoms* of a behavior pattern that is causing impairment in one or more areas of functioning. When these patterns are confirmed, a *syndrome* is deemed to be present, which is a pattern of symptoms that characterize a child's' typical functioning. Finally, these syndromes are given a formal diagnosis as a *disorder* with an accompanying label from the DSM-IV or other classification system.

Symptoms can be cognitive, behavioral, or physiological and occur singly or in combination at varying degrees of frequency, intensity, or duration. Accurate assessment and delineation of symptoms are important because they form the basis for intervention and prevention. Although diagnostic labels are useful to clinicians, they have relatively limited utility for interventions. Effective psychological intervention does not focus on disorders per se, but on the behaviors or symptoms that are causing the most impairment. Because DSM-IV disorders are polythetic and different clusters of symptoms can lead to the same diagnosis, a focus on the individual child's behaviors/symptoms is necessary for effective treatment. Accurate formal diagnosis may be helpful when prescribing medications, particularly in those cases where a physical or biological basis is suspected.

Comorbidity

An important issue for research and practice is comorbidity, which is the presence of two or more disorders in the same child. In essence, the child with comorbid conditions displays a pattern of symptoms that cannot be accounted by criteria of only one disorder. In many ways, comorbidity also applies to symptoms because it is common for some symptoms to be manifested in multiple disorders. For example, attention problems are common in anxiety, depression, and ADHD, but the reasons for them are different. In general, the *base rate*, or frequency of occurrence for all childhood disorders in the population, is relatively high, ranging from 14 to 22% (Rutter, 1989), a finding that has generally been supported in other studies. Rates vary with the type of disorder and other factors, such as SES, child ethnicity, age, and sex. However, some disorders, such as anxiety disorders, may be as high as 20% (Costello et al., 1996). The frequency of comorbidity across disorders is much higher, however, ranging from 25 to 80%, depending on the specific disorders. In some of those cases, there is an overlap of disorders that warrants multiple diagnoses. In other cases, an overlap of symptoms may not warrant multiple diagnoses. Many children who have been referred to mental health professionals have two or more comorbid disorders, which is the rule rather than the exception.

Part of the problem with comorbidity is a function of changing diagnostic approaches. In the DSM-III (APA, 1980), diagnostic decisions were characterized by a hierarchy of exclusionary criteria that discouraged multiple diagnoses. There was recognition, however, that this approach was somewhat artificial and did not accurately represent the structure of disorders and was abandoned (Sonuga-Barke, 1998).

With the publication of the DSM-IV (APA, 1994), it became possible to give multiple diagnoses, but there may be fewer syndromes present, increasing the possibility of artifactual data. The change has resulted in higher base rates and greater informant agreement, although it remains unclear the degree to which comorbidity exists (Mash & Dozois, 2003). There is ample research evidence, however, to suggest that there are "true" cases of comorbidity, although it is unclear how they emerge. If some disorders have their beginnings in early childhood, they may present initially as general or pervasive disorders that become more differentiated over time (Cantwell, 1996). Other bases for comorbid disorders include common underlying genetic or environmental effects or that the severity of one disorder increases the risk for the occurrence of another disorder (Mash & Dozois). Although it remains unclear the type and extent of comorbid conditions, it is clear that they do exist and develop over time.

The Course of Typical Development

To understand psychopathology from a developmental perspective, one must have a knowledge base of what is considered "typical" development. Although the word "normal" is often used to describe expected developmental patterns, it implies that there are rather clearly defined behaviors, stages, or milestones to which behaviors can be compared to determine if pathology exists. In this text, the word "typical" will be used in lieu of "normal" to emphasize that development implies a wide range of behavior in severity, time of onset, frequency, and intensity that must be considered on the basis of the child's developmental level and not only age. By emphasizing "typical," it is hoped that the practitioner will develop an appreciation of the wide range of variability of child and adolescent behavior and that, often, it is difficult to distinguish psychopathology from typical behavior and development.

Children develop in multiple areas, including neurological, cognitive, language, social, emotional, motor, and academic spheres. Significant deviations from typical patterns in one or more areas put the child at increased risk for psychopathology, including anxiety and depression. To understand if psychopathology exists rather than being a manifestation of typical development requires knowledge of what behaviors are expected at each age or developmental level. Some psychopathology patterns emerge at about the same age, but others may develop later, depending on factors such as environmental stress, parenting factors, and health issues. It is beyond the scope of this chapter to summarize all of the aspects of typical development of children and adolescents. Nevertheless, it is important that the clinician has a strong knowledge base about all major areas of typical child development including neurological development, brain–behavior relationships, and language, cognitive, social, emotional, family, motor, and academic development. Having this background when considering psychopathology from a developmental perspective is essential for the following reasons: (a) it helps clinicians to distinguish between typical development and psychopathology; (b) it reduces the possibility of asserting that psychopathology is present when it is not; (c) it reduces the possibility of concluding that observed behavior patterns are typical when, in fact, they are indicative of psychopathology; (d) it assists when making projections about developmental trajectories of children; and (e) it forms a basis to know when psychopathology remits to a normal level over time or occurs as a function of intervention or prevention. The clinician should remember that deviations in typical development may place a child at greater risk for psychopathology. For example, a child with epilepsy or chronic illness is at greater risk of developing academic and behavior problems (Huberty, Austin, Huster, & Dunn, 2000) as a result of psychological stress associated with the condition. By knowing about typical development and what conditions are more likely to increase the risk for psychopathology, the psychologist or other mental health professional is better prepared to understand and treat the individual child or youth.

Implications of Developmental Psychopathology for Clinical Practice

There are four primary clinical practice areas in serving children with emotional and behavioral problems: (a) assessment, (b) intervention, (c) consultation, and (d) prevention. These areas are addressed in subsequent chapters in Sects. 1.3 and 1.4 that focus on practice issues in anxiety and depression. The author believes that a developmental psychopathology perspective provides a highly useful framework for providing these four levels of practice.

Assessment

Clinical assessment is a complex process that requires a multimethod approach to develop a comprehensive description of the strengths, needs, and patterns of children with social, emotional, and behavioral problems. The clinician must have a broad understanding of typical child development and the range of variation that is considered "normal." However, "normal" behavior is a relative concept that varies as a function of numerous variables, including culture and family contexts. Consequently, the clinician must be cautious about determining that a disorder exists when the behaviors are variations of typical age-related behavior or are variants of cultural and family variables. The cornerstone of clinical assessment is a comprehensive developmental history that includes gathering as much information as possible about the genetic, biological, social, cultural, family, and school contexts. Selection and use of other assessment methods must be appropriate for the child's age or developmental status.

Intervention

A developmental psychopathology approach to intervention has four assumptions: (a) assessment has accurately identified the problem areas; (b) the problems are developmentally atypical in terms of intensity, frequency, or duration; (c) intervention is needed; and (d) the interventions chosen are appropriate to the problems and are delivered consistent with the child's developmental level. A developmental perspective to intervention not only contributes to alleviation of current symptoms but also seeks to alter negative developmental trajectories, prevent worsening of symptoms, reduce the likelihood of onset of comorbid disorders, and decrease the impact on social, personal, and academic functioning.

Consultation

Indirect services to children occur in the form of consultation with adults who have responsibility for their care, including parents and teachers. As an indirect service, consultation includes helping others to develop approaches to serve children who present emotional and behavioral problems. Consulting with parents often involves helping them develop strategies that they can apply at home and in the community. Consultation for children's emotional and behavioral problems occurs frequently in schools, where professional staff such as school psychologists work with teachers to develop and implement classroom-based interventions. An important element of consultation is to provide the consultee with information about typical behaviors that are expected at various ages and developmental levels. By having a good understanding of typical development, realistic expectations are formed that serve as a basis for effective consultation.

Prevention

Prevention of emotional and behavioral disorders has received substantial research and practice emphasis in the past two decades. From a developmental psychopathology perspective, prevention efforts are intended to prevent the onset of problems as early as possible, prevent the development of problems in children considered at risk, and reduce or prevent the onset of disorders in those who show clear indications of emotional or behavioral problems. In children who have established disorders, the goals of prevention include focusing on preventing an increase in symptom severity, reducing the likelihood of the development of comorbid disorders, and inhibiting or preventing correlated problems, for example, dropping out of school. Approaches to prevention require using curricula and methods that are developmentally appropriate and target risk factors and enhance protective factors. A more thorough discussion of prevention of anxiety and depression is presented in Chap. 13.

Implications of Developmental Psychopathology for Anxiety and Depression

This book uses the developmental psychopathology framework as a "lens" to view child and adolescent depression, which the author believes is valuable in assessment, intervention, consultation, and prevention. Anxiety and depression lend themselves quite well to a developmental perspective, given that they tend to emerge over time in relatively predictable ways and the possible pathways into adulthood are generally well understood. The developmental perspective will help the clinician to develop treatments for the immediate behavior problems, as well as to prevent or alter negative trajectories. As the chapters address the various topics, principles of developmental psychopathology will be infused and used as a framework for discussion. The reader is encouraged to view the contents of the chapters from a developmental perspective to help improve outcomes for children who have or are at risk for anxiety and depression.

Chapter 2
The Developmental Psychopathology of Anxiety

Developmental Considerations

Anxiety is one of the basic human emotions (Plutchik, 1980) and is present in all persons at some time, often on a daily basis to some degree. Concerns about taking a test or being late for an appointment often indicate anxiety in everyday life. Anxiety has a well-defined progression that is recognizable in infancy and progresses through childhood as an indicator of developmental progress. Anxiety and fear are related and often are used interchangeably. Arguably, anxiety has been described as reflecting concerns about subjective, anticipatory events, while fear has been considered to be in response to objective threatening events. Gray and McNaughton (2000) suggested that fear is a defensive response to a real threat, while anxiety is a defensive response to a perceived threat. This chapter will focus primarily on anxiety as a subjective experience of future events, although it is well known that children may have fears of specific stimuli, such as large animals, loud sounds, and unfamiliar people.

One of the first developmental signs of anxiety in children occurs at about 7–8 months of age when infants demonstrate *stranger anxiety* and become upset when held or approached by unfamiliar people. They may cry, cling to parents, and be difficult to soothe until returned to familiar persons. Developmentally, they are beginning to differentiate among people, compared to the earlier period when being handled by unfamiliar persons, does not, by itself, cause distress. At about 12–15 months old, children typically develop *separation anxiety*, which is distress about being separated from caregivers. Reactions in separation anxiety are similar to stranger anxiety, as the child shows crying, clinging, and using available words to prevent the parent from leaving. At this point in development, the child has developed some concerns that parents will not return. Developmentally, stranger anxiety and separation anxiety are predictable, and, when they occur as expected, indicate that some aspects of development are progressing normally. Both of these reactions typically have dissipated by about the end of the second year of life as the child

T.J. Huberty, *Anxiety and Depression in Children and Adolescents:*
Assessment, Intervention, and Prevention, DOI 10.1007/978-1-4614-3110-7_2,
© Springer Science+Business Media, LLC 2012

acquires more language, social, and adaptive skills. Although anxiety can become a clinical problem, it also is a marker for typical development and it may also reflect alertness to danger that is adaptive.

If these reactions occur in a developmentally inappropriate manner at older ages, however, they may be signs that a problem is emerging. For example, it is not uncommon or of great concern that a child becomes anxious about going to kindergarten the first day and has some initial difficulty being away from parents. Within a few days, however, the anxiety usually dissipates and the child enjoys being in school. If the problems persist or the child shows continued difficulty with separation or adapting to new situations, they may be signs of problems such as social anxiety, generalized anxiety, or issues with family dynamics, such as overprotective parenting (Chorpita & Barlow, 1998). Similarly, excessive or persistent separation anxiety into childhood and adolescence is not developmentally appropriate for most children and almost always is associated with some social adjustment problems. If the child has another disorder, such as Asperger's syndrome, social anxiety may be a part of the pattern and require appropriate intervention. In these cases, anxiety is not developmentally appropriate for the child's age, but is a symptom of a larger psychopathology condition. In cases such as these, a secondary diagnosis of an anxiety disorder may be appropriate.

Thus, anxiety is a basic human emotion that has some developmentally predictable onsets, occurrences, and trajectories. As long as they remain within typical developmental parameters, there usually is little reason to be concerned, and support and management of the situation is sufficient. When anxiety becomes severe in terms of frequency, duration, and intensity and is not appropriate for the child's developmental level, then consideration should be given to the possibility of an anxiety problem that should be investigated. As will be discussed later, anxiety is a risk factor for other problems, including depression, and early identification and treatment are essential for altering or preventing negative developmental trajectories.

Characteristics of Anxiety

The central characteristic of anxiety is *worry*, which has been defined as "an anticipatory cognitive process involving repetitive thoughts related to possible threatening outcomes and their potential consequences" (Vasey, Crnic, & Carter, 1994, p. 530). The key terms in this definition are that anxiety is a *cognitive process*, the presence of *repetitious thoughts*, involves the child *anticipating negative outcomes*, and that a primary feature is that the situation is perceived as *threatening*. These components are central to understanding anxiety and developing and implementing interventions, especially from cognitive–behavioral and behavioral treatment perspectives. Highly anxious children and adolescents have a tendency to worry excessively about a wider range of things and to perceive them as being more threatening than do their peers. Anxious children have a *threat attributional bias*, which reflects a greater tendency to attribute potential threat to more situations. In some situations, the child may realize that the anxiety is irrational because it is not likely to occur but nevertheless cannot control the excessive worry.

For example, the author worked with a 12-year-old boy who was demonstrating a high degree of separation anxiety about his parents flying on an airplane while he was left at home with relatives. During the clinical interview, he stated that he was extremely fearful that the plane would crash and his parents would be killed. He recognized that the likelihood of the plane crashing was very small, but for him it was a rational concern, and he could not control the anxiety. Therefore, the initial impression of developmentally inappropriate separation anxiety was a repetitive, anticipatory, and irrational fear of an anticipated catastrophic, but highly unlikely event. With some cognitive–behavioral therapy and family counseling, the situation was resolved rather quickly, with the boy reducing his anxiety to a reasonable level and the parents going on their trip and returning safely.

Trait and State Anxiety

Spielberger (1973) describes two types of anxiety that children, adolescents, and adults can experience. *Trait anxiety* refers to a tendency to have a high degree of anxiety that is generalized and pervasive across a wide range of situations. Trait anxiety is on a continuum from low to high, with high levels being related to impaired performance. It may be considered a personality trait, as it tends to characterize typical functioning of the person. High trait anxiety may not be shown in all situations or to the same degree, but the overall tendency toward generalized anxiety remains present. As a personality trait, anxiety cannot be expected to be eliminated but can be reduced to a manageable level. High levels of trait anxiety are associated with impairments in personal, social, and academic functioning (Huberty, 2008) and are the basis for the majority of anxiety disorders. Often, the "triggers" for a trait anxiety reaction are not apparent and emanate from the person's interpretation of the event.

State anxiety is the tendency to experience high anxiety in specific situations, such as public performances, taking tests, or a dangerous situation. Unlike trait anxiety, the "triggers" of state anxiety usually are readily identifiable. In these cases, the anxiety dissipates after the event has ended or the danger has passed. State anxiety is experienced by everyone at some time and may become debilitating without meeting criteria for an anxiety disorder. For example, some people are very socially competent, are not trait anxious, and do well in almost all areas of their lives, but have intense anxiety about public speaking. In general, treatment of state anxiety problems is much easier and more likely to be successful than is treating trait anxiety. People with high state anxiety are not necessarily prone to high trait anxiety, but highly trait anxious children are more likely to experience high state anxiety (Spielberger, 1973). This relationship is understandable because highly trait anxious people see more situations as threatening and having greater

Table 2.1 Characteristics of anxiety

Cognitive	Behavioral	Physiological
• Concentration problems	• Motor restlessness	• Tics
• Memory problems	• "Fidgety"	• Recurrent, localized pain
• Attention problems	• Task avoidance	• Rapid heart rate
• Oversensitivity	• Rapid speech	• Flushing of the skin
• Problem-solving difficulties	• Erratic behavior	• Perspiration
• Worry	• Irritability	• Headaches
• Cognitive dysfunctions	• Withdrawal	• Muscle tension
– Distortions	• Perfectionism	• Sleeping problems
– Deficiencies	• Lack of participation	• Nausea
• Attributional style	• Failing to complete tasks	• Vomiting
problems	• Seeking easy tasks	• Enuresis

Source: Huberty (2008)

possibilities for negative outcomes. Situations that create high state anxiety may be more problematic for state anxious children because they are likely to feel less competent to cope with stress, increasing their overall anxiety.

Characteristics of Anxiety

Manifestations of anxiety typically occur in one of three ways, either singly or in combination: cognitively, behaviorally, and physiologically. Table 2.1 summarizes these symptoms, some of which also appear in other problems, such as depression and ADHD.

Cognitive Symptoms

Cognitive symptoms include difficulties with memory, concentration, problem solving, and attention. Cognitive problems in anxiety also are seen as *distortions* and *deficiencies* (Kendall, 1992). *Cognitive distortions* occur when the child distorts incoming information, causing errors in thinking and problem solving. For example, a socially anxious adolescent may enter into a social situation and people begin laughing. Whereas a nonanxious youth may not think of this laugher as being directed at him individually, the anxious person is more likely to interpret the situation as threatening and that the people are laughing about him. The information is distorted and an incorrect conclusion is made about the situation that is not founded on accurate data. Cognitive distortions occur frequently in anxious children, causing attributional errors, irrational beliefs, and feelings of lack of competence (Kendall).

Cognitive deficiencies occur when thought processes are impaired due to anxiety and lead to lowered performance. When an anxious student is taking a test, she may be concerned about failing, lack of preparation, or other factors and not be able to concentrate on the task. These interferences lead to deficiencies in thought processes, causing impaired outcomes. If this interference occurs frequently, it may reinforce the child's feelings of low competence, failure, or lack of ability, creating more anxiety and perhaps increasing the probability of developing a mood disorder. Interventions for cognitive symptoms often focus on altering irrational beliefs using cognitive–behavioral techniques. Compared to cognitive distortions where information is altered based on incorrect interpretations, deficiencies relate to impaired effective problem-solving skills that are associated with anxiety.

Children with generalized anxiety disorder tend to have three kinds of cognitive distortions that increase the likelihood that they will worry: *catastrophizing*, *overgeneralizing*, and *personalizing* (Weems & Watts, 2005). *Catastrophizing* occurs when anxious children expect disastrous outcomes from events most of their peers would consider to be rather mild. For example, a boy who has to give a book report in class might anticipate that he will forget what to say, make numerous errors, "block" on what he wants to say, and that he will be humiliated and laughed at by classmates. *Overgeneralizing* might occur in situations where a negative outcome is expected in other situations. A child who experiences extreme social anxiety in a group of unfamiliar people is likely to anticipate that anxiety will occur in similar situations, and increase the tendency to avoid them. *Personalizing* occurs when a child takes personal responsibility for a negative event when it was not her fault, such as blaming herself for her parents' divorce. These types of distortions occur frequently in children with various anxiety disorders and often are the target of cognitive–behavioral interventions. Children with anxiety also tend to have an internal locus of control and believe that outcomes are the result of their own shortcomings rather than task difficulty or other extraneous factors. They also may have low self-efficacy and belief in their own ability, which causes them to worry more (Weems & Watts). Over time, they may resort to withdrawal and other avoidance behaviors to reduce the possibility of making errors and facing embarrassment.

Behavioral Symptoms

Behavioral symptoms are the most easily observed indicators of anxiety. Some of these behaviors (e.g., withdrawal) are voluntary and are intended to help reduce anxiety. Other behaviors, such as motor restlessness, are involuntary and indicate a high level of arousal. Symptoms such as withdrawal or lack of participation may be interpreted by others as lack of motivation, laziness, or disinterest in social or academic situations. Interventions for behavioral symptoms of anxiety may include behavioral approaches, such as self-monitoring, exposure to anxiety-producing situations, social skills treatments, and practice of newly learned coping skills.

Physiological Symptoms

Physiological symptoms are involuntary and reflect a high state of physiological arousal and distress. Some symptoms, such as flushing of the skin, can occur in situations such as public presentations and cause embarrassment and self-consciousness. Symptoms such as headaches and stomach discomfort can be highly unpleasant and cause medical referrals. Some symptoms may be chronic and unob-servable, such as rapid heart rate and muscle tension. There is evidence that resting heart rate is positively correlated with depression and anxiety in children, i.e., anx-ious and depressed children tend to have higher resting heart rates than nonanxious or nondepressed children, suggesting that they may experience a rather constant state of arousal compared to their peers (Lorber, 2004). Interventions may include relaxation training and antianxiety medications coupled with cognitive–behavioral and behavioral treatments.

Positive and Negative Affect

Research has established a high degree of comorbidity between anxiety and depres-sion, often making it difficult to distinguish them. A primary distinction between anxiety and depression is in the area of affect. Clark and Watson (1991) described a *tripartite* theory of emotion and its relation to anxiety and depression in adults, pro-posing three factors: positive affect (PA), negative affect (NA), and physiological hyperarousal (PH). Clark and Watson found that NA is related to both anxiety and depression. Low PA is specific to depression, and high PH is specific to anxiety disorders. Evidence suggests that both PA and NA are temperamental constructs and serve as risk factors for both anxiety and mood disorders (Lonigan & Phillips, 2001; Mineka, Watson, & Clark, 1998; Watson, Clark, & Harkness, 1994).

Subsequent research has found that the tripartite model generally applies to chil-dren and adolescents as well (Chorpita, Albano, & Barlow, 1998; Joiner, Catanzaro, & Laurent, 1996). Lonigan, Carey, and Finch (1994) found that self-report measures measuring low PA significantly differentiated between children with anxiety and depressive disorders, with depressed participants showing significantly less PA. Later research found that measures of PA and NA in children and adolescents were consistent with the adult model. It appears, however, that PH is not consistent across all anxiety disorders and is related primarily to panic disorders but not to other anxi-ety dimensions or disorders (Chorpita, 2002).

If both anxiety and depression are present, anxiety most likely precedes depres-sion. Cole, Peeke, Martin, Truglio, and Ceroacynski (1998) followed 330 children over three years and found that, after depression scores were controlled for, high levels of anxiety predicted depression, but not the reverse. These findings support Gray's (1982) view that the behavioral inhibition system may be the major risk factor for both anxiety and depression that has a temperamental, biological basis.

Conceptualizing the Development of Anxiety Disorders

Anxiety disorders are complex in their development and maintenance over time and represent the transactions among multiple contextual factors. Vasey and Dadds (2001) developed a model that presents the variables and transactions that contribute to development, maintenance, and amelioration of anxiety disorders (Fig. 2.1).

The model is consistent with principles of developmental psychopathology with its emphasis on protective and risk factors, predisposing factors, and the development of cumulative risk over time that are influential in the onset and maintenance of anxiety disorders. Predisposing and protective factors contribute to cumulative risk over time and reflect the balance among them, which affects the likelihood of the onset of anxiety disorders. Cumulative risk is dynamic, however, i.e., it changes

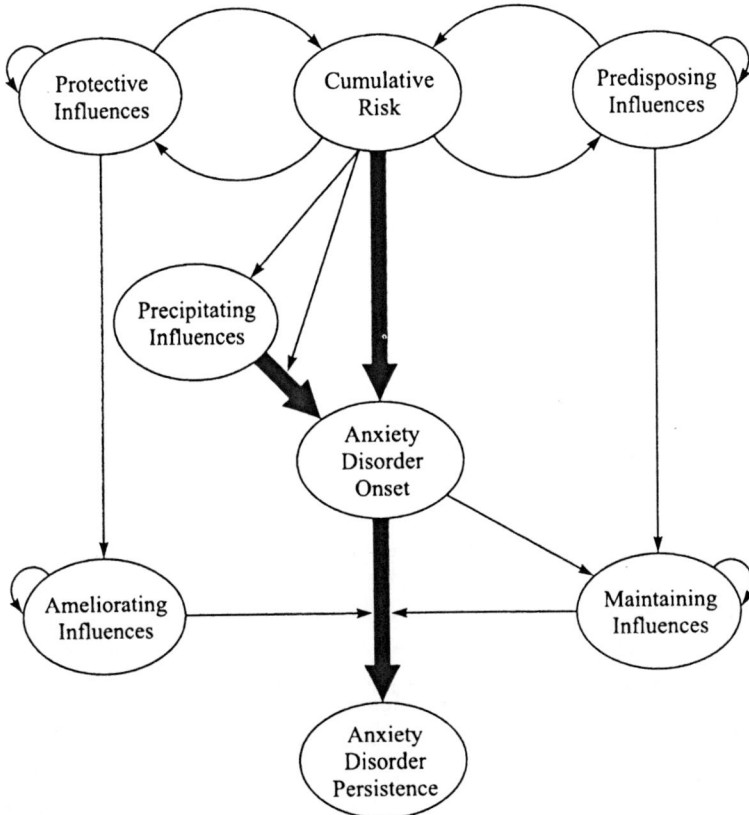

Fig. 2.1 Major categories of influence, their transactional relations, and their role in the development, maintenance, and amelioration of anxiety disorders across time. *Source:* Vasey, M. W., & Dadds, M. R. An introduction to the developmental psychopathology of anxiety (2001). In M. W. Vasey & M. R. Dadds (Eds.), *The developmental psychopathology of anxiety* (p. 13). Oxford, UK: Oxford University Press. Copyright 2010. By permission of Oxford University Press, Inc.

over time, resulting in variations in likelihood of onset. Vasey and Dadds suggest that there are nine factors that may predispose or protect a child against developing an anxiety disorder: (a) genetic factors, (b) neurobiological factors, (c) temperament, (d) emotion regulation skills, (e) cognitive biases and distortions, (f) early control experiences, (g) parental responses, (h) extent of experience with common conditioned stimuli for phobic anxiety, and (i) level of exposure to feared stimuli.

Vasey and Dadds (2001) described the transactional nature of developmental pathways to anxiety disorders as being composed of four elements:

1. Predisposing factors (e.g., genetic risk)
2. Two pathways for the onset of anxiety disorders (respondent and operant conditioning)
3. Factors that maintain or intensify anxiety (e.g., avoidance)
4. Factors contributing to desistance of anxiety (e.g., competence)

This model simultaneously considers the roles of five factors: (a) protective mechanisms, (b) predisposing factors, (c) precipitating factors, (d) ameliorating influences, and (e) maintaining influences. Of particular note is the concept of cumulative risk and precipitating event pathways. The cumulative risk pattern suggests that anxiety disorders gradually develop over time, due to predisposing factors, such as inhibited temperament. These predispositions continue to interact with other factors to increase anxiety, leading to withdrawal and avoidance that complicate the situation by preventing the child from developing coping and adaptive skills. The precipitating pathway occurs as a result of a specific stimulus event, such as a trauma, either by two forms of conditioning. The first one is *respondent conditioning* where anxiety develops from exposure to a formerly neutral stimulus which becomes a trigger for anxiety symptoms. For example, a child might be bitten by a dog and then becomes fearful of all dogs.

The other precipitating event pathway follows the *operant conditioning* paradigm where anxiety develops following an aversive event. An example of this pathway is when a child might try to make friends and is rejected or ridiculed. The event is interpreted as aversive and punishing, leading to fear and anxiety. Thus, avoidance becomes a strategy for similar aversive events, and if unavoidable, anxiety results. Over time, ineffective coping measures are used that further impede the development of adaptive coping. The model corresponds well with an approach that includes genetic, biological, cultural, family, social, and school contexts.

Vasey and Dadds (2001) suggest that any one of these factors may not be necessary for an anxiety disorder to develop but that most anxious children probably have at least one that is related to a pathway toward an anxiety disorder. Due to the self-recursive nature of these factors, anxious children likely will have a combination of several of them en route to the development of an anxiety disorder. Vasey and Dadds suggest that the model cannot easily account for specific forms of anxiety that develop from protective and risk factors or account for all pathways that are influenced by a child's level of development. They also state that the model cannot depict the possible variations in signs and symptoms of anxiety disorders at various points in the developmental sequence. Children who have high behavioral inhibition and negative affectivity may be more likely to be exposed to environmental risks but also are more likely to avoid situations where they could learn to cope with and master these stressors. Consequently, parents may be inclined to engage in behaviors that reinforce these avoidance behaviors in an attempt to help the child avoid distress. Children who have low self-efficacy or low perceived control may give up more quickly than other children when challenges arise even when they might be successful. The reader is referred to Vasey and Dadds for a more complete discussion of the model, which is an excellent conceptualization of the complexity of the development and maintenance of anxiety disorders.

Contextual Influences and the Development of Anxiety and Anxiety Disorders

Genetic Context

There is substantial evidence that genetics plays a role in general tendencies toward the development of anxiety disorders in children, as well as a higher probability toward specific disorders, such as social anxiety disorder. Studies of adult female twins found a significant, although modest, genetic contribution of 30–50% for social anxiety disorder (Kendler, Karbowski, & Prescott, 1999; Kendler, Neale, Kessler, Heath, & Eaves, 1992). Similar rates of heritability exist for most anxiety disorders, although the evidence suggests that genetic effects are more likely to create a tendency toward generalized anxiety patterns rather than for specific anxiety disorders (Eley, 2001; Last, Hersen, Kazdin, Orvaschel, & Perrin, 1991). There is some evidence that persons with first-degree relatives who have a specific anxiety disorder are four to six times more likely to develop the same disorder than those without such relatives (Hetema, Neale, & Kendler, 2001). The remainder of the variance in the development of anxiety disorders is related to a combination of moderate shared (general family) and large nonshared (specific individual) environmental factors (Gregory & Eley, 2007). There is considerable evidence that anxiety is a phenotype or observed pattern that can be seen as a personality trait, symptom, or an anxiety disorder. As a personality trait, anxiety is related to behavioral inhibition (Robinson, Kagan, Reznick, & Corley, 1992), anxiety symptoms (Thapar & McGuffin, 1995; Topolski et al., 1999), and anxiety disorders (Bolton et al., 2006). Topolski et al. (1997) found some slight sex differences in heritability estimates in trait anxiety, with ranges of 0.23 to 0.45 for boys and from 0.42 to 0.57 for girls. This sex difference may help account for the consistent findings that adolescent girls are two to three times more likely to develop anxiety disorders than are adolescent boys.

Understanding the specific genetic mechanisms underlying anxiety disorders currently is limited, especially in children. Panic disorder has been studied the most in adults, with some results implicating specific genes, but the results are not conclusive. It is likely that genetic contributions to anxiety and anxiety disorders are due to combinations of genes interacting in various ways rather than to specific, individual genes. Of particular interest is that parents report greater genetic influences and less shared environmental influences on anxiety than do their children who report the opposite pattern (Eaves et al., 1997; Thapar & McGuffin, 1995). This finding suggests that perhaps parents observe more stable anxiety patterns as traits, whereas children report more of their current state anxiety. Developmental level may be a factor in self-reports because younger children tend to be less reliable reporting their subjective affective states than do older children and adolescents. This research trend has implications for how clinical assessment is conducted, the weight given to the findings, and for the development and implementation of interventions.

Biological Context

There is significant evidence that specific neural structures are implicated in anxiety by affecting the ability to regulate mood. The septo-hippocampal area of the brain appears to be implicated in anxiety disorders and neuropsychological functioning. Gray and McNaughton (2000) discuss that antianxiety drugs primarily affect the behavioral inhibition system and the septo-hippocampal area. With changes in septo-hippocampal functioning, anxiety states tend to lessen. The hippocampus and amygdala have been implicated in both anxiety and depression in children. In a study of children with depression, MacMillan et al. (2003) found larger left and right amygdala/hippocampal volumes, but this larger volume was related more to the severity of anxiety than to the severity of depression. These findings are consistent with frequent research findings and clinical experience that anxiety and depression in children are highly comorbid.

Using functional magnetic resonance imaging (fMRI), Thomas et al. (2001) found that anxious children had much greater amygdala activity when shown fearful faces, while depressed children had decreased response to the same images. Children with high levels of anxiety tend to be hypervigilant to potential threat, which may have a partial basis in chronic higher amygdala activity. These types of studies investigate the contributions of neural structures and neuropsychological functioning to anxiety disorders. It is possible, however, that environmental factors can affect neural functioning as well. Exposure to extreme stress may affect hippocampal functioning by reducing volume. Vermetten, Vythilingam, Southwick, Charney, and Bremmer (2003) found that treatment of patients having posttraumatic stress disorder (PTSD) with the medication paroxetine showed a decrease in symptoms, improved verbal declarative memory, and increased hippocampal volume. At a clinical level, these types of findings emphasize the importance of early identification and prevention efforts for anxiety to reduce the likelihood of effects on neuropsychological functioning.

Temperament

Temperament is one of the most studied areas of child development and psychopathology and is considered a relatively stable trait with biological underpinnings that emerge early in childhood. Inhibited temperament has been shown to be related to the presence of anxiety as a personality trait as well as a risk factor for the development of anxiety disorders. Some researchers have investigated the links between temperament and anxiety on a biological basis by looking at biological substrates of motivation (Gray, 1982). Gray suggests that there is a "behavioral inhibition system" (BIS) that involves the septal area, the hippocampus, the Papez circuit, neocortical aspects of the septo-hippocampal system, prefrontal cortex, hypothalamic activity, and the locus coeruleus. This system underlies a reactive motivational system that is activated by novelty and signals for punishment and nonreward. When the BIS is activated, attention narrows, gross motor behavior is inhibited, increased vigilance and scanning occurs, caution increases, increased central nervous system arousal occurs, and the hypothalamus is activated in preparation for action, such as "fight or flight." During the activation of the BIS, the anxious child engages in processing of information from a threat perspective. These findings suggest that some children may have neurologically based biological predispositions to anxiety reaction that are more readily activated in perceived threatening situations. Environmental influences remain important in the initiation of anxiety reactions, however, because they may serve as cues which highly vigilant, to which anxious children attend and interpret as threatening.

The concept of inhibition has been investigated from a behavioral and developmental perspective for anxiety, without specific focus on anxiety disorders. Kagan (1989) discussed "behavioral inhibition" (BI) as a specific temperamental style in infants, which is related to sociability and approach–avoidance patterns in the presence of stressful circumstances. BI is shown in several behaviors, including remaining close to parents, limited physical activity, faster heart rate, pupil dilation, muscle tension, and general distress. Kagan, Reznick, and Snidman (1988) discussed the course of inhibited and uninhibited children and suggested that 15% of European American children are predisposed to be inhibited as infants. As they develop, behavioral patterns of shyness and fearfulness emerge as preschoolers, and they become quiet, cautious, and introverted in the early school years. At the other end of this continuum, as many as 30% of European American children are described as being "behaviorally uninhibited" (BUI) and are highly sociable, outgoing, and are not distressed by novelty. Both groups tend to maintain these patterns over time after the preschool years. Conversely, BI and BUI patterns at 14–20 months of age do not predict behavior at four years of age, suggesting that there may be a "window" where these patterns emerge and predict later behavior. These differences appear to be more qualitative than quantitative and have implications for understanding the developmental trajectories of anxiety disorders into childhood and adolescence.

High BI appears to be a relatively enduring temperamental trait that persists throughout life (Kagan, Reznick, & Snidman, 1987; Kagan et al., 1988). As high

BI children get older, they have fewer friends, show less initiative in social situations, are less likely to participate in school, and tend to avoid difficult tasks. High BI children appear to have qualitatively different social and personal characteristics than do their typical peers and those children who are described as being merely "shy."

As research on BI has emerged, questions have been asked about the possible association of BI with the development of anxiety disorders. Some studies have shown associations with social anxiety disorder, particularly if BI remains stable during early childhood (Biederman, Hirshfeld-Becker et al., 2001). In children with social-evaluative concerns or social anxiety disorder, BI has shown significant correlations with several physiological measures of anxiety, including heart rate, morning salivary cortisol, and activation of neurological processes associated with withdrawal and avoidance (Beidel, 1988; Davidson, 1994; Heimberg, Hope, Dodge, & Becker, 1990; Kagan et al., 1988). One study using fMRI in infants with high BI showed a modest correlation with amygdala functioning in adults when they were exposed to novel social stimuli (Schwartz, Wright, Shin, Kagan, & Rauch, 2003). This finding is consistent with research suggesting that high BI may be associated with increased risk for social anxiety disorders over time. Other research has established that high BI children are more likely to develop anxiety disorders (Biederman, Rosenbaum, Chaloff, & Kagan, 1995; Biederman et al., 1990; Caspi, Henry, McGee, Moffitt, & Silva, 1995). It should be noted, however, that having high BI does not necessarily lead to behavioral and social dysfunction or anxiety disorders. In the Biederman et al. study, about two-thirds of BI children did not develop anxiety disorders. With a prevalence rate of about 15%, BI occurs more often than anxiety disorders at any given time.

Cultural Context

Because anxiety is a universal human emotion, anxiety is experienced by all children in every culture, although its manifestation and mode of expression may vary considerably. The majority of research on anxiety has been conducted on anxiety patterns in European American children, but research comparing clinical groups is limited. Many of the studies of anxiety across cultures have used self-report measures that have been translated from English, raising questions about comparability of findings. Fornesca, Yule, and Erol (1994) reviewed studies of cross-cultural anxiety and reported that self-reported fears were generally similar across the USA, Portugal, Italy, Turkey, Australia, the Netherlands, Northern Ireland, China, and the UK, although scores were somewhat lower in the Dutch sample and higher in the Portuguese group. The authors suggested that perhaps one of the reasons for these differences is that Latin cultures show a tendency to express fears more openly, while Dutch culture tends to be associated with more control and concealment of emotions.

Anxiety symptoms appear to be more prevalent in societies that value inhibition and deference, compliance with social expectations, and social evaluation, such as in Asian countries (Ollendick, Yang, King, Dong, & Akande, 1996). Weisz et al. (1987) compared American children with Thai children using parent self-report measures. He found that Thai children demonstrated more internalizing behaviors than did the American children. The finding was consistent with the hypothesis that Thai social expectations to maintain emotional control would be associated with a greater prevalence of internalizing behaviors. Ivanova, Achenbach, Rescorla et al. (2007) conducted a study across 23 societies using the *Child Behavior Checklist Youth Self-Report* scale (Achenbach & Rescorla, 2001) and found that the patterns of child behavior problems generally are consistent across those cultures. The anxious–depressed syndrome showed a median item loading of 0.63 across the groups, with "feeling worthless" and "worries" showing the highest loadings of 0.72. These loadings suggest that these two items are consistent across cultures and mirror the literature that feelings of low self-worth and worrying are common in anxious–depressed children. The results were also consistent with earlier findings of parent and teacher ratings of children's emotional and behavioral problems. Although there does appear to be consistency of the anxious–depressed syndrome across multicultural societies, it is not clear whether interventions used in one culture for anxiety and depression are efficacious in all cultures.

In a study investigating the association among anxiety, school performance, and social functioning, Li and Zhang (2008) found that Chinese adolescents who were more academically successful had lower levels of anxiety and were more popular than their low-achieving counterparts. This finding may be related to research suggesting that Chinese children and adolescents perceive significant pressure to perform well in school (Chen et al., 1995).

Although there is ample research to indicate that patterns of anxiety are reasonably consistent across cultures, less is known about the nature, emergence, developmental trajectories, and outcomes for anxiety disorders across cultures. Nevertheless, the clinician should assume that anxiety disorders do exist across cultures and should be prepared to address them while simultaneously considering culturally unique factors, such as attitudes toward emotional expression, parenting, social expectations, and conceptions of psychopathology. Even if an anxiety disorder is identified, cultural expectations and attitudes toward mental health issues and interventions may vary across societies, affecting the delivery of services.

Social Context

The social context represents some of the most salient aspects of anxiety because impairments in social functioning are often the consequence of high levels of anticipatory worry. In the majority of anxiety disorders, some degree of social impairment occurs, although it may be brief, such as in a public performance, or more extended, such as with social phobia/social anxiety disorder. Because many anxiety disorders are associated with perceptions of social competence, acceptance, and performance, many interventions are directed toward addressing the social consequences of anxiety.

As discussed earlier, stranger anxiety and separation anxiety are common occurrences in children and indicate that development is progressing as expected. Muris, Merkelbach, Gadet, and Moulaert (2000) found that children aged four to six reported being separated from parents as being a major worry, but older children did not identify parent separation as a primary concern. These findings support the notion that there is a normal amount of separation anxiety in younger children that dissipates over time. However, the distinction between this typical developmental trend and pathological separation anxiety is the degree of social impairment. In early childhood, anxiety tends to be focused on meeting people, entering new situations, and being concerned about appearing incompetent in front of others (Spence, Rapee, McDonald, & Ingram, 2001). A related construct seen in a small group of children is extreme shyness, which tends to be highly consistent over time (Fordham & Stevenson-Hinde, 1999). These authors found that extreme shyness was significantly related to higher levels of trait anxiety, lower ratings of self-worth, and less adequate friendship quality. Thus, extreme shyness places these children at higher risk of developing social phobia/social anxiety disorder, again depending to a large extent on environmental influences.

As children develop into adolescence, social concerns tend to create more anxiety. During this period, increased concerns about social evaluation emerge, especially with girls. In a study of two cohorts of 15-year-olds, 40–45% of girls worried most about school performance and weight (29 and 38.3%), while boys were concerned about school performance (39.1 and 35.6%) and unemployment (35.6 and 25%) (West & Sweeting, 2003). Highly anxious children tend to have a variety of social and interpersonal problems, depending on the nature or severity or the symptoms. They tend to be perfectionistic, self-conscious in social situations, have delayed or impaired social interaction skills, and are sensitive to perceived criticism or evaluation of their ability. Withdrawal is seen often, as the children attempt to control or minimize the anxiety. They may be awkward when initiating or entering social situations, may think that others are evaluating them, and are hypersensitive to perceived criticism by others. Highly anxious children tend to "catastrophize" social situations and anticipate that negative occurrences are more likely to occur than is probable. They may engage in repetitious, ritualistic, or ruminative behaviors in an effort to reduce anxiety. Because anxious children tend to have an attributional bias for threat, they may interpret mild or innocuous social situations incorrectly and see them as personal affronts or references. Social skills may be delayed or impaired, making it more difficult to cope with the demands of social situations, which may be compounded by difficulties in correctly perceiving subtle interpersonal cues and social nuances. Behavioral and physiological symptoms such as fidgeting, flushing of the skin, excessive perspiration, or frequent seeking of reassurance may result in teasing, embarrassment, or social rejection, leading to more anxiety and reduced social coping skills.

Family Context

There is ample evidence that family factors, including parenting, are highly related to the development and maintenance of anxiety disorders. Although much of the research has focused on the influence of parents on children, the influence of the child on family functioning also is of interest. Rather than focusing only on the influence of family and parenting factors on the child, the anxious child also has effects on family functioning that have implications for clinical practice.

Parental Psychopathology

As stated earlier, some anxiety disorders and behavioral inhibition appear to have heritable bases that are transmitted across generations, primarily as general tendencies toward anxiety patterns (Eley, 2001). Because these associations show modest relationships of 30–50%, however, the remaining effects come from environmental factors, including family functioning and parenting. Nevertheless, it is important to understand family histories of anxiety-related problems in clinical assessment and intervention of anxious children in order to establish the historical context of the development of disorders. Knowledge of the historical family context is useful in determining how the developmental trajectory began and was maintained over time.

A substantial research base exists regarding the association of parenting factors with the development and maintenance of anxiety and anxiety disorders. Two research approaches have been used in studies: (a) whether children with anxiety disorders have a parent with some form of psychopathology or (b) whether children with parents who have psychopathology are more likely to develop anxiety disorders. In the first type of studies, the results have been rather inconsistent. Some studies have found that parents who have children with anxiety disorders are more likely to meet criteria for anxiety disorders, while others have not found this relationship (Malcarne & Hansdottir, 2001). An example of the second group of studies is shown by Turner, Beidel, and Costello (1987) who found that children of anxious parents were seven times more likely than children of parents without psychopathology to develop anxiety disorders and twice as likely compared to children of parents who had dysthymia. Weissman, Leckman, Merikangas, Gammon, and Prusoff (1984) found some evidence of increased rates of separation anxiety disorder (SAD) in parents with depression and panic disorder but not in parents with depression and agoraphobia, depression and generalized anxiety disorder, depression only, or a nonclinical control group. Malcarne and Hansdottir concluded that these studies suggest that parental anxiety or depression may be a risk factor for childhood anxiety and may implicate genetic influences, but the mechanisms of this relationship are unclear.

Parenting

Whereas the previous discussion addresses issues of parental psychopathology that may have some origins in genetic and biological factors, the role of parenting relates more to interpersonal and family relationships with childhood anxiety. Highly anxious children become distressed about issues of control and being able to predict outcomes. Chorpita and Barlow (1998) suggest that parents of anxious children tend to have an overcontrolling, intrusive, or overprotective parenting style. Parents who use overcontrolling parenting styles limit their children's exposure to anxiety-producing situations and reinforce their avoidant behavior. Limiting exposure to negative situations does not give the child the opportunity to develop coping skills, and maladaptive anxiety coping behaviors are reinforced. Kendall (2008, personal communication) described these parents as "helicopter parents" who "hover" over their children and are overprotective. These behaviors may also be modeled as well, which a child may imitate over time. Learning of behaviors that reduce or avoid anxiety tends to be self-reinforcing and is likely to be repeated in similar circumstances. This pattern has been shown in research by findings that anxious children tend to choose avoidant solutions compared to children who are defiant and oppositional (Barrett, Rapee, Dadds, & Ryan, 1996). As children age and enter into more social situations where parents cannot protect them as well, they may develop a perception of uncontrollability. Chorpita, Brown, and Barlow (1998) found that a high degree of parental control mediated family environment and was related to anxious symptoms in children.

Recent research has demonstrated that parenting has a significant influence on children exposed to trauma. Smith, Perrin, Yule, and Rabe-Hesketh (2001) found that both exposure to trauma and parental distress were related to posttraumatic stress symptoms in 9–14-year-old Bosnian children. Spell et al. (2008) found that 11% of children exposed to Hurricane Katrina showed PTSD symptoms, and 12% showed clinically significant levels of internalizing problems. Higher levels of maternal distress following exposure to the disaster were associated with higher levels of child internalizing and externalizing symptoms, regardless of the degree of the children's exposure to the hurricane. These findings suggest that it was not the disaster per se that affected the children but the degree of the mother's psychopathology, i.e., better mental health of parents was a protective factor for children with less exposure to disaster.

Inadequate affection by parents has been found to be associated with anxiety in children, usually in conjunction with a controlling maternal parenting style (e.g., Gerlsma, Emmelkamp, & Arrindell, 1990). Parents of anxious children showed more intrusive and critical behavior when working together on a puzzle task (Hudson & Rapee, 2001), lending support to the notion that parenting style is associated with the development and maintenance of anxiety. In this latter case, it is possible that this kind of parenting style might be shown when these parents are working with the children on schoolwork and similar tasks. Other research has found that parents of anxious children emphasize the threatening aspects of ambiguous situations that lead to misinterpretations of events, again reinforcing avoidant behavior (Barrett et al., 1996).

Overall, however, the association between broad parenting styles and childhood anxiety may be unclear due to methodological problems, and there may not be a meaningful relationship with childhood anxiety (Wood, McLeod, Sigman, Hwang, & Chu, 2003). There is some suggestion that specific behaviors have an effect on the development of anxiety in children, but the data are unclear. From a clinical perspective, however, it may be an area for consideration with individual cases.

School Context

The association of anxiety with school factors can be viewed from social and cognitive perspectives, which can operate singly and in combination to affect academic performance. To a great extent, highly anxious children demonstrate symptoms in a variety of situations, with the specific circumstances having great influence on the type, frequency, and intensity of behaviors. The school setting provides the greatest opportunity for social interaction and the development of children's interpersonal skills and relationships because there are many other children and adults present on a daily basis, and they attend school for many hours. For the anxious child, however, school can be a place where demands and social pressures may contribute to increased anxiety, an increase in maladaptive coping behaviors, and negative effects on learning and performance.

Social Factors

Children with high anxiety or anxiety disorders are more likely to have social problems that may create a developmental pathway for generalized or social anxiety disorders. Many of these social concerns are about being evaluated, and schools provide many opportunities for formal and informal evaluation of social, physical, and academic skills. Anxious children tend to show involuntary shifting of attention away from positive feelings and circumstances and focus on negative aspects of situations and perceived threat. These children are unable to use problem-focused coping techniques (Mellings & Alden, 2000) and instead use rumination and avoidance strategies that have little anxiety-reducing effect (Garnefski, Legerstee, Kraaij, Van Den Kommer, & Teerds, 2002). When faced with the complex social challenges of the school setting that include working in small groups and performing in public, highly anxious children may be perceived as being socially inept, incapable, or disinterested.

Social factors may appear in instructional situations as well. Highly anxious children volunteer less in class, are uncomfortable participating in or leading small groups, show discomfort in public performances (e.g., giving speeches, displaying skills), avoid difficult tasks, seek easy tasks, react poorly to criticism, and lack normal levels of assertiveness. Signs of perfectionism may be seen, as anxious children attempt to control their anxiety by creating a structured and predictable environment. These situations demonstrate the interaction between academic and social aspects of anxious children because these behaviors may have an effect on others' perceptions and acceptance in a social context. Because they may have fewer social interactions, anxious children have less opportunity to develop social skills.

Cognitive Factors

As indicated in Table 2.1, some cognitive characteristics of anxiety are manifested in learning situations in the school setting. A major effect of anxiety on learning and performance is on attention. In instructional tasks, children must be able to attend to relevant cues, directions, and stimuli while minimizing the effect of competing stimuli. This *selective attention* is essential for effective information processing and problem solving. The association between anxiety and attention has been considered from the direction between them. It is possible that underlying neurological processes cause difficulties in the regulation of attention and predispose children toward anxiety and anxiety disorders (MacLeod, Rutherford, Campell, Ebsworthy, & Holker, 2002). The alternative view is that anxiety might influence the ability to attend. For example, children who experience trauma show difficulties in attending to threat stimuli even if they do not self-report anxiety (Dalgleish, Moradi, Taghavi, Neshat-Doost, & Yule, 2001).

Although determining which, if either, of these directions is operating is not feasible in schools and clinical settings, the result is that anxious children have difficulty in selective attention and overall attention to tasks. Concentration may be impaired, interfering with the ability to evaluate and select from multiple possibilities and to give a correct response. Attention may also be a factor in the frequent observation that anxious children have difficulties with memory and may report that they cannot recall information when taking tests and performing other tasks. Anxious children often appear to be "daydreaming," which may be due to difficulties with attending and recalling information. Chronic difficulties performing in the classroom likely will lead to increased feelings of incompetence and the tendency to interpret more situations as threatening.

Developmental Pathways of Anxiety Disorders

Although the developmental pathways of anxiety disorders may appear to be relatively predictable, many factors within the various contexts of development can interact in multiple and complex ways and lead to similar (equifinality) or numerous (multifinalilty) outcomes. Individual vulnerabilities, risk factors, protective factors, and resilience contribute to the various pathways of anxiety disorders. Thus, the developmental courses of anxiety disorders vary significantly across children. Nevertheless, an understanding of common pathways is helpful to the clinician to work with children and parents by increasing understanding of possible trajectories of untreated and treated problems.

There is sufficient research evidence that many anxiety disorders can lead to significant negative social, emotional, personal, and socioeconomic outcomes, especially if untreated. Even if treated, some disorders with early onset, high chronicity, severe symptomatology, and high comorbidity often show residual effects or relapse in adolescence and adulthood. Woodward and Ferguson (2001) found significant correlations between anxiety disorders in 14–16-year-olds and risks for mental health, educational, and social problems when they were 18–21 years old. Mental health problems included anxiety and depressive disorders, academic underachievement, suicidal ideation, early parenthood, and alcohol, drug, and nicotine dependence. When factoring out social and family variables and personal disadvantages, the association between the number of anxiety disorders and these variables was nonsignificant. The results suggest that the outcomes were more related to risk factors and life circumstances rather than anxiety disorders alone. Nevertheless, multiple anxiety disorders increased the risk for anxiety disorders, depression, illicit drug use, and not attending college. Sonntag, Wittchen, Hofler, Kessler, and Stein (2000) found associations between cigarette smoking and social fears and social phobia in young adults and adolescents. These findings indicate that the adolescents and adults began using cigarettes to reduce feelings of anxiety. The findings also point to the possibility that, in some cases, onset of smoking may be at least partially attributable to an undetected anxiety disorder.

Research has established a high degree of comorbidity of anxiety and depression and that, if both patterns are present, anxiety likely preceded depression. Early anxiety is associated with later onset of depression, which increases the risk of suicidal ideation or attempts (Pawlak, Pascual-Sanchez, Rae, Fischer, & Ladame, 1999). Nelson et al. (2000) found increased risk for suicidal thoughts and attempts and alcohol use in adolescents with comorbid major depression and social phobia. Such findings are not surprising, given the comorbidity between anxiety disorders and depression and indicate that clinicians should consider the possibility of suicide in anxious and phobic children and adolescents, not only depressive disorders. Thus, anxious children likely are at higher risk for suicide than many clinicians may assume.

Specific Anxiety Disorders

Anxiety disorders are rarely identified in infancy and preschoolers. It is known that infants and young children show stranger anxiety and that separation anxiety from parents is common from about age one to four (Dashiff, 1995). Fears of the dark, animals, and monsters are seen frequently in toddlers and preschoolers (Campbell, 1986). Extreme shyness may be an indicator or of anxiety, but children typically do not meet diagnostic criteria for a specific anxiety disorder before school entry age. Anxiety may accompany other problems, such as stressful environments, illness, and some developmental disorders. The majority of anxiety disorders have their beginnings after entry into school, although some early signs associated with inhibited behavior and temperament may indicate a higher probability of the development of an anxiety disorder during childhood or adolescence (e.g., Kagan et al., 1997, 1998). For example, children who show high levels of inhibition as preschoolers are more likely to develop generalized anxiety disorder and social anxiety disorder.

Separation Anxiety Disorder (SAD) is the only anxiety disorder specifically designated for children in the DSM-IV. Children can be diagnosed with any anxiety disorder in the DSM-IV using the same criteria that are applied for adults. In the DSM-III-R (APA, 1987), Overanxious Disorder (OAD) was included as a childhood anxiety disorder, and several research studies focused on it. The disorder was not included in DSM-IV, however, due to lack of support that it was a separate disorder, and it was subsumed under generalized anxiety disorder (GAD) in the DSM-IV. SAD has a basis in typical development in that the majority of children have concerns about separation from parents into early school years. The distinction between separation anxiety and SAD is the degree to which it is developmentally appropriate and excessive. With older children, the presence of chronic or severe separation anxiety alone can be an indicator of SAD. In these situations, there will be signs of notable, if not clinically significant, separation anxiety that may require intervention. It may be difficult to distinguish between SAD and social phobia/social anxiety disorder without careful observation, clinical assessment, and detailed developmental and symptomatic history.

The other anxiety disorders in DSM-IV can occur in children and adults, and the criteria are applicable to all ages and both genders. A typical distinction between children and adults is that children are not required to recognize the nature of their anxiety. Young children typically have not achieved a developmental level to be able to reflect and report on their subjective mood states and cognitive processes. Because the majority of anxiety symptoms are extremes of typical behaviors, differentiating them from anxiety disorders can be challenging. The developmental pathways of anxiety disorders vary in their outcomes and comorbidity. In Table 2.2, the primary anxiety disorders experienced in childhood and adolescence are summarized by typical age of onset, primary symptoms, comorbidity, and developmental outcomes.

Clinical Implications of a Developmental Psychopathology Perspective on Anxiety Disorders

Anxiety disorders are among the most common childhood emotional problems and are comorbid with other disorders, especially depression. Children with anxiety disorders are at significant risk for social, personal, and academic problems in childhood and adolescence, as well as problems associated with substance abuse. A developmental psychopathology perspective on childhood disorders, including anxiety, suggests that they can develop in multiple ways through the interactive effects of biological and psychological vulnerabilities with environmental factors, including parenting, socialization, and culture. To attempt to separate these factors and place the emphasis primarily on the child is likely to lead to misconceptualization of clinical problems and inadequate assessment and treatment. Therefore, the contextual

Table 2.2 Anxiety disorders of childhood and adolescence

Anxiety disorder	Typical age of onset	Primary symptoms	Comorbidity	Developmental pathway
Separation anxiety disorder (SAD)	8–12-years old but can occur at any age	Procrastination; refusal to leave home or go to school; reluctant to develop friendships; refuses to stay away from home; avoidance; somatic complaints; specific fears; wanting to sleep with parents; mild somatic complaints may progress to more severe physical reactions, such as vomiting or panic reactions	Generalized anxiety disorder secondary to SAD in about 1/3 of cases; 1/3 have onset of depressive disorder within a few months after onset of SAD; rarely associated with suicidal ideation	Onset acute and early, usually after a major stressor, such as a move or death of a parent; course varies and symptoms tend to recur when stressors occur; complete remission may take years and relapse be sudden; no gender differences in prevalence; girls at greater risk of panic disorder and agoraphobia
Generalized anxiety disorder (GAD)	10–13 years of age, but can occur in preschoolers and early childhood	Uncontrollable worry about general daily functioning, the future, social, and academic competence; overestimate likelihood of negative outcomes; underestimate ability to cope with challenging situations; highly self-conscious; perfectionism; intensity of worry distinguishes GAD from typical behavior somatic complaints	Separation anxiety and attention deficits in younger children and more depression and anxiety in older children	Long-term course with childhood onset; symptoms tend to be stable and likely to be present at some level into adolescence and adulthood; increased risk for mood disorder; some evidence of increased risk for alcohol use in adolescence, perhaps to help control worry

(continued)

Table 2.2 (continued)

Anxiety disorder	Typical age of onset	Primary symptoms	Comorbidity	Developmental pathway
Obsessive–compulsive disorder (OCD)	10–12 years of age although can occur at younger ages but rarely before school age	Recurrent and intrusive obsessions and compulsions; are time-consuming (more than 1 h per day) and cause stress or impairment; child and adult symptoms are similar and children tend to report obsessions about germs and illness; repetition of behavior, such as hand washing; concerns about religious, sexual, and moral issues; ritualistic behavior in excess of typical child patterns; in over 90% of cases, symptom pattern changes over time; may cause problems with schoolwork due to failing to complete tasks in a timely manner and frequent rechecking; must distinguish from nonsymptomatic typical childhood rituals that begin about age 2 and dissipate by about age 9; with primary criterion being degree of distress if the ritual is prevented or interrupted	Increased risk of other anxiety disorders (e.g., GAD) and mood disorders; early age of onset associated with ADHD and phobias; coexisting mood disorders more common in older children; panic disorders; as many as ¾ of OCD patients report panic attacks; seen in as many as 50% of cases with tic disorders, but only a small percent of Tourette's disorder cases have OCD	One follow-up study (Wewetzer et al., 2001) of children with OCD onset at 12 years of age and 11 years later found 36% still had OCD and 71% had some form of disorder. 70% of OCD subjects had at least one other disorder (most often, anxiety or depression). 12.7% had paranoid personality disorder, and 25.5% had obsessive–compulsive personality disorder. Untreated OCD is associated with a chronic course of impairment and comorbid disorders into adulthood

Social phobia (social anxiety disorder)	Diagnosis usually first made in early teen years, but history often indicates onset of shyness and inhibition before age 10	Extreme self-consciousness and social discomfort; socially avoidant; physiological reactions in social settings; low self-esteem; prefer company of adults rather than peers; unlike GAD, is specific to social situations	Other anxiety disorders, especially GAD; depression; specific phobia; comorbid ADHD and learning disorders range from 10 to 15%	Effects are multidimensional and are noticed in school-related spheres, such as frequent absences, test anxiety, poor performance, and fear of evaluation; attention deficits to tasks; school dropout; fewer friends and social supports; less likely to marry; male developmental trajectories more affected than are females; as adults, seen as aloof, having lack of poise, timid, and socially awkward; greater chance of substance and alcohol abuse and suicidal ideation
Specific phobia	Can occur at any age, with onset primarily related to age and type of stimulus or situation; increased frequency occurs between 10 and 13; fear of animals occurs before age 7; fear of blood at age 9; dental phobia at about age 11; natural environment phobias (e.g., thunderstorms) tend to onset at about age 12	Increased physiological symptoms; panic reactions or attacks; attempts to escape or avoid the situation; avoidance responses may include crying, tantrums, hiding, flight; if unavoidable, child shows high distress	Comorbid patterns not well established, but children with separation anxiety disorder or social anxiety disorder may be at greater risk of developing specific phobia; may be related to onset of panic attacks or panic disorder and traumatic events	Developmental pathways are related to age of onset and type of phobia; in many cases, remission occurs over time; in absence of other psychopathology, pervasive impairment over time is less likely

(continued)

Table 2.2 (continued)

Anxiety disorder	Typical age of onset	Primary symptoms	Comorbidity	Developmental pathway
Posttraumatic stress disorder (PTSD)	Can occur at any age, but the types of stressful events can be determinants; type I: rapid, sudden onset due to specific traumatic event, such as death or illness; type II: gradual, continuously developing trauma associated with chronic, long-term stress, such as child abuse, dangerous environments, exposure to violence	Reexperiencing traumatic events through dreaming and thinking; extreme stress; sleep problems; hypervigilance; concentration problems; exaggerated startle response; lack or loss of interest in important activities; avoidance of places or circumstances that may trigger memories of events; trauma-specific reenactment of specific events; restricted affect; "numbing" of responsiveness	Other anxiety disorders and depression; may have some obsessive thoughts or repetitive behaviors but do not meet criteria for OCD diagnosis; is differentiated from other anxiety disorders by the recognition of specific events or chronic stress as triggers	Developmental course depends to a great extent on whether the trauma is a single event or chronic exposure to stress and when it occurred. Children tend to adapt and resolve reactions to single events, while children exposed to chronic trauma have more difficulties, including depression and anxiety; girls tend to show more PTSD symptoms than do males; may be long-term effects of chronic stress into adulthood and contribute to problems in personal functioning, including substance abuse
Panic disorder	Panic attacks have been reported to be relatively common in adolescents, with about 40–60% of adolescents reporting them, but occur less frequently in children (Ollendick et al., 1994); panic disorder occurs two to three times more often in females than males with onset most likely between late adolescence and the mid-30s; median age of onset about 24 years of age (Burke et al., 1990)	Physiological symptoms including heart palpitations, sweating, trembling or shaking, chest pain or discomfort, dizziness; cognitive and affective symptoms include fears of dying, loss of control, depersonalization, and feelings of unreality; person tends to have high anxiety sensitivity and associate many behaviors and physical signs as warnings of impending panic attack; symptoms tend not to be age-related	Agoraphobia, OCD, depression, substance abuse, personality disorders, GAD, specific phobia, social phobia; comorbid disorders are more common in adolescence and adulthood; some evidence of co-occurrence of panic attacks and refusal to eat in children and adolescents due to fear of vomiting (Ballenger et al., 1989; Bradley & Hood, 1993)	Although onset is in late adolescence to adulthood, children with GAD and phobias are more likely to develop panic disorder; presence of agoraphobia is associated with greater impairment and persistence; desire to prevent panic attacks may cause avoidance of some situations; more adverse outcomes in adults with onset prior to age 17; average time from onset of symptoms to treatment ~12.7 years (Moreau & Follet 1993)

approach described in Chap. 1 as applied to anxiety problems in this chapter provides a useful perspective upon which to conceptualize and work with childhood anxiety disorders. In developing a clinical approach within a developmental framework, the clinician is better able to assess all relevant variables and develop interventions that are appropriate for the child's cognitive, social, emotional, and behavioral level.

A particular challenge in working with childhood anxiety disorders is that, because anxiety is a normal and pervasive emotion, differentiating it from psychopathology can be difficult. Some anxiety is expected at certain ages and developmental levels and in specific circumstances (e.g., meeting new people, performing in public). The clinician must be careful not to "pathologize" normal variations of anxiety as being clinical problems. Nevertheless, the clinician has the task of conducting a thorough developmental and clinical assessment that addresses as many of the contexts as possible, which will have effects on how intervention is developed and implemented.

Because anxiety is highly associated with vulnerability to stress, particular attention must be given to identifying and treating stressors that put a child at greater risk of developing or exacerbating an anxiety disorder. These stressors may include parental psychopathology, learning disabilities, parenting styles, socioeconomic factors, and social relationships. Some of these stressors may be difficult, if not impossible, to alleviate (e.g., socioeconomic factors) but nevertheless should be considered as potential contributors to the development and maintenance of anxiety disorders.

Conclusion

The developmental psychopathology of anxiety is a complex, multifaceted, and progressive problem with onset of some symptoms in early childhood. Anxiety disorders are associated with a wide range of trajectories and problems if left untreated. Research has established substantial relationships of anxiety with deficits in social, personal, and academic functioning extending into adolescence and adulthood, including increased risk for depression and substance abuse. Assessment and intervention must consider not only the child's current functioning but also negative developmental trajectories and outcomes and emphasize strategies to alter them.

Chapter 3
The Developmental Psychopathology of Depression

Unlike anxiety that is a normal developmental experience and progression from infancy through adulthood, depression and other mood disorders are not typical and do not occur in all persons. Of course, all people have feelings of being "blue" or have depressive reactions to life events at times, most of which dissipate. Nearly all adolescents present as being "moody" and irritable at times, which is part of their biological, cognitive, social, and emotional development. For the most part, symptoms of depression are more severe manifestations of typical behaviors, such as feeling "down" or "blue," which all persons experience at some time. The similarity between anxiety and depression is that a disorder emerges when typical behaviors become intense, chronic, or otherwise developmentally inappropriate and impair functioning. There is significant comorbidity between the conditions, and the severity of specific symptoms varies depending on whether the primary pattern is anxiety or depression. The primary distinction between them from a developmental perspective is that mood disorders are more episodic, which, over time, require smaller environmental stressors to serve as a stimulus for episodes to occur (Pennington, 2002). Conversely, anxiety disorders tend to develop more slowly over time and become relatively stable behavioral patterns and traits.

Interest in childhood depression has increased over the past two to three decades, despite the knowledge that adult depression has been known for centuries. The Freudian perspective suggested that young children could not experience depression because they lacked the intrapsychic processes such as insight and self-reflection seen in adults. Freud hypothesized that depression was the result of loss that leads to internalized anger through the superego. Because he did not believe that young children had a well-developed superego structure, depression was therefore impossible.

Another conceptualization of the idea that depression could not exist in children was that, if a child showed depressive symptoms, they were presumed to be transient in nature, but not true depression (Kaslow & Rehm, 1991). However, not all children show depressive symptoms, demonstrating that they are not typical developmental occurrences. Another model suggested that depression is "masked"

T.J. Huberty, *Anxiety and Depression in Children and Adolescents:*
Assessment, Intervention, and Prevention, DOI 10.1007/978-1-4614-3110-7_3,
© Springer Science+Business Media, LLC 2012

in children by other disorders, such as conduct disorder, i.e., that behavior prevents the detection of the underlying depression. However, that view has not been confirmed in research. It is true that depression is often comorbid with externalizing behaviors, but the depression is not "masked" but part of a larger clinical picture of distress and clinical disturbance. Thus, research has established that depression can and does occur in children and adolescents, although the symptoms and expression may vary as a function of developmental level. For example, some symptoms of depression seen in adults, such as feelings of helplessness, hopelessness, and low self-esteem, may not occur in children, due to their relative lack of cognitive and emotional maturation.

The fact that there are some qualitative differences in the expression of depression in children and adults has contributed to some inconsistent and diverse opinions about mood disorders in children. The criteria for mood disorders in children in the DSM-IV are applied to children, although children may show signs of irritability and "crankiness" as primary symptoms. The fact that it is well recognized that children may not have the developmental capacity to experience some symptoms of depression and therefore express them differently raises questions whether adult criteria should be applied. This issue is particularly relevant for the diagnosis of bipolar disorder, which has shown an increased frequency in children during the last two decades. For example, children who have been given a diagnosis of bipolar disorder often do not meet the majority of criteria listed in the DSM-IV but nevertheless are given the diagnosis based largely on mood lability. Although the nature of depression and mood disorders in children is not clearly understood, there is little doubt that they do exist and require careful assessment and empirically based interventions.

Characteristics of Depression

Unlike anxiety where there is a central cognitive characteristic of worry, there is not a single primary cognitive feature in depression, although several occur simultaneously, such as "all-or-none" thinking and learned helplessness. However, many depressed children do worry about many aspects of their lives, including social and academic spheres. Also, because anxiety and mood disorders are comorbid, worry is often seen in syndromes. Worry is not necessarily the pervasive characteristic, however, but is part of the larger clinical picture. Even though depressed children may manifest worry, it is qualitatively different from the worry associated with anxiety that is more associated with concerns about social evaluation (Huberty, 2008). Although depressed children may have concerns about social evaluation, most often it is not the primary stressor.

Like anxiety, depression is manifested in cognitive, behavioral, and physical symptoms. As discussed in Chap. 2, there is considerable comorbidity of symptoms between anxiety and depression in the area of negative affect. There are also some important differences between them in the cognitive area, particularly regarding the

Table 3.1 Characteristics of depression

Cognitive	Behavioral	Physiological
• "All-or-none" thinking	• Depressed mood	• Psychomotor agitation or retardation
• Catastrophizing	• Social withdrawal	• Somatic complaints
• Memory problems	• Does not participate in usual activities	• Poor appetite or overeating
• Concentration problems	• Shows limited effort	• Insomnia or hypersomnia
• Attention problems	• Decline in self-care or personal appearance	• Low energy or fatigue
• Internal locus of control	• Decreased work or school performance	
• Negative view of self, world, and future	• Appears detached from others	
• Automatic thinking	• Crying for no apparent reason	
• Negative attributional style	• Inappropriate responses to events	
• Negative affect	• Irritability	
• Feelings of helplessness	• Apathy	
• Feelings of hopelessness	• Uncooperative	
• Low self-esteem	• Suicide attempts	
• Difficulty making decisions		
• Feels loss of control		
• Suicidal thoughts		

role of cognitions and belief systems in depression. The primary symptoms are presented in Table 3.1.

An examination of Table 3.1 shows that there are some similarities and important differences between anxiety and depression across the three areas. In the behavioral area, withdrawal, less participation, and decreased performance appear to be common to both syndromes. However, the reasons for these behaviors may be quite different. For example, the depressed child who shows withdrawal likely does so due to lack of energy to put forth effort, while the anxious child withdraws to minimize anxiety. In cases where both anxiety and depression are present, both factors may be operating simultaneously. To others, however, the behaviors may appear similar. A teacher, for example, may interpret the similar behaviors of the anxious and depressed child as being uninterested, "lazy," and unmotivated in the classroom. In the physiological area, there are likely to be more signs of hypoarousal, slowed motor responses, and few or no signs of physiological distress, such as perspiration, flushing of the skin, and rapid pulse seen in anxiety.

Cognitively, there are some similarities between anxiety and depression because both conditions present with attention, concentration, and memory problems. Depressed children often have difficulty attending in school, but it is likely due to lack of interest and energy, while the anxious child is inattentive due to being distracted by his own thoughts or stimuli in the environment. For similar reasons, anxious children have difficulty concentrating, while depressed children tend to have less interest in tasks and lack energy to focus when studying, taking tests, or following directions. Some important differences in the cognitive area are related to processes associated with dysfunctional schemas or belief systems.

Negative Cognitive Triad

Aaron Beck (1987; Beck, Rush, Shaw, & Emery, 1979) is credited as being one of the earliest proponents of cognitive models of depression and developed one of the most influential theories of depression regarding adult depression that has been extended to children and youth. He proposed that depressed persons have a "negative cognitive triad" that includes having a negative view of themselves, the future, and the world. In this model, depressed people may see the world as unfair or hostile and that the future is hopeless. Associated with this triad is Beck's view that depressed people have systematic cognitive biases and errors in thinking that include idiosyncratic and incorrect interpretations of events. This thinking pattern becomes a typical mode of processing information that is automatic, repetitive, and negative and increases one's susceptibility to depression. He proposed that depressed people develop negative cognitive schemas or internal cognitive structures that serve to incorrectly filter and process incoming information. As these errors and biases continue, more dysfunction and depression are presumed to develop. These cognitive schemas and the associated thinking errors are the basis for cognitive–behavioral therapy that will be discussed in Chaps. 9 and 11. It is not clear, however, if negative thoughts directly cause depression. It is more likely that depression causes negative thoughts (Pennington, 2002). However, the negative outcomes of dysfunctional thinking may exacerbate depressed mood and adjustment problems.

All-or-None Thinking

Another cognitive characteristic of depressed persons is "all-or-none" thinking. This type of cognitive dysfunction occurs when the depressed person can perceive only one encompassing solution and others are not considered. This pattern shows the relative inflexibility and rigid thinking style of depressed people. They are deficient in the ability to view multiple perspectives or alternatives or how to evaluate options and select one from several. One of the goals of cognitive therapy is to improve cognitive flexibility and decrease all-or-none thinking and other cognitive distortions.

Learned Helplessness

Seligman (1975) proposed a theory of learned helplessness that emerged from research on animals' responses to stress. As most psychology students know, research with dogs that were exposed to inescapable shock ultimately succumbed to the stress and stopped attempting to escape when their efforts were ineffective. Later, when placed in a situation where they could escape shock, the dogs did not try because they had learned to be helpless and showed behaviors similar to clinical depression. From a learning perspective, the dogs learned that their efforts did not provide the desired response (escape from shock) and continued the helpless behavior in future similar situations. Seligman applied these findings to conceptualizing depression, particularly with regard to perceptions of control in the experience of persons with depression. Of course, it cannot be assumed that dogs have the ability to experience control from a cognitive perspective, as do humans. The fact that they did not try to escape in a nonshock situation, however, suggests that the dogs learned that prior escape was impossible and exhibited the same behavior in a similar, albeit nonshock situation.

When applied to humans, however, it was not clear whether control was a causal factor in depression in adults. If the theory can be applied to human depression from a learning perspective, helplessness can perhaps be explained by the perception that one's life circumstances are beyond personal control and that efforts do not provide the desired response. Either one's efforts do not lead to positive outcomes (reinforcement) or lead to negative outcomes (punishment). Therefore, the future appears to be out of one's control, efforts do not lead to positive outcomes, and there is nothing one can do to change the circumstances (helplessness). If the model is accurate when applied to depression, depressed mood, lack of energy, and continued lack of effort to change circumstances correspond with the concept of feeling helpless. The idea that the concept of control can be applied to adolescents and adults is reasonable because they can understand and express feelings about the control they have over circumstances. For young children, however, who may not have yet attained the cognitive capacity to understand and express feelings of control, it is less clear whether they experience depression as a lack of control similar to adolescents and adults.

Attributional Style

In 1978, Abramson, Seligman, and Teasdale presented a reformulation of the learned helplessness theory by focusing on the concept of negative attributional style (NAS). The person with NAS explains or "attributes" negative outcomes to personal shortcomings and positive outcomes to be beyond individual ability or control. Over time, persons with NAS accumulate evidence that negative outcomes are their fault and that they cannot control their lives, leading to low self-esteem, feelings of helplessness, lowered motivation, and increased the risk of developing depression. As NAS becomes more pervasive and depression develops, a feedback loop and cycle develop, leading to increased accumulation of negative attributions and feelings of lack of control. Although NAS has been associated with depression in many studies, it is not clear if it is the cause of depression or is a susceptibility factor. Other factors, such as genetic predisposition or environmental variables, may be the primary causes that lead to the development of NAS. Nevertheless, despite that the learned helplessness theory and NAS do not fully explain the development and maintenance of depression, both concepts have significantly increased understanding and treatment of the various manifestations of mood disorders.

A variation on the NAS and learned helplessness concepts is the notion that repeated exposure to negative life events leads to cognitive vulnerability to depression. Rose and Abramson (1992) suggest that depressed children have a hopefulness orientation and explain negative events as being a function of circumstances. For example, a child might not do well on a test in school and attribute it to failure to prepare and think "Well, I did not do well because I did not study hard enough and I will do better the next time." At this point, he feels a sense of control over outcomes and is hopeful and expectant that the future will be better. With repeated failure, however, the hopeful beliefs are not confirmed, and he may develop the belief that his efforts are not producing positive outcomes and that there must be something wrong with him. Thus, belief systems change from "I didn't prepare well" to "I am a dumb person and cannot ever do well," representing a shift from a hopeful to a hopeless belief structure. Rose and Abramson proposed that this type of belief system will generalize to other negative life events, increasing cognitive vulnerability to depression. They also proposed that this vulnerability is particularly salient in cases of children who experience emotional maltreatment. Over time, these children conclude that they are worthless, and it is their fault that they are being mistreated. These belief systems are inaccurate and irrational, but they may be logical to the developing child, given their circumstances. Depressed persons with NAS tend to have an *internal locus of control* where they believe that the reasons for negative outcomes are due to their own failures. Also, these attributions are *stable* and resistant to change and are *global*, perceived to affect all areas of one's life.

Scar Hypothesis

Lewinshohn, Steinmetz, Larson, and Franklin (1981) proposed the "scar hypothesis" that formerly depressed people develop psychological changes after remission of a depressive episode that increases vulnerability for future depression, including NAS. If the hypothesis is true, it suggests that depressive episodes leave residual effects that increase vulnerability to recurrence. These residual effects might help explain why people who have depressive episodes are likely to have additional episodes (Kraemer, Stice, Kazdin, Offord, & Kupfer, 2001). Some studies have found that increases in depressive symptoms are related to the development of NAS (Gibb, Wheeler, Alloy, & Abramson, 2001; Nolen-Hoeksema, Girgus, & Seligman, 1992; Rohde, Lewinshohn, & Seely, 1994) and competence (Hoffman, Cole, Martin, Tram, & Seroczynski, 2000). These findings suggest that, for some children, there is continuity and an accumulation of psychological deficits that result from repeated depressive episodes.

More recently, Beevers, Rohde, Stice, and Nolen-Hoeksema (2007) conducted a prospective study of the scar hypothesis. They took the position that earlier studies had methodological limitations, including not collecting data prior to, during, and after depressive episodes. The researchers followed a large sample of female adolescents for seven years, 49 of whom had experienced a major depressive episode and recovered. The sample was compared to a random sample of 98 female adolescents who had no history of depression on 13 psychological, social, and psychiatric, and life event variables. All 13 variables were elevated before, during, and after the episode, with some increasing during the episode. The authors found no support for the scar hypothesis, but that several variables may be elevated at various times around a depressive episode, which may increase the risk for recurrence. Although the scar hypothesis may not have received support in this study, the findings suggest that several factors may operate to maintain depressive symptoms and increase the likelihood of another episode. There are significant implications for intervention because clinicians may be able to identify these variables to prevent or lessen the number or severity of future episodes.

Contextual Influences and the Development of Depression and Mood Disorders

Genetic Context

As with anxiety, family history is a strong predictor of depression in children, but disentangling it from the contribution of genetics is problematic. Behavioral genetic studies of children, adolescents, and adults have found modest heritability (Rice, Harold, & Thapar, 2002; Sullivan, Neale, & Kendler, 2000). When parents rate their youth's depressive symptoms, heritability estimates range from modest to high (30–80%). Conversely, when youth rate their own depressive symptoms, the range is much greater (15–80%) (Rice, Harold, and Thapar, 2002). Interestingly, heritability is more associated with depressive symptoms after age 11, while environmental factors but not genetics are linked with depression before this age. These findings suggest that genetic effects may vary as a function of the age of the children. Other studies have found modest heritability estimates of about 30% (e.g., Eaves et al., 1997; Kendler, Neale, Kessler, Heath, & Eaves, 1992; Silberg et al., 1999). The majority of evidence suggests that depressive symptoms rather than specific disorders are heritable, similar to the findings about anxiety (Eley, 2001). It is highly likely that multiple genes transmit several risk factors that increase the likelihood of the development of depressive disorders, whereas environmental variables have significant influences on which specific disorders emerge.

Children of depressed parents are three times more likely to have a depressive episode than are children of nondepressed parents (Beardslee, Versage, & Gladstone, 1998) and have a 40% probability of having a depressive episode before the age of 18 (Weissman et al., 1987). Overall, the genetic contribution to childhood depression is about 30–50% in children's self-reports, while the evidence for environmental effects is mixed. Onset below the age of 20 is associated with a greater likelihood of depression in family members, although it is unclear whether the relationship is due to genetics or factors associated with shared environmental influences (Rutter et al., 1990).

Biological Context

Research on the biological context of depression has been based largely on adults and has focused on brain structures and neurotransmitters. Specific biological structures comprise a neural circuit that has been shown to be related to vulnerability to depression (Davidson, Pizzagalli, Nitschke, & Putnam, 2002). As with anxiety, the amygdala is implicated in depression as a region in the subcortex that mediates fear, anxiety, and emotional memory. The amygdala is part of a neural circuit that includes the prefrontal cortex, mesolimbic dopamine system (MDS), and frontal brain activity. The MDS has a role in mediating reward and pleasure, while the prefrontal cortex is a contributor to control of behavior, affective flexibility, and approach/withdrawal. There is some evidence that prefrontal cortex dysfunction and left frontal underactivity create a stable predisposition to depression (Davidson et al.; Tomarken & Keener, 1998). Infants and children of depressed mothers at high risk for depression have shown evidence of left frontal underactivity, suggesting another path to biological vulnerability to depression.

The hypothalamic–pituitary–adrenal axis (HPA) regulates human stress responses and dysfunction and has been implicated as another biological vulnerability to depression (Meyer, Chrousos, & Gold, 2001). When a person experiences stress, the hypothalamus releases peptides that stimulate the pituitary gland, which causes release of cortisol from the adrenal glands. Cortisol is a stress hormone regulated by the HPA, and some evidence suggests that improper regulation of cortisol is associated with depression in adults, although the evidence is less conclusive in children and youth.

Norepinephrine (NE) is a neurotransmitter that has been found to be related to depression and mood disorders. Low levels of NE are associated with depression, and high levels are linked to mania (Pennington, 2002). Levels of the neurotransmitter serotonin are clearly linked with depression. Lower levels of serotonin are found in depressed persons, and high levels are found in suicide victims. The fact that selective serotonin reuptake inhibitors (SSRIs) have been shown to be effective as pharmacological treatments supports the link between serotonin levels and depression. Pennington cautions, however, not to assume that the actions of neurotransmitters alone explain the development and manifestation of mood disorders but rather that they are related to activity in the larger biological arousal/motivation system. It is possible that these patterns may be genetically transmitted, acquired prenatally, or result from the outcomes of stress precipitated by impairment of a depressed mother in a child's early development.

Temperament

There is substantial evidence that genetically/biologically based temperamental influences create a vulnerability pathway for depression in children and adolescents. Depression has been linked to the concept of "negative emotionality" or neuroticism, which refers to the degree to which a person perceives the world as hostile, threatening, or stress inducing. People who self-report high levels of neuroticism describe themselves as anxious, depressed, angry, having low self-adequacy, and being under greater stress (Watson, Clark, & Harkness, 1994). Consequently, people with high levels of neuroticism or negative emotionality are more prone to being affected by a greater number of stressors (Kendler, Gardner, & Prescott, 2003) and lack the resilience to cope with daily hassles and more severe situations (Roberts & Monroe, 1994). It is noteworthy that highly anxious children also have some of these characteristics, reflecting the comorbidity of anxiety and depression.

An interesting, recent study regarding the association among neurological functioning, temperament, and depression was conducted by Shankman et al. (2011). The study involved investigating the association of high negative emotionality (NE; sadness, fear, anger) and low positive emotionality (PE; anhedonia, listlessness, and lack of enthusiasm) with resting EEG activity in frontal and posterior parts of the brain in 329 preschoolers. When PE was high, NE was associated with more relative right activity, whereas when PE was low, NE was not related to posterior asymmetry. The differences were related to variations in EEG activity in the right posterior regions, which are implicated in emotional processing and arousal. However, the differences were found only in girls, which suggest that, for some girls, there is an association among PE, NE, and some neurological functioning that increases the risk for depression. The results may be related to many findings that adolescent girls and women tend to have more frequent diagnoses of depression and mood disorders. It is possible that some girls may have biologically based predispositions to depression that are related to NE, PE, and some aspects of neural functioning.

Cultural Context

The association of depression with various cultural and ethnic groups has been studied in adults and children, but the number of studies and the diversity of samples in children are lacking. In one of the largest studies to investigate this relationship, Roberts, Roberts, and Chen (1997) found few comparable rates of depression in nine different ethnic groups of children in grades six to eight, except for higher rates in those of Mexican descent. Costello et al. (1996) found few differences in depressive patterns between European American and African American adolescents. Another study found that African American girls did not show the same increase in depression often shown from preadolescence to adolescence compared to European American girls (Hayward, Gotlib, Schraedley, & Litt, 1999).

The impact of socioeconomic status (SES) on the development of depression has been well documented and is about the same for adults and children. When depressive symptoms rather than depressive disorders are the variables of study, there is a link between low SES and depression (Offord et al., 1992). Costello et al. (1996) found that low income was associated with higher depression and other disorders in children, with the poorest children having over three times greater prevalence for any disorder. These findings suggest that SES exerts a considerable influence on the development of depression and other disorders. However, findings of higher incidence among ethnic or cultural groups may be confounded with SES that includes low income, unfair treatment, and racism (Clark, Anderson, Clark, & Williams, 1999).

A recent meta-analysis of studies by Mendelson, Rehkopf, and Kubaznsky (2008) comparing Latino and non-Latino Whites in the USA on depressive symptoms found a significant but clinically nonmeaningful difference. There was no difference between the groups on lifetime prevalence of depressive disorders. Latino women showed slightly higher rates of depressive symptoms than did non-Latino women. The authors posited that cultural differences in socialization may be a factor in the magnitude of this difference and that the traditional Latino values of strength and authority for males (*machismo*) and submissiveness for females (*marianismo*) may cause Latinas to express distress through internalizing ways, such as depression. These findings suggest that clinicians should consider the role of culture, cultural values, and level of acculturation when working with children of different ethnic backgrounds when considering assessment and treatment for depression.

Social Context

Children and adolescents with depression tend to have many social and interpersonal problems, including lack of competence. A behavioral explanation of these deficits is based on reinforcement theory that the depressed person has deficits in the ability to respond to positive events. Lack of positive feedback results from competence deficits interferes with the ability to form interpersonal relationships and to appreciate positive experiences (Lewinshohn, 1974). Cole, Martin, Powers, and Trujillo (1996) explain depression from a competence-based approach where negative feedback is internalized as negative self-perceptions. Transaction theories explain depression and social deficits as dysfunctional and bidirectional because the depressed person both reacts and contributes to interpersonal problems including social impairment, problem-solving deficits, and difficulties regulating emotion (e.g., Joiner, Coyne, & Blalock, 1999).

Depressed children are more withdrawn, show less imitative behavior and affect, elicit negative reactions from others, and demonstrate frequent needs for reassurance compared to their nondepressed peers. The need for reassurance appears to play a role in social transmission of depressive symptoms, as high reassurance-seeking persons are more likely to develop depression, such as when interacting with a depressed roommate or partner (Katz, Beach, & Joiner, 1999). Excessive reassurance needs interact with negative events to increase the likelihood of the development of depressive symptoms over time (Joiner & Metalsky, 2001). Excessive reassurance may be applicable only to early adolescence, however, and, in one study, was associated with increased depressive symptoms following increases in hassles or parental depression (Abela, Zuroff, Ho, Adams, & Hankin, 2006). As adolescents get older, they appear to need less reassurance.

In social situations, depressed children tend to use less active and problem-focused coping, have higher levels of passive or ruminative coping, and feel helpless when challenged (Nolen-Hoeksema, Girgus, & Seligman, 1992; Rudolph, Kurlakowsky, & Conley, 2001). Avoidance, withdrawal, decreased assertiveness, and passivity are observed frequently when depressed children are confronted with socially stressful situations. Irritability, anger, and aggression may be seen in response to stress and challenge. In a school setting, depressed children are likely to be seen as being lazy, uninterested, noncompliant, and unmotivated to participate in social and academic activities.

Another variable associated with social functioning and depression is dependency. As stress increases, depression also tends to increase and is accompanied by high levels of dependency in adults. Less information is available for children and youth, however. Some research suggests that dependency and depression are related in adolescence, but not in young children (Abela & Taylor, 2003). It may be that greater levels of dependency are normal in younger children; thus, a possible association with depression may not be easily identified. Moreover, dependency in young children may be adaptive while being a vulnerability factor in older adolescents.

Family Context

The family context has been found to be highly influential in the development and maintenance of depressive symptoms and disorders. The majority of research has focused on family dynamics and the association of depression in parents with depression in children. Variables found to be associated with child and adolescent depression include family atmosphere, relationships among family members, and family stressors. Factors such as marital and family discord appear to contribute to the development or worsening of depressive symptoms in children and youth (Kashani, Burbach, & Rosenberg, 1988; Kaslow, Deering, & Racusin, 1994; Sheeber, Hops, Alpert, Davis, & Andrews, 1997). Negative family life events, chronic stress, abuse, and low family support have been implicated in the development of child depressive symptoms (e.g., Davis, Sheeber, Hops, & Tildesley, 2000).

Much research has focused on the role of parental psychopathology in the development of depression and other disorders in children. Although there is a parental genetic influence on the development of depression in children, there is clear evidence of a substantial effect of parental depression on children. Most of these studies have focused on mother–child interactions, including those involving infants in nonclinical samples. Two general patterns have been found: (a) withdrawal, lack of engagement, flat affect, and unresponsiveness (Field, Healy, Goldstein, & Guthertz, 1990) and (b) hostility and intrusiveness (Cohn, Matias, Tronick, Connell, & Lyons-Ruth, 1986). Lovejoy, Graczyk, O'Hare, and Neuman (2000) conducted a meta-analysis of the association of maternal behavior and childhood depression and found that depressed mothers showed more negative behaviors, disengagement, and fewer positive behaviors. The negative behaviors were more salient with currently depressed mothers rather than those with lifetime diagnoses. The specific mechanisms of these effects are unclear but likely involve negative modeling and aversive behavior.

Depressed children generally have more negative perceptions of family than do nondepressed children. Depressed children perceive less family support, acceptance, parent availability, and attachment. These perceptions appear to persist, as studies of young adults indicated that they recalled poor maternal care, less affection, and nurturance, as well as more punitiveness, rejection, and overprotectiveness (Blatt & Homman, 1992). The possible consequences of these behaviors include children being less effective problem solvers, showing fewer positive behaviors, and being less communicative.

Parental behaviors and dysfunctional family interactions increase children's vulnerability to depression in several ways, including modeling of negative feedback, learning ineffective social interaction skills, developing poor problem-solving skills, and showing impaired ability to regulate mood (Garber & Flynn, 1998). As depressed children accumulate these deficits, they become less able to cope with social and academic demands and experience continued difficulties, increasing the risk for worsening depression or other disorders.

Insecure Attachment

Several studies have shown that insecure attachment is related to the development of depressive symptoms in adults, adolescents, and children. In a prospective study, Hammen et al. (1995) found that depressive symptoms increased over a one-year period in high school-age girls and that the depression–attachment relationship was moderated by severity of interpersonal stressors. Similar findings have been found in children that are consistent with a vulnerability–stress perspective. Abela, Zinck, Kryger, Zilber, and Hankin (2009) found that higher levels of insecure attachment in children corresponded with increases of depressive symptoms subsequent to increases in parents' depressive symptoms.

School Context

Because school is the primary social and learning environment for most children, it is important to understand how depressed children function in these settings and cope with the various demands. Like anxiety, depression is associated with social problems and difficulties with learning, task performance, and engagement in the schooling process. Using a competency-based model of depression, Cole, Martin, and Powers (1997) proposed that childhood depressive symptoms reflect feelings of low self-competence. Consequently, maladaptive beliefs result from perceived failures in primary life areas, including social and academic spheres. Failure in social or academic pursuits decreases feelings of self-competence, thereby increasing the risk for depression. Patterson and Stoolmiller (1991) suggest that academic and social problems are stressors that have direct effects on the development of dysphoric moods.

Social Factors

In the school setting, teachers have reported that depressed children have diminished prosocial skills and show more aggressiveness (Rudolph & Clark, 2001). They also are described by peers and teachers as being less popular, socially rejected, or isolated than their nondepressed peers (Rudolph & Clark; Rudolph, Hammen, & Burge, 1994). In the school setting, children often participate in small groups and interact where the interpersonal effects of depression can be seen more readily. Depressed children tend to elicit more negative feedback in small group interactions, partly due to excessive needs for reassurance. Due to being less assertive and participatory, depressed children are less likely to participate in classroom activities, ask questions, and initiate interactions. Because schools are social environments, depressed children are more likely to show avoidance and less assertiveness when confronted with demands, conflict, or negative reactions from others. These behaviors are related to the difficulties depressed children have with affect regulation and impaired emotional coping skills.

Depressed children also tend to be victims of bullying and relational aggression, most of which occurs in the school setting. Children who are bullied or experience relational aggression typically are not well integrated into social networks. Similarly, rejected or socially isolated children are more likely to develop depressive symptoms. Being bullied and physically victimized and experiencing relational aggression (e.g., teasing, social ostracism) are associated with depression in both girls and boys (Crick & Bigbee, 1998; Prinstein, Boergers, & Vernberg, 2001). LaGreca and Harrison (2005) found that relational aggression predicted depressive symptoms better than physical aggression in adolescents of both genders.

Cognitive Factors

Depressed children also have difficulty with the academic demands of school and making expected achievement gains and tend to have negative academic self-concepts. Some studies have used grades as performance criteria in evaluating the association between achievement and depression. Results have shown negative correlations between grades and depressive symptoms (Forehand, Brody, Long, & Fauber, 1988). Ialongo, Edelsohn, Werthamer-Larson, Crockett, and Kellam (1996) found that depression was associated with lower achievement and concentration problems in children as young as first grade. There is little evidence that depressed children have a tendency toward having lower cognitive ability; therefore, academic achievement difficulties are presumed to be related to the effects of depression on feelings of competence, concentration and memory difficulties, inability to sustain effort, and learning-related behaviors, such as participation and initiative.

Interactions of Social and Cognitive Factors

Although many studies have focused on social and cognitive factors in the school setting regarding depressed children, the interaction among these factors is an important consideration, as well. In a recent study, Schwartz, Gorman, Duong, and Nakamoto (2008) looked at the interaction of peer relationships and academic achievement as predictors of depressive symptoms in children. The study follows longitudinal research showing that academic and social problems have independent effects on the prediction of depressive symptoms in children (Cole, 1991; Patterson & Stoolmiller, 1991). Schwartz et al. found that low grade point average (GPA) predicted depressive symptoms, but only for children who had few friends. Children with few friends had more depressive symptoms, but this effect was less for those with high GPAs. The authors concluded that competency in one domain can moderate the risk in the other domain. Thus, not only do social and academic factors operate singly in the school setting, they can also combine to create a complex risk pattern for the development of depressive symptoms. These findings have implications for intervention and prevention of depression, i.e., intervening with children who struggle academically can help prevent depression and vice versa.

Developmental Pathways of Depression and Mood Disorders

Similar to anxiety disorders and most psychopathologies, earlier onset of depression and mood disorders is associated with increased intractability, greater maladjustment, resistance to treatment, and long-term course through adolescence and into adulthood. The majority of depressive disorders begin in middle to late adolescence, with rare occurrences in preschool children (<1%) and school-age children (1–2%). While DSM-IV-TR (APA, 2000) lists one anxiety disorder as unique to children (separation anxiety disorder), there are no depressive disorders specific to children. In general, onset of depression and mood disorders occurs after age 11, with most beginning in middle to late adolescence. Although depression and mood disorders tend to respond relatively well to treatment, often there are residual symptoms and risk for recurrence remains. Table 3.2 summarizes the typical age of onset, primary symptoms, comorbidity, and developmental pathways of the primary mood disorders of major depression, dysthymia, and bipolar disorders. Other depressive disorders exist, such as seasonal affective disorder, psychotic depression, and cyclothymia, but these disorders are uncommon in children and adolescents and are not included.

Table 3.2 Depression and mood disorders in childhood and adolescence

Mood disorder	Typical age of onset	Primary symptoms	Comorbidity	Developmental pathway
Major depression	Age 11 or later, most often in middle to late adolescence	Depressed mood: loss of interest in pleasure or most activities; loss of weight not attributable to illness or dieting; hypersomnia; insomnia; psychomotor agitation; loss of energy; fatigue; feelings of worthlessness or guilt; concentration problems; recurrent thoughts of suicide; absence of positive affect; irritability; anger; withdrawal; low self-esteem; feelings of hopelessness; internal locus of control that is global and stable	Social phobia: general-ized anxiety disorder; disruptive behavior disorders; substance use, including smoking and alcohol use (primarily in adolescents); academic underachievement	Relatively young age earlier onset indicates more protracted, severe, or recurrent course; early onset more predictive of lifelong course; early onset of anxiety disorders increases risk of depressive disorders; early onset conduct disorder may increase risk of depression due to social isolation, interpersonal conflicts, and social maladjustment; childhood onset tends to predict significant disorder but not necessarily recurring depression and instead leads to emotional and behavioral regulation problems
Dysthymia	Late childhood to early adolescence; adolescents who show dysthymia and later develop depression usually have first depressive episode 2–3 years after onset of dysthymia	Chronically depressed mood, with some symptoms common to depression: appetite problems, insomnia or hypersomnia, low energy, fatigue, low self-esteem, concentration difficulties, hopelessness; flat affect; "blah" feelings; limited social interac-tions; no history of depressive episodes; may be seen by self and others as more of a personality style; highly self-critical; person may not realize the presence and significance of the mood problems	Depression and mood disorders; "double depression" (coexisting dysthymia and major depression)	Gradual and slow onset compared to relatively rapid onset of depressive episodes; chronic course; if "double depression" is present, impairment is greater and is more resistant to treatment than depression alone; symptoms are less severe than major depression and cause less impair-ment; suicidal ideation less common in dysthymia; increased risk for recurrent or chronic mood disorder into adulthood

(continued)

Table 3.2 (continued)

Mood disorder	Typical age of onset	Primary symptoms	Comorbidity	Developmental pathway
Bipolar disorder	Variable in children, with controversy about bipolar manifestations in young children; likely rare in classic form in young children; at least 25% of cases have onset in middle to late adolescence; some early symptoms may show in childhood or be mistaken for symptoms of other disorders, for example, ADHD	Bipolar I: persistent, expansive, or irritable mood; high level of energy; insomnia; "racing thoughts," distractible, talkative, risky behavior, grandiosity; at least one manic or mixed episode; Bipolar II: symptoms are similar to Bipolar I, except that person must have or had at least one major depressive episode and at least one hypomanic episode, but no manic episodes	ADHD; conduct problems; substance use, including smoking and alcohol use; anxiety disorders: separation anxiety disorder, social phobia, specific phobia; psychosis; use of alcohol and drugs can elicit a manic episode in adolescents prone to bipolar symptoms or disorder	Usually sudden onset of manic episode in some adolescents; some may present with depressive disorders prior to manic or hypomanic episodes; severely depressed children and youth may change from depression to mania in about 25% of cases; with treatment, recovery from episodes tends to be rather rapid; even under control, mood variations greater than normal are likely to persist into adulthood

Specific Depression and Mood Disorders

Major Depressive Disorder

Major depressive disorder (MDD) is the most common mood disorder, occurring in up to 20% of adolescents (Cole et al., 2002; Garber, Keiley, & Martin, 2002). In childhood, the prevalence rate of MDD is about the same for boys and girls. At adolescence, however, the prevalence rate increases to about 3–7% (Costello, Mustillo, Erkanli, Keeler, & Angold, 2003), with girls showing about twice the rate of boys. An increase in the prevalence of depression from late childhood to early adolescence has been observed in the last several years, primarily due to an increase in depression in girls. Some evidence suggests that as many as 28% of girls and 14% of boys have experienced MDD or dysthymia by age 18, although the overall prevalence has not increased significantly over the past several years (Costello, Erkanli, & Angold, 2006).

Not only do girls have more depressive disorders, they are likely to show more symptoms, more severe symptoms, and greater risk of self-harm and suicidal thoughts. For girls, MDD episodes are likely to last longer, are more impairing, and are more likely to lead to a variety of mood problems. Keenan and Hipwell (2005) suggest that gender differences are attributable to three factors: (a) girls tend to demonstrate excessive empathy and may take on ill-placed responsibility for the problems of others, (b) girls tend to show excessive compliance and may defer their own needs to please others, and (c) some girls tend to have more difficulty regulating their emotions, have fewer coping strategies, and tend to overcontrol and hide their feelings, leading to an increased risk of developing mood problems. It is likely, however, that a combination of biological and environmental factors contributes to the higher prevalence rate in girls.

Untreated depressive episodes tend to last from 8 to 13 months in children and from 3 to 9 months in adolescents. About 90% of children and 50–90% of adolescents recover from these episodes, although relapse tends to occur within two years in about 60% of cases. About 72% of cases have a relapse within five years (Birmaher, Arbelaez, & Brent, 2002; Simons, Rohde, Kennard, & Robins, 2005). Brendgen, Wanner, Morin, and Vitaro (2005) report four patterns of mood symptomatology in children and youth:

1. Fifty percent show very low levels of depressive symptoms and are at low risk for developing mood disorders, with boys comprising a large majority of the group.
2. Thirty percent show consistent but moderate levels of symptomatology throughout childhood and adolescence, with little impact on daily functioning; boys comprise the majority of this group.
3. Ten percent show chronic high levels of symptoms starting in late childhood and persisting through adolescence. Most of the members of this group are girls with histories of early parent–child conflict and difficulties with mood regulation.

4. Ten percent show low levels of symptoms in childhood that increase significantly in adolescence. This group is comprised primarily of girls with difficult temperaments, parent–child conflict histories, and who experience peer rejection and social alienation.

These data show that about 20% of youth will have significant mood problems and are four times more likely to experience mood disorders in adulthood compared to others their age (Harrington, Fudge, Rutter, Pickles, & Hill, 1990). If the 30% who show subsyndromal symptoms are included, the combined data suggest that up to 50% of youth have significant symptomatology that warrant screening and interventions to treat current problem and prevent the worsening or onset of a disorder.

Dysthymia

Dysthymia is a mood disorder characterized by a chronically depressed mood on most days for at least two years. The level of impairment is generally mild, and people with dysthymia do not show the rapid onset of mood problems seen in major depression. For some children and youth, dysthymia is of such chronicity that it often appears more like a personality pattern or trait than an obvious disorder. The developmental course is more long term and chronic than major depression and has a gradual onset.

There is a question on whether dysthymia is a distinct disorder or a less severe form of major depression. Goodman, Schwab-Stone, Lahey, Shaffer, and Jensen (2000) analyzed data from the Methods for the Epidemiology of Child and Adolescent Mental Disorders (MECA) study regarding the association between major depressive disorder (MDD) and dysthymia in children and youth. Groups were formed that met criteria for (a) MDD alone, (b) dysthymia alone, or (c) MDD and dysthymia combined. The average age of onset for the MDD only group was 12.6, while average ages of onset for the dysthymia only and the combined group were 10.0 and 10.5, respectively. Thus, there was nearly a 3-year difference between the onset of dysthymia or MDD–dysthymia and MDD alone. The results indicated no support for differentiation of MDD and dysthymia on sociodemographic, clinical, or family and life event variables. Youths who had both diagnoses, however, showed significantly less competence and were more impaired than those with either disorder alone. Those with both MDD and dysthymia ("double depression") had comorbid disorders, especially generalized anxiety disorder. The authors hypothesized that youths with both disorders may have a higher genetic loading for affective disorder and be inherently more predisposed to severe depressive pathology. Some significant family variables were that parents of the dysthymia group tended to use harsher punishment and children with both disorders received less parental supervision. Although these findings do not provide support for differentiation of MDD and dysthymia, they do indicate that dysthymic mood can have an onset as early as five years of age (based on a standard deviation of 4.8 years).

Bipolar Disorder

Bipolar disorder, formerly termed manic–depressive disorder, has been well established in adults. In children and youth, however, bipolar disorder is controversial when adult criteria are applied to childhood symptoms. By definition, bipolar disorders are recurrent and cyclical between manic or hypomanic symptoms and depressed mood. Children rarely show these types of cycles, and onset is not sudden as occurs in adolescents and adults. Also, usually there are no periods of relatively good functioning between episodes. Irritability, rage, and aggressiveness are more likely to be symptoms in younger children, accompanied by destructiveness, noncompliance, and uncontrolled behavior. Mania episodes in young children are rare, as are severe depressive episodes seen in adolescents and adults.

Many of the behaviors deemed to be bipolar symptoms in children are similar to those seen in ADHD, conduct disorder, and oppositional defiant disorder. There is some support for overlap of symptoms of ADHD and bipolarity in children. Biederman (1998) and Faraone, Biederman, Mennin, Wozniak, and Spencer (1997) have reported very high rates of ADHD in young children diagnosed with mania and elevated levels of mania in children diagnosed with ADHD. These findings suggest a comorbidity of ADHD with bipolar disorder and perhaps that the former may mask the latter (Biederman). It is also possible that a genetic subtype of ADHD and bipolar comorbidity may exist (Faraone, Biederman, Mennin, Wozniak, & Spencer, 1997).

These findings and clinical experience indicate that differentiating bipolar disorder from other co-occurring conditions and variation in typical development can be challenging. In a school-based survey study, the rate of bipolar disorder in children was about 1%, with the majority being Bipolar II type, and about 5.7% showed hypomanic symptoms (Lewinshohn, Klein, & Seeley, 1995). These findings are similar to rates found in adult populations. The current evidence suggests that Bipolar I disorder is extremely rare in children, although clinicians and others often disagree.

Bipolar disorders are thought to have strong genetic bases, perhaps the most significant of all child mental disorders. Evidence of a genetic basis has been found in twin and family studies, suggesting a link between parents with bipolar disorder and affective disorders in their children. Lapalme, Hodgins, and LaRoche (1997) conducted a meta-analysis of studies involving bipolar disorders and found that about 52% of children with parents who had bipolar disorder met criteria for some mental disorder, compared to 29% of children of parents without a disorder. Of these parents, 26% had some form of affective disorder, and 5.4% had specific bipolar disorder. Of the parents who had no disorder, none of the children had bipolar disorder. As with other disorders, however, it seems likely that the specific manifestations of the disorder in the children were affected by parental behavior. From a developmental course perspective, fewer or milder episodes seem to predict a more benign course, perhaps affecting the rather rapid increase of using mood-stabilizing drugs in children as preventive measures. More severe symptoms are associated with significant difficulties in mood regulation, disruptive behavior, interpersonal difficulties, and academic problems.

These findings suggest that, although there is evidence of bipolar disorders in children and adolescents, it is challenging to differentiate them from other disorders and developmental variations in mood and behavior. Thus, considerable care in assessment must be taken to improve differential diagnosis and reduce the possibility of misdiagnosis. Diagnostic accuracy is especially important if medication is considered as a form of treatment.

Clinical Implications of a Developmental Psychopathology Perspective on Depression and Mood Disorders

Although anxiety and depression share common characteristics and show comorbidity in children and adolescents, they differ in their developmental characteristics. Whereas anxiety has typical developmental markers that are expected and also has adaptive qualities, depression has no normal developmental progression and is not associated with adaptive functioning. Children and youth may show sadness at times, but they do not appear at specific times and most often show onset when a confluence of risk factors converges. Although many adolescents show sadness, irritability, and "moodiness" at times, the vast majority of them do not develop depression and, in fact, show good psychological adjustment during their teen years.

The vulnerability–stress model of psychopathology applies to depression and mood disorders that often begin with exposure to negative events that create risk. Stressors in a child's life may occur as a series of negative events. A single negative event can raise initial levels of negative affect that include a variety of negative emotions, including anger, depression, and anxiety (Watson, 2000). Over time, these emotions contribute to the development of cognitive distortions, NAS and impaired personal and social functioning that may require treatment. Moreover, depressed children are more likely to have dysfunctional families that may also have to be considered in case conceptualization and treatment. Thus, the clinician should assess the role of past and current stressors from a developmental perspective that may have direct relevance to understanding the distorted cognitions of depressed children and adolescents that exacerbate and maintain depressive behavior. This approach is especially relevant if the mode of treatment is to be cognitive–behavioral in nature, which is the most well-established and efficacious psychotherapeutic method. In Chaps. 9 and 11, methods of assessment and intervention are discussed in more depth.

The contextual approach described in Chap. 1 and this chapter provides a framework for conceptualizing child and adolescent depression. Depression has well-established genetic and biological bases, although they may not be evident in clinical practice except through inferences from developmental history. The research literature on whether culture is significantly related to the development of depression is varied, although it does exist in some form in virtually all cultures. Family functioning (including consideration of parenting and parental psychopathology), social factors, and schooling are highly related to depression and should be considered during assessment, case conceptualization, and treatment.

Conclusion

Like anxiety, depression has rather well-understood developmental trajectories if untreated that can persist into adulthood and have significant impairing effects on social, personal, and academic functioning. Unlike anxiety, depression is associated with a higher risk of suicidal ideation and attempts, particularly as the symptoms worsen. Early identification and intervention for depressive symptoms from a developmental perspective offer the best opportunity to work with depressed children and to prevent negative trajectories and to facilitate positive ones.

Chapter 4
Emotion Regulation

The Case of Aaron

Aaron is a 10-year-old, fifth-grade boy who has average cognitive ability and is capable of achieving at grade level, as shown by his standardized achievement test scores and classroom performance. He often does not complete his schoolwork, and the work he does complete is at a level below his ability. His current classroom placement is a self-contained classroom for students with emotional disturbance due to frequent episodes of aggressive behavior, noncompliance, temper outbursts, and angry verbal exchanges with peers and adults. His behavior cannot be managed effectively in the general education classroom, and he often needs an adult aide to monitor and accompany him. Most of the time, his behavior appears unprovoked and he often complains that other students or adults are causing him to misbehave. On one occasion, he is sitting at his desk, but is not working on his assignments. The teacher stops to ask if he needs help and gives positive encouragement to work. Almost instantly, he gets out of his seat and becomes enraged, yelling profanity, and claiming that the teacher is "picking on me" and that he does not have to do what he is told. He attempts to leave the classroom and two teachers and an aide restrain him physically and put him in a "time-out" room, where he hits the walls and remains enraged for nearly a half hour.

Aaron has many difficulties with becoming angry, showing inappropriate behavior and mood, and has deficits in controlling his emotions, particularly anger. Psychological assessment indicates that he has unregulated mood problems, depression, social anxiety, conduct problems, aggressiveness, and high levels of trait anger. His angry emotional outbursts appear to be unprovoked in most cases, and he is unable to control them himself. Aaron demonstrates problems with *emotion regulation*, a pattern of impairments in the ability to prevent becoming angry, controlling his behavior, and using alternative strategies to cope with perceived stress or negative stimuli.

T.J. Huberty, *Anxiety and Depression in Children and Adolescents:*
Assessment, Intervention, and Prevention, DOI 10.1007/978-1-4614-3110-7_4,
© Springer Science+Business Media, LLC 2012

The Concept of Emotion Processing

Emotions are central to human functioning and serve an adaptive function necessary for psychological and physical survival. They arise as a result of stimuli or situations and appear as motivational systems that help the child to achieve goals. Research conducted over many years has consistently found that there are seven basic human emotions: anger, joy, empathy, fear, sadness, shame, and guilt (Chaplin & Cole, 2005). Other psychologists have proposed a greater number of emotions, some of which may be combinations of other emotions, such as distress and contempt.

Most models of emotion processing contain components that work in a linear manner to explain what happens when emotion is activated and the consequences of emotional reactions (e.g., Gross & Thompson, 2007). These models include appraisal of a situation as a key cognitive component that has a significant influence on the type and intensity of the emotion. Figure 4.1 demonstrates an emotion processing model that begins with situations encountered by the person and ends with the manifestation of responses.

In this model of emotion processing, a situation occurs that draws the attention of the person, which leads to immediate cognitive appraisal of the nature of the stimulus. During the appraisal process, a conclusion is reached almost immediately regarding whether the situation is positive and pleasant, neutral with little or no positive or negative valence, or negative or threatening. Almost simultaneously, a basic or complex emotion is activated, such as anger, happiness, or distress. The experienced emotion leads to cognitive, behavioral, or physiological responses or a combination of them. Cognitive responses might include worry, inattention, or concentration difficulties. Behavioral responses could include aggression, withdrawal, or immobilization. Physiological responses might be increased heart rate, flushing of the skin, or muscle tension. The model is recursive, i.e., the outcomes of the emotion process may affect how the person processes and responds to similar situations in the future.

Models such as this one can be useful in understanding, assessing, and treating emotion regulation problems. Children and youth with emotion regulation problems may have difficulties in attending to the situation properly, correctly appraising the cues, identifying and recognizing appropriate emotions, or responding appropriately. Understanding what situational cues may provoke emotional reactions is useful in altering or preventing circumstances that serve as stimuli. For a person to have an

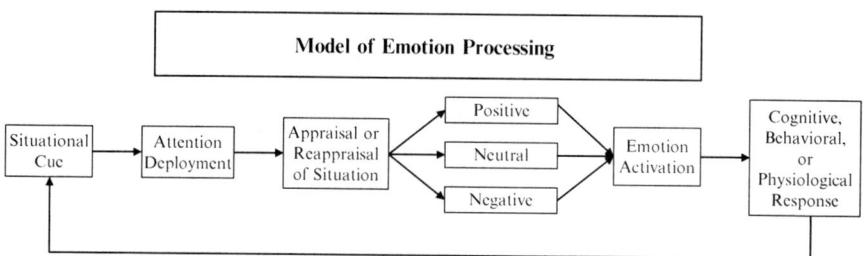

Fig. 4.1 Model of emotion processing

emotional reaction, attention to the situation is necessary for the appraisal process to begin. Impairments in attention can have clinical significance because children with emotion regulation problems may attend to the wrong stimuli or have psychological problems that interfere with attention. The appraisal component is important for intervention, because a child's evaluations of situations may not be accurate, leading to misinterpretation of the situation. This cognitive perspective is the basis for various cognitive–behavioral treatments that focus on faulty thinking patterns, irrational beliefs, and attributional style problems. As the appraisal process ends, an emotion is activated, such as anger or anxiety, based on the person's evaluative conclusions. Finally, cognitive, behavioral, and physiological responses are demonstrated that reflect the type and intensity of the experienced emotion. The consequences of these responses may "loop" back so that when other situations occur, attention, appraisal, and emotions are affected, which may alter subsequent cognitive, behavioral, or physiological responses. Situations may also be reappraised upon recurrence, based on response and outcomes or consequences of those responses. Such models are termed "recursive" because they loop back from responses to future situations. The recursive nature of this model has implications for clinical interventions because one of the goals of cognitive–behavioral treatment approaches is to help the client to improve appraisal abilities of situations, which may change emotion activation, emotion regulation, and the type of response.

Interventions are often targeted toward the responses, with the effects also affecting the emotion processing sequence when future situations are presented. Interventions may alter whether situational cues are recognized and attention is alerted. If attention does occur, the child may change the appraisal process that results in another emotional experience or a different or less intense response. For example, let us assume that a child becomes highly anxious when meeting new people such as occurs in social anxiety. Prior to treatment, the child is highly anxious when encountering new people, is attentive to cues, appraises the situation as threatening (negative), and experiences fear. To reduce the anxiety, the child withdraws which is effective in reducing the anxiety temporarily, reinforcing withdrawal behavior. In future situations, the pattern is repeated. With treatment, however, the child learns to cope with social anxiety so that when future situational cues occur and attention is alerted, the appraisal process leads to a neutral or more positive evaluation, fear is lessened, and he or she does not withdraw and at least stays in the group. As the child becomes more able to cope with situations, the recursive aspect of emotion processing models is altered as social anxiety lessens and the child become more socially adept with less social anxiety.

Returning to Aaron's Case

When Aaron became angry and aggressive, the emotion processing model presented in Fig. 4.1 suggests that the cue from the teacher to work alerted his attention, his appraisal process led him to conclude that he was being threatened or coerced, anger was activated, and his observed response was primarily behavioral with verbal and physical aggression, as well as cognitions indicating a negative attribution toward others. The consequence of being physically managed and controlled was also negative, so that the effects are more likely to be repeated in future situations, which corresponds to the recursive nature of emotion processing. The response of segregating him, although perhaps necessary in the situation, did not teach him new skills. He did not learn new approaches to solve problems or to appraise situations, so that similar behaviors are likely to recur in similar circumstances. Interventions should focus on a number of areas, including helping him to learn to regulate his emotions through self-monitoring, anger management training, and mood stabilization techniques. His current pattern of being unable to regulate his emotions needs to be altered so that future episodes do not occur or are at least are reduced in frequency, duration, or intensity.

The Concept of Emotion Regulation

A central developmental task for children and adolescents is learning how to manage or regulate emotions as they get older and encounter new situations. At young ages, children experience emotions such as anger and anxiety, but have few skills to manage them, resulting in less regulated expression. Although regulation of emotions at a high level is not expected of infants and preschool children, increased mastery of emotional expression is expected as they become older. Thompson (1994) defines emotion regulation as "the extrinsic and intrinsic processes responsible for monitoring, evaluating, and modifying emotional reactions, especially their intensive and temporal features, to accomplish one's goals" (p. 27). As early as the ages between two and five, children show increases in cognitive, motor, and language skills that permit them to regulate their emotions much more effectively, compared to infancy (Kopp, 1989; Thompson). As children and adolescents develop emotion regulation skills, they learn how to recognize, label, and express emotions in socially acceptable ways. They also learn that emotions such as anger are normal, but that they must learn how to express them appropriately and regulate their reactions to situations. The ability to regulate emotion is essential to social and psychological functioning, and failure may lead to a variety of problems, including development of psychopathology.

Emotion vs. Emotion Regulation

A vast literature exists regarding emotion regulation, although much of it is conflicting, due in large part to variations in definitions and conceptualizations of emotion and emotion regulation. Cole, Martin, and Dennis (2004) note that studies of emotion regulation have had various foci, including how emotions regulate other psychological processes, individual differences in emotional self-regulation, emotional regulation as a trait, and as a transitory change in state that can be momentary. Cole et al. also state that most studies do not define emotion regulation, do not distinguish between emotion and emotion regulation, and interpret associations between emotion valence (positive or negative) and factors of interest (e.g., adjustment) as providing support for the concept of emotion regulation without demonstrating the presence of a regulatory process. Although there is definite interest in establishing the emotion regulation concept, definitional and methodological variations and challenges present difficulties in construct validation.

The issues and problems associated with defining and differentiating emotion and emotion regulation are far too complex to address in this limited space. Thus, the discussion is limited to some issues regarding clinical assessment and treatment, which will be elaborated upon regarding anxiety and depression. A basic problem is that there is no standard definition of "emotion," and the term often is confounded with "emotion regulation." For example, a child who is showing a negative emotion may also be considered simultaneously to be having difficulty regulating emotions. Thus, a question arises regarding at what point emotion begins and ends and when emotion regulation begins. Cole, Martin, and Dennis (2004) suggest that emotions are considered to be the result of appraisal processes that also are self-regulatory. Thus, distinguishing between emotion and emotion regulation is complicated by how each is viewed by researchers, and, ostensibly, by clinicians. Nevertheless, Cole et al. suggest that emotion regulation occurs following activation of an emotion.

Another issue of research and clinical significance is that emotion regulation emerges within the child over time as a function of maturation and learning. Although children do develop emotion self-regulatory skills, experience and environmental situation also have a regulating effect. For example, if a child becomes upset and is comforted by a caring adult, that adult imposes external regulatory influence. Over time, the child learns that when distress occurs that cannot be self-managed, seeking out the comfort of a caring adult will provide relief from distress and help to regulate emotion. Thus, emotion can be viewed as both regulating and being regulated (Cole, Martin, & Dennis, 2004). From a clinical perspective, clinicians are interested in emotion and emotion regulation as a basis for understanding the development of emotional and behavioral problems and how to address them through assessment and interventions. Indeed, interventions often include helping children to learn to identify their emotions and develop skills to regulate them when problems occur. They learn about both positive and negative emotions and how they are related to consequences and outcomes.

Thus, for the purposes of this book, the model presented in Fig. 4.1 can be modified to incorporate the concept of emotion regulation as the next step after a child experiences emotion subsequent to an appraisal process with the recognition that the distinction is arbitrary and difficult to separate from emotion itself. Figure 4.2 represents a variation of Fig. 4.1 to include emotion regulation as the next step in a linear process of appraisal. Based on the nature of the regulation process and the conclusions reached by the child, one or more of the three types of response classes occur: cognitive, behavioral, or physiological. Following the responses, there may be one

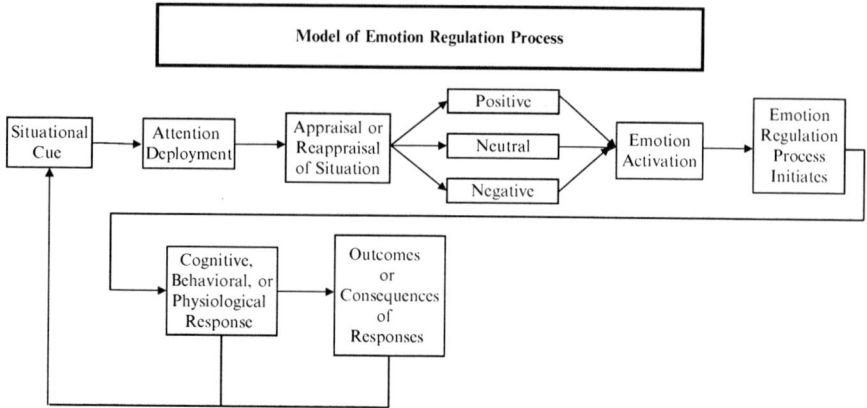

Fig. 4.2 Model of emotion regulation process

or several outcomes, such as increased or decreased anger or anxiety, resolution of a situation, or achieving a desired goal. The outcomes or consequences can be natural sequelae to the appraisal and regulation process or the result of environmental events, such as acceptance or nonacceptance by others. From both the responses and the outcomes/consequences, the child uses the information when future situations are encountered, making the model recursive similar to Fig. 4.1. As in Fig. 4.1, the recursive nature of the model applies upon initial appraisal or reappraisal.

Emotion as a Mediator or a Moderator

Introducing emotion regulation between emotion activation and cognitive, behavioral, and physiological responses raises the question of whether it is a mediator of emotion or a moderator. If it is a mediator, it provides a link between emotion and response and acts as a facilitator or mechanism for a response to occur. If it is seen as a moderator, then emotion regulation has a role in altering the appraisal process, activation of emotion, and response in a recursive model. Emotion regulation can occur in one of three forms: (a) as an involuntary process that occurs as the neurological system makes attempts to regulate emotion and return the person to a balanced state, (b) a voluntary process in which the child exhibits behaviors that are attempts to regulate emotion, such as clinging to a caregiver when experiencing distress, or (c) regulation imposed externally, such as by a parent who attempts to calm a child who is having a temper tantrum. Although children have little awareness and appreciation of the involuntary, biological emotion regulation processes, they likely are aware of their own actions and those of others to some degree. As experience is gained from both voluntary and external regulation, the child may be able to reappraise situations in the future, which will affect the activation of emotions.

From this perspective, emotion regulation is more than a mediator between emotion activation and response, but can change how situations are evaluated and managed, especially in a recursive model. Many therapeutic interventions are targeted at helping children to develop skills to regulate and mange their emotions, thus making emotion regulation more of a moderator. In Aaron's case, there likely was neurological activity that could only be inferred. His behavioral response to the perceived threat or challenge to him was intended to maintain the situation and not have to comply. The response of a "time-out" room was an attempt to moderate his behavior and return him to his pre-episodic state and was necessary to control aggressiveness and to prevent injury or destructive behavior. In the situation, however, Aaron likely learned little from the experience about how to regulate his emotions and deal with similar situations in the future. From a clinical perspective, intervention efforts could be made to help him learn how to regulate his behavior more effectively and to help the teachers learn how to avoid similar situations and to develop proactive strategies to handle them more effectively in the future. Thus, emotion regulation in this situation is more of a moderator than a mediator. For the purposes of this book, emotion regulation will be viewed primarily as a moderator of emotion activation.

Potential clinical implications exist from a model that includes emotion regulation and outcomes of the appraisal process. Some cognitive–behavioral interventions focus on helping children to identify emotions and to develop strategies to regulate them, such as anger and anxiety. Interventions also target cognitive responses such as worry, behavioral responses such as withdrawal, and physiological symptoms (e.g., muscle tension). As children learn new emotion regulation and coping skills, they are less likely to show the same intensity, frequency, and duration of symptoms when confronted with a new or stressful situation. An emphasis on outcomes or consequences of the child's response can become a treatment focus by working with parents, teachers, and others with regard to help the child regulate emotion and cope with situations. Thus, treatment in the form of family therapy, consultation, and psychoeducational approaches can lead to improvements in outcomes, potentially altering the child's appraisal and emotion regulation process that will result in more appropriate cognitive, behavioral, and physiological responses.

Emotion Regulation in Multiple Contexts

Genetic Context

There is little doubt that genetics play a major role in many aspects of human behavior, and their association with emotion regulation is no exception. At a basic level, genes control the regulation of neural and biological functions, including those that influence emotion regulation. Their role in neurotransmitter function has been studied with regard to emotion regulation. The neurotransmitters serotonin and dopamine appear to have major roles in emotion regulation and are controlled by specific gene systems. The serotonin system has been implicated in the generation and regulation of emotional behavior, while the dopamine system is related to reward processing and traits (Hariri & Forbes, 2007).

Other work has been done with regard to genetics and personality and behavioral variables and heritability estimates. The personality dimension of introversion–extraversion in adults has been found to have heritability estimates of 40 to 50% with about the same amount of variance being accounted for by nonshared environmental variables (Jang, Livesley, & Vernon, 1996; Viken, Rose, Kaprio, & Koskenvuo, 1994). Research investigating genetic effects is often conducted with twin studies, but such studies are few regarding emotion regulation, and many of those studies are with infants. Some studies of emotion regulation have focused on *effortful control*, which refers to the degree of effort a child may exhibit to control and regulate emotions. Effortful control has been found to be associated with emotion regulation and shows similar heritability estimates.

Goldsmith, Pollak, and Davidson (2009) discuss the role of genetics in emotion regulation and draw similar conclusions that it is moderately heritable. They summarize studies that have found parent rating scale reports of emotion regulation in their children to be clearly heritable, as are measures completed by observers. They conclude, however, that there are insufficient data about more specific genetic emotion regulation links regarding (a) continuity and change, (b) the association of effortful control with clinical diagnoses and temperament, and (c) sex differences.

Thus, there is ample evidence to suggest that emotion regulation abilities have a moderate heritability basis but also that the environment is a major factor. Environmental factors could include the degree to which risk factors affect regulation ability, the role of parents and other caregivers in regulating children's emotions, and how the child responds to situations that require varying degrees of emotion regulation. Whether emotion regulation skills are transmitted intergenerationally is not well understood at this point.

Biological Context

More is known about the role of neurological and biological systems and functions in emotion regulation than is known about genetics. The brain subsystems involved in emotion regulation described by Lewis and Stieben (2004) include:

- Brain stem—mediates arousal and behavioral activation
- Limbic system—mediates coarse perception, memory, learning, and affective feeling
- Cerebral cortex—subserves higher-order perceptual processes, attention, working memory, and voluntary control

Lewis and Stieben (2004) state that emotion regulation involves the synchronization of these subsystems and that they do not involve discrete, sequential processes, but operate simultaneously and interactively to influence each other. As a unified process, emotion regulation at the neural level involves four components: (a) specific action readiness, (b) a restricted attentional focus, (c) a stable cognitive appraisal, and (d) a distinct emotional feeling. These four components are consistent with the emotion processing model presented in Fig. 4.1, especially with regard to the notion that the person must attend to a situation or stimulus, appraise it, and then experience an emotion. Lewis and Stieben state that "From a neural perspective, then, regulatory processes are intrinsic to the cascade of neural changes underlying emotion" (p. 372). These authors suggest that this perspective is congruent with the position of Cole et al. (2004) that emotion is both regulating and regulated and that emotion regulation is embedded in emotion. This perspective, then, appears consistent with the model presented in Fig. 4.2 that suggests that appraisal leads to the experience of an emotion, which is followed by attempts by the individual or others to regulate it. However, it is not assumed that a child is able to distinguish between experiencing emotion and attempts to regulate it, especially because the processes are intertwined. Young children and those with developmental or language delays may have more difficulty in recognizing and labeling emotions and regulating them. More research is needed into the nature of the association between the experience and the regulation of emotion in children, especially those with emotional and behavioral disorders.

Neurological Structures Associated with Emotion Regulation

Several neurological structures are associated with how emotion is regulated in the brain. Some structures are associated with basic, rudimentary processing, such as perceptual awareness, while others are more directly involved with management and coordination of emotion responses. A summary of the roles and functions of the brain stem, limbic system, and frontal cortex is provided, with the acknowledgement that they interact in emotion processing and regulation.

Brain Stem

As noted above, the brain stem's primary role is to process incoming stimuli, mediate arousal, and to activate behavior in response to stimulation. Along with the hypothalamus, the brain stem regulates the cortex by providing specific neurotransmitters in response to stimulation. Presumably, this action corresponds with initiating attention to stimuli at a behavioral level that is represented in Figs. 4.1 and 4.2. The brain stem is also highly involved with regulation of the sleep–wake cycle. In turn, brain stem activity is mediated by the limbic system, the latter also alerting and preparing the cortex for sensory events (Tucker, Derryberry, & Luu, 2000). The visceromotor brain stem also has links with the amygdala, which is involved with rapid emotional responses to highly salient information (Vuilleumier, 2003).

Limbic System

The limbic system is composed of several structures, many of which are involved with emotion processing and regulation. It is a more primitive part of the mammalian brain and is often considered to be the primary center for emotions. The primary limbic system structures that play a major role in emotion are:

- Thalamus—serves as a "relay station" by sending signals to the cortex and has links to other limbic system structures
- Amygdala—signals the cortex about stimuli that motivate behavior, such as fear and reward; mediates major affective responses (e.g., mood, fear, rage, aggression); mediates expression of mood; signals and alerts the person to danger; related to "fight or flight" responses; center for identification of danger
- Hypothalamus—associated with pleasure, rage, aversion, and anxiety and more involved with expression than initiation of affective states
- Hippocampus—highly involved with long-term memory, making it possible to compare new emotion-arousing situations with past occurrences that help a person to choose appropriate options
- Cingulate gyrus—involved in emotional reactions to pain and regulation of aggressive behavior, associates sensory functions of sight and smell with past pleasant emotions, and associated with anxiety and depression

Prefrontal Cortex

The prefrontal cortex (PFC) is responsible for numerous cognitive functions that involve complex reasoning, executive functions, and certain aspects of emotion processing. It is involved in specific and deliberate cognitive activities, including activation when people experience emotion (Davidson, Putnam, & Larson, 2000). An interesting inverse relationship exists between the PFC and the amygdala, in that prefrontal activity is associated with inhibition of amygdala activity (Davidson et al., 2000). Medial and lateral parts of the PFC become more activated when negative emotions are reappraised, while some amygdala locations become less active (Ochsner, Bunge, Gross, & Gabrieli, 2002). Thus, there is ample evidence that PFC activity has a direct relationship to mediation of emotional responses that are centered in the amygdala by affecting the intensity, duration, or scope of negative emotions (Lewis & Stieben, 2004). These findings have implications for the role of cognitive–behavioral therapies that focus on altering dysfunctional cognitions. Therapies may lead to improved affective and emotional functioning by activating PFC areas that, in turn, reduce negative emotions centered in the amygdala.

The anterior cingulate cortex (ACC) is a more primitive part of the PFC and has direct links with the limbic system. It is situated between subcortical motivational and prefrontal systems that are involved in planning and control. Consequently, the

ACC is associated with mediating selective attention in demanding situations that require cognitive monitoring. These findings combined with behavioral research suggest that the ACC is likely highly involved in emotion regulation and cognitive control (Lewis & Stieben, 2004). Thus, the PFC and ACC appear to be primary cortical structures that are involved with emotion processing and regulation and may also be associated with temperamental variables that are related to the regulation of emotion.

Cultural Context

The role of culture cannot be underestimated in understanding emotion and emotion regulation, due to differences in cultural beliefs about whether or how expression of some emotions is permissible. Thus, emotion regulation is highly influenced by cultural values, beliefs, and, in many situations, by parenting practices. The cultural context will have a significant role in how emotion-related phenomena are addressed by clinicians. Culture is both a mediator and moderator of emotion and emotion regulation. As a mediator, cultural values, expectations, and practices provide guidelines to children about how they are to behave and express emotion. As a moderator, these cultural factors exert a strong influence on what emotions are expressed and the degree to which intensity or frequency of emotion is permitted. These factors have significant influences on how emotion is regulated. Culture determines the desirability and undesirability of emotional responses and the likelihood of activation (Strack, Schwarz, Bless, & Kuebler, 1993). Following the model in Fig. 4.2, culture also serves as an indirect source of emotion regulation as the child attempts to express emotion in culturally acceptable ways. Parenting practices that are based on cultural values and beliefs also are external sources of emotion regulation that affect the degree and type of expressed emotion. Failure to demonstrate culturally acceptable emotion regulation may be viewed as signs of psychopathology. Cultural models demonstrate that emotion regulation is not limited to intrapersonal factors, but is also highly influenced by cultural beliefs and standards (Mesquita & Albert, 2007). These models also prescribe boundaries and contexts in which relationships, self, and goals are formed, defined, and promoted (Bruner, 1986).

Mesquita and Albert (2007) propose that culture affects emotion regulation in three ways: (a) by influencing the situations that are selected that elicit emotions consistent with cultural expectations, (b) by influencing how situations are modified and how attention is deployed toward them, and (c) by influencing how situations are appraised and subsequent emotions are regulated. With regard to situation selection, Mesquita and Albert compare American and Japanese schools and how emotions are to be expressed and regulated. In American schools, children are expected to be "happy" and meet individual goals and achievements. In contrast, Japanese culture is considered to value an orientation toward others and to promote anticipatory shame or fear. They use the example of the concept of *hansei*, where children are encouraged to find and evaluate their inadequacies and to improve them for the benefit of the group. Whereas American children are encouraged to express their emotions about their individual achievements, Japanese children are encouraged to emphasize benefits to the group and to regulate and minimize emotions relating to self.

Mesquita and Albert (2007) use the terms *situational modification* and *attentional deployment* to reflect how cultural factors influence emotion regulation. They assert that cultural practices exert influence on individuals to modify situations and direct their attention in ways that are consistent with cultural goals and achievements. Success in modifying situations and directing attention enhances one's ability to cope with situations and to regulate emotions. In turn, others in the environment support the person who modifies situations and directs attention to culturally supported goals. For children, this reciprocity is shown when parents provide caregiving to their children who, in turn, modify their behavior to situations, attend appropriately, and regulate their emotions. Parents and other caregivers (e.g., teachers) may direct the child's attention or modify situations toward culturally accepted goals.

Finally, Mesquita and Albert (2007) take the position that appraisal of situations always occurs within cultural parameters of self and relating to others. Appraisal is considered to be a process of making meaning from events and that making meaning always has a cultural focus. Thus, when a person appraises a situation, it is done within a cultural framework and the resulting emotional experiences have cultural underpinnings. Culture provides schemas that serve as guides for how to appraise situations. When situations are predictable, they are appraised differently than when they are unpredictable, and fate is presumed to be the determinant of outcomes. Culture also highly influences the meaning of events and their implications for self and relating to others, affecting how people perceive and act when emotion-arousing situations arise.

The three components described by Mesquita and Albert are consistent with the models of emotion and emotion regulation presented in Figs. 4.1 and 4.2. Culture affects the nature of attention to a situation and affects appraisal of the situation, which leads to emotion activation. It is also likely that culture influences how emotion is regulated and the specific cognitive, behavioral, and physiological responses that occur. The responses also may influence consequences that are culturally mediated and moderated, which affect future appraisals or reappraisals.

A construct related to the cultural context of emotion regulation is *suppression*, which is the tendency to inhibit or suppress emotion due to the expectation of social consequences. Emotion suppression is the tendency to engage in reduction of emotional expression while a person is emotionally aroused (Gross & Levenson, 1997). Most of the research has focused on suppression of negative emotion, with little attention to cultural variations. In general, suppression is associated with negative outcomes, such as avoidance, reduced sharing of emotions, lower peer-related likability, and reduced interpersonal closeness (John & Gross, 2004). The question of whether there are specific social consequences and are culture specific was tested in a study by Butler, Lee, and Gross (2007). These authors found that habitual suppression of emotions consistently was associated with negative outcomes and self-protection tendencies in Americans with Western European values. Americans with Asian values showed less negative effects with suppression, suggesting that culture both mediates and moderates emotion suppression. Thus, emotion suppression appears to have distinct cultural associates that affect emotion regulation and may have negative outcomes. Therefore, clinicians must simultaneously address issues of emotional suppression and their clinical consequences, while also being sensitive to powerful cultural influences in designing and implementing treatment programs.

Social Context

The ability to regulate emotion is important in successful social functioning and adaptation. Successful emotion regulation is related to social competence and popularity (Eisenberg et al., 2004) and high levels of empathy and prosocial behavior (Eisenberg et al.). Conversely, lack of effective emotion regulation skills is seen in children with impulsiveness and acting before thinking (Arsenio & Lemerise, 2004). The ability to inhibit negative behavior and to demonstrate positive behavior is related to adaptive skills and is linked with social competence. Conversely, young children who lack effortful control and show high reactive undercontrol are seen as being less socially competent and function at a low level in social situations (Caspi, 2000; Caspi, Henry, McGee, Moffitt, & Silva, 1995). Thus, children who are able to regulate their emotions positively and cope well with situations are more likely to be socially accepted, seen as socially competent, interact well with others, and have friends. Children without good emotion regulation skills and show impulsiveness are more likely to have social difficulties and be socially marginalized, as other children overtly or covertly reject them.

Although separating cultural and social contexts is difficult and often they are intertwined, a consideration of how social factors such as socioeconomic status (SES) is important to understanding emotion regulation in children and adolescents. A primary consideration with regard to social variables is the extent to which there is an association between SES and emotion regulation. It is well known that children who live in poverty and lower SES environments are at greater risk of developing emotional and behavioral problems. However, most of these children do not develop serious psychopathology, despite their circumstances. Of interest is whether variables such as SES and poverty are associated with emotion regulation difficulties. In general, the associations of effortful control as a method of emotion regulation with developmental outcomes are similar across SES levels (Eisenberg et al., 2003).

Studies of low-income, ethnic minority children generally have shown that they use some of the same strategies to regulate emotion as do middle-income children (e.g., Ingolsdby, Shaw, Owens, & Winslow, 1999; Maughan & Cichetti, 2002). A common strategy used by children to regulate their emotions is to distract themselves from a situation. Evans and English (2002) found that low-income children use self-distraction as an emotion-regulating mechanism in a manner similar to higher-income children. Self-distraction is an example of effortful control, where the child engages in specific attempts to activate or inhibit behavior as needed (Rothbart & Bates, 2006).

Family Context

The role of the family, including parenting, is associated with effective emotion regulation in children and adolescents, beginning in infancy. Family effects on emotion regulation are the beginnings of the socialization process long before children interact with the environment and peers. As early as a few days or weeks of age, infants begin showing rudimentary emotional states, primarily through distress caused by stimuli such as loud noises or a state of contentment when physiological needs are met. When infants become distressed, parents typically will attempt strategies to soothe them, such as holding, rocking, or stroking. As children age, they typically develop increased emotion regulation skills and rely less on parents and other caregivers. In the early years, the family, particularly parents, exerts much influence over the development of child's emotion regulation skills, which serve to help the child cope with new situations.

Most often, parents use direct intervention methods to help their children learn to regulate their emotions. Physical contact to soothe distressed infants and small children is a common technique. Other techniques include modeling of behavior, distracting the child in times of distress or unhappiness, and encouraging the use of words and language to express emotions rather than exhibiting negative behavior. Parents also influence the regulation of positive emotions in infants by smiling, imitating, and other facial expressions designed to elicit smiling and other behaviors. Eisenberg et al. (2001, 2004) found that the social competence of children is influenced by how mothers communicate positive and negative emotions in the home setting. These findings and others demonstrate that a family environment characterized by positive emotions among family members is associated with the development of effective emotion regulation in children. Conversely, parents who are critical, denigrating, or dismissive of their children's feelings contribute to increased difficulty of their ability to regulate their emotions. This pattern is magnified when children express negative emotions because behaviors exhibited by parents and others communicate that the feelings are inappropriate, the child is not competent, or that the relationship is not close. These behaviors can worsen the negative emotions and interfere with the child's attempts to develop emotion regulation skills (Thompson & Meyer, 2007).

It is clear that children respond to the evaluations of others, especially parents and teachers with whom they spend much time, and negative input from these adults increases the probability of more negative emotions and impairment in development of regulation skills. When parents and other caregivers are unable to manage their own emotions and help children to regulate their emotions, children do not develop the ability to develop emotion-coping strategies. Consequently, they may exaggerate or inhibit negative emotions (Burge et al., 1997). Therefore, the influence of parents, family members, and other adults on the development of children's emotion regulation skills cannot be underestimated and may become a focus of intervention for addressing emotional and behavioral problems.

School Context

Apart from being with family members, children spend many of their waking hours in school and school-related activities. Consequently, schools present both opportunities and challenges to the development of emotion regulation skills. As settings where children are challenged to learn increasingly complex material while navigating social relationships, they are exposed to conditions that can create feelings of happiness, success, positive self-esteem, and self-efficacy. At the same time, they are also exposed to situations that may create frustration, negative self-evaluation, and negative mood if they face academic and social challenges that are difficult to surmount. Thus, schools can create conditions requiring regulation of both positive and negative emotions.

Three areas have the most relevance with regard to emotion regulation and schooling for children: (a) academic learning and performance, (b) social functioning in the school setting, and (c) the student–teacher relationship. Singly or in combination, these factors can have a significant influence on a child's success in school.

Academic Learning and Performance

Children who struggle academically face greater challenges with regard to emotional development and regulating their emotions relative to their learning difficulties. Children who show early signs of academic problems are at greater risk for continued problems and dropping out of school before graduation. Children who have adequate emotion regulation skills appear to do better on cognitive tasks (Phillips, Bull, Adams, & Fraser, 2002), whereas lack of these skills is associated with problem in working memory, attention, planning, and concentration (Blair, 2002). One study found a positive correlation between scores on standardized achievement tests and parents' ratings of their kindergarten children's emotion regulation abilities (Howse, Calkins, Anastopolous, Keane, & Shelton, 2003). Impaired emotion regulation skills may affect a child's ability to pay attention to a teacher's instruction and to complete academic tasks. Good emotion regulation skills reduce the chances of behavioral problems that can interfere with task completion, accuracy, and motivation to perform. Chronic academic problems can also lead to frustration and increase difficulties with regulating emotions and exhibiting appropriate behavior.

Social Functioning at School

Because children spend so much time at school and interact with many children on an almost daily basis, multiple opportunities exist for the development of social skills. For children who have difficulties with emotion regulation, social relationships at school can be difficult and challenging, especially if they are accompanied by academic problems. Risks for social rejection, ostracism, conduct problems, and aggression increase as impairments in emotion regulation increase. Because there is high comorbidity between academic and behavioral/emotional problems, emotion regulation is an important consideration in social problems at school (Dodge & Petit, 2003). Children with emotion regulation problems may show a range of behaviors, ranging from withdrawal and other internalizing symptoms to aggression, temper tantrums, defiance, and other externalizing patterns. These children may be marginalized or develop social relationships with peers who have similar difficulties. With fewer models of appropriate emotion regulation, they are less likely to observe and learn effective ways to manage their emotions. Children who are able to manage their emotions and not be disruptive in the school setting are more likely to be successful on academic tasks and in relationships with peers and adults. Peers also exert influence to regulate emotions by their reactions, acceptance, and willingness to include other children in social relationships. Children such as Aaron are less likely to be accepted by peers and tend to be marginalized.

Student–Teacher Relationships

An important factor in the regulation of positive and negative emotions is the relationship that children have with their teachers. A positive student–teacher relationship creates an environment where the teacher supports the child in various learning and social tasks. Consequently, the child feels supported and cared for and is better able to regulate both positive and negative emotions. A positive student–teacher relationship is a protective factor that reduces the risk of behavioral problems in the classroom (Pianta, Steinberg, & Rollins, 1995). A relationship that is characterized by warmth and closeness is associated with reduced aggression (Hughes, Cavell, & Jackson, 1999), while one that is conflictual and controlling increases risk for future behavioral problems (Pianta, Steinberg, & Rollins, 1995). Underlying these findings is the notion that the child who is able to regulate emotions will exhibit positive social behaviors and social competence.

For a positive student–teacher relationship to emerge that helps children to regulate emotions appropriately, it is a mutual, reciprocal process. The teacher must demonstrate behaviors such as encouragement, recognition of effort as well as performance, praise, positive approaches to discipline, and ability to direct and redirect the child's attention and behavior in positive ways. The child must be able to demonstrate age-appropriate social skills, follow directions, work well with other children, and inhibit impulsive and aggressive behavior. If the student–teacher relationship is positive, then the teacher becomes a facilitator of emotion regulation skills for the child, who develops increased social competence. If either of these types of patterns does not occur, the relationship is likely to be conflictual and result in the child being impaired in the ability to acquire and exhibit emotion regulation skills. If the teacher finds it difficult to manage emotion-related behaviors of the child, punitive disciplinary actions and angry and critical behavior may occur (Coie & Koeppl, 1990). In particularly difficult cases, the child may be referred for special education services for students with emotional or behavioral problems. The child may be evaluated for eligibility for special education services and, if found eligible, may be given services on a continuum ranging from classroom consultation to placement in a separate classroom or facility. This process is described in more detail in Chap. 14.

Emotion Regulation in Anxiety

The ability to regulate emotions is a central issue in the development and maintenance of anxiety disorders in children and adolescents. The contextual approach in emotion regulation described above applies to anxiety and the management of anxious cognitions and feelings. A core feature of anxious children is that they are in a relatively constant state of hypervigilance and are attempting to regulate their anxious emotions through cognitive (e.g., self-talk), behavioral (e.g., withdrawal), or physiological (e.g., deep breathing) means. All persons have a limited capacity to attend to events, and anxious children and adolescents have an attentional bias to threat, i.e., their attention is biased toward seeing situations as threatening or dangerous, and their ability to attend appropriately is impaired. Anxious children also tend to interpret ambiguous situation as threatening compared to nonanxious children, which is significantly related to the level of trait anxiety (Chorpita, Albano, & Barlow, 1996).

The processing of emotion corresponds with the model presented in Fig. 4.2 in terms of how anxious children process stimuli and regulate their emotions. Because anxious children tend to be hypervigilant, they spend more of their time scanning and evaluating the environment than their peers. Thus, it is more likely that their attention will be alerted to the presence of threatening stimuli. Like all children, anxious children engage in appraisal processes of these situations and determine if they have positive, neutral, or negative valence. Because they tend to see more situations as threatening, anxious children are more likely to conclude that situations are negative, which elicits fear as an emotion. Then, they engage in emotion regulation to control their fear and anxiety, leading to cognitive, behavioral, and physiological symptoms, such as worry, tension, and withdrawal. The process cycles again so that when similar situations occur, the child may or may not be better able to manage anxious emotions and cognitions. Using an attentional bias for threat and fear as being the dominant emotion, Fig. 4.2 can be adapted specifically for anxiety. In Fig. 4.3, the model has been changed from attention deployment to attentional bias for threat to indicate that the anxious child's attention is typically more oriented toward threat. Therefore, appraisal is likely to lead to a negative conclusion represented by the solid lines, which leads to activation of fear. The activation of fear will lead to a variety of attempts to regulate it, either individually or by others. If the strategies are effective, then future situations may not be as likely to have an attentional bias for threat and the outcomes of the appraisal process may not be as negative. If the emotion regulation strategies are not effective, then the process is likely to repeat in a similar manner.

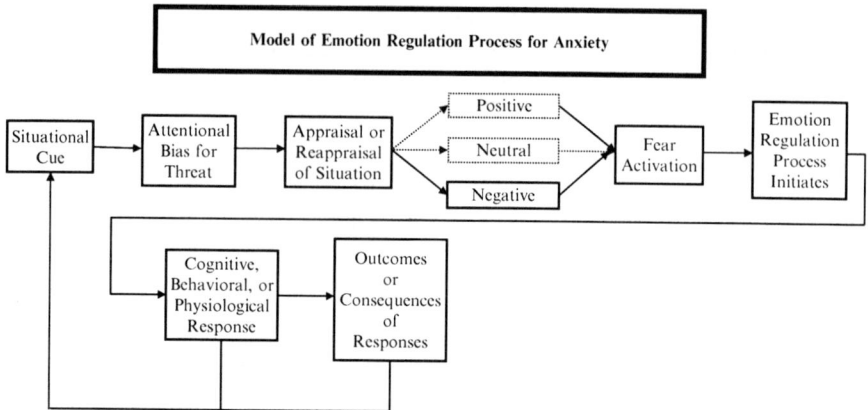

Fig. 4.3 Model of emotion regulation process for anxiety

The concept of fear is important to understanding anxiety and attempts to regulate it. Foa and Kozak (1986) suggest that anxiety disorders are based in specific pathological fear structures that mediate stimuli and responses. For example, children with generalized anxiety disorder (GAD) have a fear structure that is broad-based and can be triggered by a variety of stimuli. Children and adolescents with panic disorder or symptoms have a fear structure that is characterized by excessive attention to bodily and physiological sensations. In these situations, unexpected physiological symptoms, such as a choking sensation or shortness of breath may signal a fear structure of impending death. Consequently, physiological symptoms of tachycardia, perspiration, and flushing of the skin may occur, accompanied by high levels of anxiety and worry. In cases of specific phobia, a fear structure is created of specific situations and circumstances, which, if avoidable, do not elicit a fear response. However, if the situation is not avoidable, then a fear response is highly likely to occur. In all of these cases, attentional bias for threat and ingrained fear structures tend to precipitate and maintain anxious responses.

Dysregulation of fear is related to the development and maintenance of anxiety disorders. Fearful children tend to stop specific behaviors (inhibition), attempt to escape, or avoid situations by withdrawal. These behaviors indicate that the child is not regulating fear emotions well and is likely to repeat them in future situations if stress reduction does not occur. In these situations, it is the underregulation of fear that is associated with anxiety disorders, especially GAD that is characterized by excessive worry. Children with social phobia/social anxiety have excessive fear of negative evaluation that they cannot regulate, leading to anticipation of humiliation, embarrassment, or social ridicule. In both of these cases, withdrawal is a primary method to cope with the fear, although avoidance does not lead to effective coping skills and anxiety persists. In some cases, tendencies toward high degrees of fearfulness present as temperamental variables that cause stress on the child, leading to underdevelopment of effective coping skills (Lonigan, Vasey, Phillips, & Hazen, 2004; Rothbart, Posner, & Hershey, 1995).

Although anxiety is most often associated with the underregulation of fear, there is also the possibility that fear can be overregulated. When this pattern emerges, the child minimizes fear and does not allow it to become overwhelming. Overregulation of fear is associated with externalizing traits such as antisocial behavior, impulsiveness, and failing to anticipate consequences of actions (Barkley, 2004). In extreme externalizing disorders such as conduct disorder, the overregulation of fear is associated with lower levels of empathy, sympathy, and autonomic arousal.

Implications for Clinical Assessment

Emotion regulation of anxiety has significant implications for clinical assessment. Although general assessment methods are discussed in Chap. 7 and assessment of anxiety is presented in Chap. 8, consideration of emotion regulation in anxiety with emphasis on fear is an important factor in planning and conducting clinical assessment. Most assessment instruments do not assess fear directly, but emphasize behavioral symptoms and subjective self-reports of primary characteristics. Some measures address fears directly, such as the *Fear Survey Schedule for Children-Revised* (Ollendick, 1983). The assessment of fear should focus on the following:

1. Events and circumstances that elicit fear responses
2. Determining specific cues that arouse attentional bias for threat
3. Determining how the child appraises situations that lead to fear activation
4. Determining the valence or intensity of the fear emotion
5. Assessing the overall level of impairment
6. Determining what the child does to cope with activated fear emotions in cognitive, behavioral, and physiological responses

Much of the assessment of these areas must be done in a clinical manner, because there is no published instrument to address all of them simultaneously. Clinical interviews, observations, clinician ratings, parent and teacher ratings, and, as appropriate, self-ratings by the child can be used to gather this information. Comparing these sources of information can yield valuable data for the development of interventions. Although it is beyond the scope of this chapter to provide extensive detail about this type of assessment, some general guidelines may be useful. The first two areas can be assessed by observations of the child and interviews with the child, parents, and others. From the data generated, events and circumstances that elicit the most frequent or severe activation of fears are identified and prioritized. Interviews with the child will help to determine how he or she appraises situations, i.e., what are the specific aspects of situations that cause negative evaluation. Point #4 can be assessed with informal rating scales, such as having the child or others rate on a scale of "1" to "10" the level of intensity of activated fear. Similarly, for point #5, the child or others can rate how much impairment is apparent in those situations where fear is activated and can be compared to the level of reported intensity. Finally, observations and interviews can be used to determine what cognitive, behavioral, or behavioral symptoms occur upon fear activation.

Implications for Intervention

The primary goal of interventions for anxiety disorders is management of the principal symptoms of worry and hyperarousal that are associated with the activation of fear. Most intervention programs focus on addressing these patterns through cognitive, behavioral, and physiological methods. Cognitive approaches focus on helping children to recognize their fears, understand the links with behavior and physiological responses, and altering dysfunctional cognitive structures associated with fear. Behavioral approaches may include methods such as self-reinforcement, self-monitoring, and practice of alternative responses. Physiological approaches include relaxation training and systematic desensitization methods that focus on exhibiting behaviors that are incompatible with anxiety. These methods are discussed in more detail in Chap. 10. In part, intervention methods for anxiety focus on helping the child improve the ability to regulate activated fear emotions.

Emotion Regulation in Depression and Mood Disorders

Although anxiety and depression share some common features, there are some important differences with regard to how emotion regulation is used and manifested in children who have one or the other pattern. Although anxiety tends to be associated with the primary emotion of fear, depression is more of a chronic mood pattern that may not show clearly identifiable emotion activation. Durbin and Shafir (2008) suggest that there are three primary emotion regulation patterns that are associated with depression: (a) rumination, (b) high levels of dispositional emotion regulation, and (c) suppression of emotion.

Rumination is a cognitive style that is characterized by repetitive thinking about depressed mood and its causes and consequences. Frequent rumination appears to be associated with an increase in depressive symptoms even after accounting for initial levels of depressive mood. Ruminative thoughts are intrusive, difficult to control, and cause increased depression and impairment in functioning. Durbin and Shafir (2008) cite research that adolescent girls and women appear to engage in rumination more often than males and tend to talk about and focus more on negative feelings with their peers. They suggest that this pattern may help explain why depressed adolescent girls tend to have more social support from peers than do boys, despite having more internalizing symptoms. Worry may accompany rumination, but does not present as the major cognitive component of depression.

Dispositional emotion regulation refers to the notion that depressed persons may have a tendency to engage in excessive or rigid emotion regulation strategies that can increase the risk for depression and mood disorder. These strategies could involve rumination, worry, negative self-talk, self-deprecation, and distraction efforts. Durbin and Shafir suggest that many of the self-regulation strategies that depressed children and adolescents use involve considerable expending of effort that may deplete available resources for other regulation attempts.

Suppression of emotion involves a person making direct efforts to regulate emotion by controlling its expression and minimizing reactivity to situations. In an effort to appear to be functioning adequately and to appear to be in control, depressed people may try to inhibit emotion, specifically depressed mood and related symptoms. This strategy does not appear to be effective (Durbin & Shafir) and may impair the ability to interact socially, solve problems, and develop coping skills to use in subsequent situations.

Durbin and Shafir conclude that overregulation of emotion by any of these or other methods may require so much effort that opportunities to learn appropriate and effective skills necessary for the development of social cognition, interpersonal skills, or cognitive abilities are limited. As an example, they cite Abe and Izard (1999) who suggest that experiencing anger may help a child to develop appropriate skills in perspective taking, assertiveness, social rules, and even shame and guilt that can have a positive effect on developing knowledge of moral behavior and social standards. Durbin and Shafir conclude by positing that dispositional overregulation can interfere with the development of skills necessary for psychological and social adjustment.

Regulation of emotions associated with depression and mood disorders can be conceptualized in the model presented in Fig. 4.2. Compared to anxiety in which the primary emotion that is aroused is fear, there are several strong emotions that can emerge in depressed children, including sadness, anger, and guilt. Depressed children tend to have a negative attentional and attributional bias, in that they focus on negative rather than positive situations and circumstances. When they engage in self-talk that might precipitate emotion activation, their appraisals have a negative valence, which leads to negative cognitive, behavioral, and physiological symptoms. As with anxiety and other emotions conceptualized in Fig. 4.2, a negative cycle of emotion processing continues unless altered by factors such as maturation, changes in circumstances, efforts by caregivers, or therapeutic interventions.

Implications for Clinical Assessment

Whereas the primary focus of clinical assessment of anxiety is on worry, activated emotions in depression and mood problems may be more varied and complex. Of particular focus are the three components described by Durbin and Shafir (2008), i.e., rumination, dispositional overregulation, and suppression of emotion. Typical clinical instruments do not assess these areas directly and must be done in a clinical manner, similar to that described above for anxiety. Rumination can be assessed by conducting a clinical interview that focuses on (a) what areas or circumstances is associated with frequent rumination and (b) which ruminations occur most often. Self-ratings and information from daily logs and similar documents can be used to determine the degree of intrusiveness of the ruminations and the degree of impairment caused by the inability to control them. The six points presented above regarding anxiety can also be used as a general guide for assessing ruminations and associated symptomatology. Assessment of dispositional overregulation and suppression of emotion is more challenging and is beyond the scope of this discussion. In general, however, tendencies toward dispositional overregulation should be assessed as a temperamental variable and since the onset of symptoms. Similarly, suppression of emotion may be both temperamental as well as a strategy that has emerged to cope with depressive symptomatology and can be assessed to some extent through clinical history, interviews, and observation.

Implications for Intervention

The primary goal of the treatment of depression is alleviation and reduction of symptoms that are interfering with functioning. Assessing emotion regulation dysfunction may lead to more effective interventions, which will include helping the child to become aware of and begin to alter distorted cognitions. Efforts should be made to reduce the tendency toward rumination, which may interfere with the ability to problem-solve and participate effectively in treatment. By reducing rumination, the child may have more psychological resources to devote to problem solving, learning of appropriate social behaviors, and developing appropriate levels of anger expression, assertiveness, and perspective taking.

Conclusion

Although emotion regulation is a valid and valuable area for research, its implications for clinical assessment and intervention are not fully understood. However, an understanding of how a child or adolescent responds to situations, the emotions that are activated as a result of appraisal processes, how the child and others attempt to regulate them, and the outcomes in the form of symptoms are important considerations for clinicians. By including a focus on emotion regulation in assessment and treatment planning, the clinician may be able to implement various interventions more effectively with improved outcomes.

Part II
Differential Diagnosis

Chapter 5
Differential Diagnosis of Anxiety Disorders

Historical Context of Child and Youth Anxiety Disorders

Although anxiety is a basic human emotion that affects adults and children alike, clinical and research emphasis on child and adolescent anxiety disorders is relatively recent. Perhaps the first famous case of an anxiety disorder was Freud's (1955) case study of "Little Hans" who presented with a phobia. Freud conceptualized and treated Hans from a psychoanalytic perspective with emphasis on unconscious processes that had an underlying psychosexual basis associated with oedipal impulses. Conversely, the case of "Little Albert" by Watson and Raynor (1920) demonstrated that, using behavioral principles, a stimulus that originally did not elicit fear (i.e., white rats and white furry stimuli) could be paired with an unpleasant stimulus (i.e., loud sound) to elicit a fear response. Since Freud's seminal work, conceptualization of anxiety, fear, and phobic reactions has changed from a primarily psychoanalytic perspective to one that emphasizes cognitive, behavioral, and physiological responses. A cognitive–behavioral perspective emphasizes the interactions among these three components that contribute to the development and maintenance of anxiety symptoms that interfere with functioning. From a behavioral perspective, anxiety and fear may be caused by or exacerbated by the presence of aversive or stressful situations that the child cannot avoid or control.

The diagnosis of childhood anxiety disorders has seen the most clinical and research emphasis in the last two to three decades. In the *Diagnostic and Statistical Manual of Mental Disorders* (DSM; American Psychiatric Association, 1952), anxiety disorders were termed as phobias and called *psychoneurotic reactions*, but were not specific to children. In the second edition of the DSM (DSM-II; American Psychiatric Association, 1968), the related diagnostic category was termed *phobic neuroses*, but *overanxious reaction* was included as a specific category for children and adolescents. The inclusion of overanxious reaction was the beginning of the movement to recognize anxiety disorders of childhood, which also became an impetus for research on their development, assessment, and treatment that began in earnest in the 1980s with revised editions of the DSM-II.

T.J. Huberty, *Anxiety and Depression in Children and Adolescents:*
Assessment, Intervention, and Prevention, DOI 10.1007/978-1-4614-3110-7_5,
© Springer Science+Business Media, LLC 2012

The publication of the third edition of the DSM (DSM-III; American Psychiatric Association, 1980) and the revised third edition (DSM-III-R; American Psychiatric Association, 1987) included three anxiety disorders specific to children: avoidant disorder of childhood and adolescence, overanxious disorder (OAD), and separation anxiety disorder (SAD). Generalized anxiety disorder (GAD) was reserved only for adults. In addition, children and adolescents could also be given diagnoses that applied to adults, including phobic disorders, OCD, and PTSD. These changes reflected recognition of the overlap of symptoms across disorders and that multiple comorbid anxiety disorders could occur in children and youth. When the fourth edition of the DSM (DSM-IV; American Psychiatric Association, 1994) was published, avoidant disorder was subsumed under Social Phobia/Social Anxiety Disorder. Similarly, OAD was deleted from the DSM-IV as lacking sufficient evidence to support its inclusion, and it was subsumed under GAD, thereby removing the criterion between age and GAD. Thus, SAD is the only child-specific anxiety disorder in DSM-IV, and other anxiety disorder diagnoses, including GAD and various phobias, can be applied to children and adolescents. Differentiating anxiety disorders from each other and from other disorders, including some externalizing syndromes, is often a challenging task for clinicians, due to the high degree of symptom overlap.

DSM-IV Criteria for Anxiety Disorders

There are twelve anxiety disorders in DSM-IV, and all can be present in children and youth: Separation Anxiety Disorder, Generalized Anxiety Disorder, Obsessive–Compulsive Disorder (OCD), Social Phobia (Social Anxiety Disorder), Posttraumatic Stress Disorder (PTSD), Panic Disorder, Agoraphobia, Specific Phobia, Acute Stress Disorder, Anxiety Disorder due to General Medical Condition, Substance-Induced Anxiety Disorder, and Anxiety Disorder Not Otherwise Specified. For the purposes of this chapter, emphasis will be placed on seven disorders as the more common ones seen in clinical practice and for which there is a substantial research base. In Chap. 2, summarizes the typical age of onset, primary symptoms, common comorbid conditions, and developmental trajectories associated with each anxiety disorder presented here. In this chapter, attention is given to prevalence and epidemiology, specific DSM-IV criteria for each disorder, primary and secondary symptoms, comorbidity, differential diagnosis considerations, and typical assessment profiles. The chapter concludes with a discussion of how to use a developmental psychopathology approach to improve efficiency and accuracy when conducting differential diagnosis of anxiety disorders.

Separation Anxiety Disorder

As the only anxiety disorder in DSM-IV that is unique to children, the central features of SAD are excessive anxiety and fear about being separated from primary caregivers and must be inappropriate for the child's age or developmental status. Developmentally, separation anxiety is normal in children from about 6 months to 6 years of age; therefore, differentiation of typical levels from clinical levels is less clear. Children with SAD have an excessive and overwhelming fear that they will be separated from caretakers (primarily parents) by adult choice or by some catastrophic event, such as being kidnapped or a parent being killed. The development of SAD begins with mild separation anxiety as shown by requests to begin with parents constantly, wanting to sleep with them, complaining of night-mares, and not wanting to be alone. Over time, the progression of the disorder can become so severe that the child cannot separate from caregivers without significant emotional distress that is difficult to moderate. Children with SAD are not likely to be comforted with rational explanations, cajoling, or reassurances that their fears are unwarranted.

Prevalence Rates and Epidemiology

Onset of SAD is most often in preadolescents, especially at young school age level, but can occur at any age. SAD tends to occur about equally in boys and girls, and age of onset is not associated with gender in clinical samples, but girls in commu-nity samples appear to have a greater incidence of the disorder (Costello & Angold, 1995a, b; Silverman & Ginsburg, 1995). Young children with separation anxiety symptoms are more likely to report fears of harm to themselves or caregivers, have nightmares, demonstrate school refusal, and show extreme distress at separation. Older children and adolescents are more likely to report somatic complaints and school refusal, and younger children report a greater number of symptoms (Francis, Last & Strauss, 1987). Silverman and Ginsburg report prevalence rates ranging from 3 to 12% across studies, and the DSM-IV reports a prevalence rate of about 4%. The primary distinction between normal and clinical levels of separation anxi-ety is when the symptoms become so severe that the child's social, personal, family, or school functioning is impaired.

Foley et al. (2008) studied a large sample ($N=2,067$) of 8–16-year-old twins in a community-based registry to determine the relationship between SAD and func-tional impairment. The children and their parents completed two separate inter-views 18 months apart regarding current history of SAD and whether there was associated impairment. They found that SAD caused little impairment but that there was significant continuity over time with regard to age and symptom level. Older participants showed greater persistence of symptomatology than did younger children and prior symptom levels were the only significant predictors of future separation anxiety symptoms, diagnostic symptom threshold, or levels above diagnostic threshold with impairment. When controlling for prior symptom levels, neither diagnostic threshold nor severity of impairment predicted outcomes at Time 2. There were no differences between girls and boys in the degree of impair-ment. The authors concluded that current levels of impairment may guide treatment, but that symptom levels are the best indicators of prognosis and disorder severity. The authors also discuss the point that, although SAD may cause little impairment

Table 5.1 DSM-IV-TR Diagnostic Criteria for SAD

A. Developmentally inappropriate and excessive anxiety concerning separation from home or from those to whom the individual is attached, as evidenced by three (or more) of the following:

1. Recurrent excessive distress when separation from home or major attachment figures occurs or is anticipated
2. Persistent and excessive worry about losing, or about possible harm befalling major attachment figures
3. Persistent and excessive worry that an unwanted event will lead to separation from a major attachment figure (e.g., getting lost or being kidnapped)
4. Persistent reluctance or refusal to go to school or elsewhere because of fear of separation
5. Persistently and excessively fearful or reluctant to be alone or without major attachment figures at home or without significant adults in other settings
6. Persistent reluctance or refusal to go to sleep without being near a major attachment figure or to sleep away from home
7. Repeated nightmares involving the theme of separation
8. Repeated complaints of physical symptoms (such as headaches, stomachaches, nausea, or vomiting) when separation from major attachments figures occurs or is anticipated

B. The duration of the disturbance is at least 4 weeks
C. The onset is before age 18 years
D. The disturbance causes clinically significant distress or impairment in social, academic (occupational), or other important areas of functioning
E. The disturbance does not recur exclusively during the course of a Pervasive Developmental Disorder, Schizophrenia, or other Psychotic Disorder and, in adolescents and adults, is not better accounted for by Panic Disorder with Agoraphobia

Specify if:

   Early onset: if onset occurs before age 6 years

Source: American Psychiatric Association (2000, p. 125). Copyright 2000 by the American Psychiatric Association. Reprinted with permission

at the time of diagnosis, treatment of symptoms may be more cost effective because resolution of mild cases may prevent the development of more serious disorders at a later time.

Primary Symptoms

- Withdrawal
- "Clinging" to parents or caretakers
- Avoidance of other people or peers
- Procrastination in initiating activities
- "Shadowing" caretakers and refusing to be alone
- Refusal to engage in tasks without caretakers present
- Will not sleep alone or wants to sleep with parents
- Tends to occur more often during the week with children of school age
- Verbal and emotional protests about separation from caregivers

Secondary or Related Features

- Somatic complaints
- Limited or declining number of friendships
- Impaired social relationships
- Greater number of fears

Comorbidity

Although there is not a large body of research to indicate that SAD is comorbid with a wide range of disorders, about one-third of children with SAD present with secondary comorbid GAD, and one-third develop a depressive disorder several months after onset (Last, Strauss, & Francis, 1987). Suicidal ideation or attempts are uncommon in children with SAD, although some children might verbally threaten to commit suicide as a method to manipulate or coerce caretakers to remain close. There is some evidence that SAD is associated with later onset of panic disorder. This evidence is indirect and retrospective, however, as prior SAD symptoms have been reported by adults with panic disorder in longitudinal and family studies (e.g., Klein & Pine, 2002). An implication of this association is that treatment of SAD may help prevent the onset of panic symptoms or panic disorder in some individuals. An alternative possibility is that SAD is a response to various forms of distress, because children who have SAD tend to have parents who have major depression (Biederman, Faraone et al., 2001).

In addition to evaluating the symptoms and DSM-IV criteria A through D, a key element in differential diagnosis is to address criterion E to rule out competing diagnoses. The first step is to rule out Pervasive Developmental Disorder (PDD), which has an earlier onset than does SAD and is most often associated with a wide range of behavioral, developmental, and language problems that are not characteristic of SAD. A thorough developmental history and assessment of cognitive, language, and adaptive skills are necessary, and positive findings increase the likelihood of PDD rather than SAD.

The next step is to rule out psychotic disorders and schizophrenia, which, in young children and adolescents, are rare. These disorders are associated with delusions, hallucinations, disorganized speech, highly disorganized or catatonic behavior, and negative symptoms, such as flat affect, alogia (poverty of speech), and avolition (lack of motivation, desire, or drive) (DSM-IV-TR, pp. 285–286). In general, these symptoms are observed readily, and behavior ratings by parents and teachers most often show elevations on "atypicality" subscales, as well as a variety of behavior problems, including withdrawal, inattention, and social skills deficits.

The final step is to rule out Panic Disorder with Agoraphobia that is characterized by recurrent unexpected panic attacks followed by concerns about future panic attacks, concerns about the implications of future attacks, or a significant change in behavior related to the attacks. Social and specific phobias, OCD, and PTSD must be ruled out (DSM-IV-TR, pp. 402–403). Assessing panic attacks with typical psychological assessment instruments may be difficult, so the clinician will need to rely on history, clinical observation, interviews, and parent, teacher, and child reports of panic-related behaviors.

Differential Diagnosis Considerations

As noted in Chap. 2, separation anxiety is a normal developmental process during the first two years of life. Beginning in the third year, most children are able to separate from parents rather easily and enjoy being with others for brief periods of time. Even in these situations, however, some apprehension about being separated from home and parents is common, but it does not impair functioning significantly. Being "homesick" may reflect separation anxiety and may even cause some children to call parents to come home from staying overnight at a friend's house. Such situations are not uncommon and do not necessarily indicate the presence of a disorder. The "homesick" child who is planning to stay overnight with a friend faces a dilemma of wanting to be with a friend but also is apprehensive about being away from home. Older children in these situations may be concerned about being teased regarding inability to be apart from parents. Over time, however, repeated occurrences may contribute to social relationship difficulties, including developing negative feelings of competence, low self-esteem, and lowered independence.

Young Children

Young children often show separation anxiety when encountering new situations, such as beginning school, but the behaviors typically subside within a few days, and there is no significant short- or long-term impairment. If separation anxiety appears to be a long-standing pattern, it may be indicative of an undiagnosed anxiety disorder or subclinical anxiety pattern. It is important, however, to determine the reasons for the resistance to part from caretakers. In children who resist going to school, it is important to consider what is often termed *school phobia*, although the term *school refusal* has been used most often in recent years. If the child appears to be afraid to go to school, anxiety about separation from parents should be considered. If this pattern is evident, the clinician should conduct a family assessment to determine if parents are contributing to or reinforcing the behaviors. The clinician should also determine if there are perceived or real concerns that the child has about going to school, such as a realistic fear of being bullied or victimized or feeling academically inferior and not wanting to be exposed to ridicule.

Adolescents

SAD is less common in adolescents. If a separation pattern appears to emerge over a period of time, it may be a sign of depression, dysthymia, or social phobia/social anxiety disorder. Like young children, however, an adolescent may want to avoid going to school if there are concerns about being bullied or victimized, but may present as separation anxiety. In cases such as these, the issue may not be separation anxiety but an active attempt at *avoidance* of perceived or real stressors. If onset is sudden at any age, it may indicate that an event has occurred that has caused extreme anxiety. The author was consulted on a case where a teenage girl rather suddenly did not want to leave home, be with friends, or want to separate from parents. A referral was made, and it was determined that she had been assaulted at a party, but had not told anyone. In this case, separation anxiety symptoms were present, but they were indicative of a serious traumatic reaction. Key indicators were sudden onset and "classic" separation anxiety symptoms that are not common in adolescents.

Psychological Assessment Profiles

Children with SAD may show high levels of trait anxiety, withdrawal, distress, and social isolation. They may also show less elevated depressive symptoms or flattened affect and may present as sad and unhappy. They may be rated by teachers as being uncommunicative, not engaged with others, and as having social skills deficits. Parents may rate their child as having higher levels of trait anxiety and acceptable social skills and being comfortable at home.

Generalized Anxiety Disorder

GAD is one of the most common anxiety disorders affecting children and adults, with its primary characteristic being uncontrolled and excessive worrying about the future outcomes of a wide range of events and activities. In a sample of clinic referrals, Strauss, Lease, Last, and Francis (1988) found that 95% of the children were worried about future events. The degree of worry children with GAD experience is severely out of proportion to the circumstances, and often there is little or no objective evidence to warrant the excessive concerns. Although the child sees the worry as being justified, observers view it as being irrational, peculiar, or unwarranted. Parents and teachers may react with confusion, cajoling, coercion, belittling, rationally based reasoning, or minimizing, all of which are not likely to be effective and may exacerbate the symptoms. Although all children have worries, fears, and concerns about events and activities at times, children with GAD are at the extreme end of an intensity continuum. Studies have indicated that nonreferred children report as many worries as do referred children, but that the intensity of the worries

Table 5.2 DSM-IV-TR Diagnostic Criteria for GAD

A. Excessive anxiety and worry (apprehensive expectation) occupying more days than not for at
    least 6 months, about a number of events or activities (such as work or school performance)
B. The person finds it difficult to control the worry
C. The anxiety and worry are associated with three (or more) of the following six symptoms
    (with at least some symptoms present for more days than not for the past 6 months). Note:
    Only one item is required in children
    1. Restlessness or feeling keyed up or on edge
    2. Being easily fatigued
    3. Difficulty concentrating or mind going blank
    4. Irritability
    5. Muscle tension
    6. Sleep disturbance (difficulty falling or staying asleep, or restless unsatisfying sleep)
D. The focus of the anxiety and worry is not confined to features of an Axis I disorder, for
    example, the anxiety or worry is not about having a Panic Attack (as in Panic Disorder),
    being away from home or close relatives (as in Separation Anxiety Disorder), gaining weight
    (as in Anorexia Nervosa), having multiple physical complaints (as in Somatization Disorder),
    or having a serious illness (as in Hypochondriasis), and the anxiety and worry do not occur
    exclusively during Posttraumatic Stress Disorder
E. The anxiety, worry, or physical symptoms cause clinically significant distress or impairment
    in social, occupational, or other important areas of functioning
F. The disturbance is not due to the direct physiological effects of a substance (e.g., a drug of
    abuse, a medication) or a general medical condition (e.g., hyperthyroidism) and does not
    occur exclusively during a Mood Disorder, a Psychotic Disorder, or a Pervasive
    Developmental Disorder

Note: From American Psychiatric Association (2000, pp. 472). Copyright 2000 by the American
Psychiatric Association. Reprinted with permission

differentiates the groups (Muirs, Meesters, Merckelbach, Sermon, & Zwakhalen,
1998; Perrin & Last, 1997; Weems, Silverman, & LaGreca, 2000). These findings
suggest that interventions should focus on reducing the intensity of the anxiety,
which appears to be the factor that mediates the difference between feelings of
controllability and uncontrollability that children with GAD experience.

Prevalence and Epidemiology

As one of the most common anxiety disorders, GAD (including overanxious disorder) tends to have a chronic course, and onset can be at any age, with the typical age
of onset from about 10 to 18 and a prevalence rate of 3% in children to 10% in adolescents (Costello & Angold, 1995a, b). In the National Comorbidity Survey, GAD
was estimated to have a lifetime prevalence of 5.1% and a one-year prevalence rate
of 1.6% (Wittchen, Zhao, Kessler, & Eaton, 1994). GAD occurs more than twice as
often in adolescent girls (Yonkers, Warshaw, Maisson, & Keller, 1996) and shows a
persistent trajectory and a low remission rate (Yonkers et al., 1996). Early onset
(before age 19) is associated with a history of fears, avoidance, and inhibition, while
late onset in adulthood appears to be associated with an identified stressor (Hoehn-
Saric, Hazlett, & McLeod, 1993).

Primary Symptoms

- Excessive and uncontrollable anxiety
- Generalized worry and apprehension
- Pervasive across situations, although may vary
- Chronic feelings of distress
- Occurs on a daily or almost daily basis
- One or more physiological symptoms (e.g., muscle tension, nausea, sleep problems)
- Hypervigilance
- Attributional bias for threat
- Self-conscious
- Perfectionistic
- Exceedingly high standards for personal performance
- Overestimation of negative outcomes
- Expect that low frequency events will occur at a rate much greater than is likely
- Concentration and memory problems
- Difficulty maintaining attention to tasks
- Difficulty completing academic tasks in a timely manner, often due to perfectionistic behavior and making constant revisions
- Low degree of participation and volunteering in the school setting
- Absence of negative affect and presence of high physiological arousal
- Withdrawal

Secondary or Related Features

- Higher likelihood of state anxiety
- Excessive anxiety about being evaluated
- Social skills difficulties (e.g., not initiating interactions or group participation)
- Separation anxiety symptoms in younger children

Comorbidity

Williams, Reardon, Murray, and Cole (2005) suggest that GAD differs from other anxiety disorders by being more like a chronic stress reaction, due to the six DSM-IV somatic symptoms that are part of the diagnostic criteria. They cite Borkovec and Hu (1990) who found that worry helps to reduce physiological arousal. These findings were influential in helping to shift emphasis on high levels of arousal characterized by physiological symptoms to an emphasis on the worry dimension. If worry does help to reduce physiological arousal, interventions that focus on hyperarousal such as relaxation training may help to reduce the intensity and frequency of worry.

Although GAD is recognized as a distinct disorder, some authors have commented on its validity, suggesting that it is a complicating factor in several anxiety disorders and may not be a distinct disorder. This question has been raised due to the fact that GAD is nearly always comorbid with another anxiety disorder (Klein & Pine, 2002). Nevertheless, GAD is a current diagnosis in DSM-IV with stated criteria, and there is research that has established its comorbidity with other disorders. GAD has high comorbidity with depression, and children with both disorders have more functional impairment than those with either disorder alone (e.g., Masi, Favilla, Mucci, & Millepiedi, 2000). A unique aspect of GAD that differs from other anxiety disorders is its strong association with Major Depressive Disorder (MDD). Although other anxiety disorders such as OCD, PTSD, and Panic Disorder are associated with GAD, they are not as strongly related to MDD as is GAD. This association has been found in genetic studies (e.g., Silberg, Rutter, & Eaves, 2001) and in longitudinal studies (Pine, Cohen, Gurley, Brook, & Ma, 1998). Consequently, cases of "pure" GAD without depressive symptoms can be difficult to identify, especially because research suggests that the comorbidity between GAD and depression occurs in about half of cases. The best evidence to date is that anxiety disorders represent a group of distinct disorders that are highly interrelated. Frequently co-occurring anxiety disorders include GAD, SAD, social and specific phobias, OCD, PTSD, panic attacks, and panic disorders.

In preadolescent children, there is no significant difference in prevalence rates between girls and boys. At adolescence, however, girls report GAD symptoms at about twice the rate of boys. Adolescents with GAD also tend to report disturbing dreams, especially in girls (Nielson et al., 2000). Disturbed dreams may be associated with sleep disturbances and should be included in an assessment of symptomatology.

At first impression, anxiety disorders as part of the internalizing dimension of child psychopathology would seem to be unrelated to externalizing disorders. However, research has shown that co-occurrence with disruptive behavior disorders is higher than chance and should be considered as possibilities in clinical assessment and intervention. An interesting association between anxiety and conduct disorder was reported by Hinshaw, Lahey, and Hart (1993) that comorbidity of conduct problems with anxiety disorders was predictive of less intense and assaultive behavior at initial assessment. Over time, however, the comorbid group became more aggressive than those without comorbid anxiety. It is possible that the anxiety served as a protective factor for some children but was a risk factor for others. Although the reasons for these trends are not clear, Hinshaw and Lee (2003) posited that anxious symptoms appeared to be a protective factor with regard to the presence of assaultive behavior and the intensification of antisocial behavior. Conversely, social isolation and withdrawal were suggested as being associated with increased aggression and more negative trajectories.

Differential Diagnosis Considerations

As with SAD described above, procedures and considerations to rule out Psychotic Disorder and Pervasive Developmental Disorder (PDD) are necessary, with both showing anxious symptoms, but are secondary to these disorders. Psychosis in children is relatively rare in young children and typically does not onset until adolescence or later, although childhood onset is possible. Typically, PDD shows onset in the preschool years, while GAD has onset during the early to middle school years. The anxiety symptoms shown by children with psychosis or PDD are more likely to be caused by disruptions in routine, rather than the central symptom of worry about a wide range of events and circumstances.

Differentiating GAD from mood disorders can be more challenging due to the higher degree of symptom overlap. In general, children with GAD will be rated by parents or teachers as high on anxiety and lower on mood and depression scales, although the latter may also be in the clinically significant range in cases of comorbidity or subsyndromal symptoms. Children with GAD will show the core symptom of worry to a greater degree than those who have a mood disorder. Moreover, children with a mood disorder will demonstrate a relative absence of positive affect and more negative affect.

Criterion F also indicates that the clinician should rule out a medical condition that might cause physiological symptoms that mimic anxiety (e.g., hyperthyroidism). A possible differentiating criterion is whether the symptoms show comparatively sudden onset and the child does not seem to show pervasive worry or affective problems. Criterion F also requires that possible effects of prescribed medications or abused substances be ruled out. Substance abuse can cause symptoms that mimic anxiety and may require more thorough clinical assessment. Although substance abuse is more likely with adolescents, younger children may also engage in abuse of substances other than drugs, such as inhalants. The author consulted on a case of a six-year-old boy new to a school system and who showed signs of extreme anxiety and high activity. School personnel were of the opinion that he had an emotional or behavioral disorder. Upon review of his medical history, he was taking prescribed medication at inappropriate dosages, creating toxicity. After the dosages were adjusted to proper levels, the boy performed well academically and behaviorally.

Children with ADHD often show behaviors such as distractibility, inattention, concentration problems, and being "fidgety," which may be seen in children with GAD. Although comorbidity between anxiety and ADHD ranges from about 20 to 45% (Biederman, Newcorn, & Sprich, 1991) and some behaviors are similar, children with ADHD alone typically do not show the characteristic pervasive chronic worry of anxiety, and the onset is most often at preschool levels. Careful comparison of symptoms and clinical assessment often will help to determine the correct diagnosis or if there are comorbid conditions.

Psychological Assessment Profiles

Children and adolescents with GAD typically show high levels of trait anxiety on self-report and multidimensional measures of anxiety, along with fears of evaluation and high social self-consciousness. They also tend to score high on measures of perfectionism, which may be nearly as high as general trait anxiety. Due to the comorbidity with mood disorders, many children with GAD show mild to moderate levels of mood problems, although they may not meet criteria for a mood disorder. Observations often will show the primary symptoms in numerous settings, although some symptoms may be more pronounced than others. Children with GAD show signs of inattention, lack of concentration, and short-term memory difficulties. In the school setting, these behaviors may be mistaken for attention deficit or learning problems. These children are likely to show some positive affect, but also will appear to be "keyed up" or "wired."

Obsessive–Compulsive Disorder

OCD is a complex disorder that involves the interaction of repetitive and intrusive thoughts (obsessions) with repeated and ritualistic behaviors (compulsions). The DSM-IV-TR (APA, 2000) defines obsessions as recurrent thoughts, feelings, or images that are intrusive and unwanted and cause significant levels of distress and anxiety. Although the obsessions are recognized by the child as undesirable, inconsistent with goals and values, and uncontrollable, they are inescapable and the child engages in behaviors (compulsions) designed to neutralize the thoughts, lessen the distress, or prevent a dreaded consequence (APA, 2000). The child also worries that if the behaviors are not performed or if they are prevented or interrupted, catastrophic consequences will occur. Older children are more likely to recognize the irrational nature of their symptoms but are unable to stop either the obsessions or the associated compulsions. There are three OCD symptom subtypes: (a) harming/religious/sexual obsessions and checking compulsions, (b) contamination obsessions and washing/cleaning compulsions, and (c) symmetry/ordering of specific obsessions and counting/repeating/checking compulsions (Baer, 1994; Mataix-Coles, Rauch, Manzo, Jenike, & Baer, 1999; Summerfelt, Richter, Antony, & Swinsion, 1999). The child must show impairment for a formal diagnosis of OCD to be applied.

Prevalence Rates and Epidemiology

Estimates of prevalence rates of OCD have shown variability across samples. Whitaker et al. (1990) found a weighted lifetime prevalence of 1.9% in a sample of nonreferred 9th to 12th graders. Girls showed a rate of almost three times that of boys (weighted prevalence of 1.8% vs. 0.6%, respectively). Last and Strauss (1989) found a prevalence rate of 10.5% in children and adolescents who were being treated in an outpatient clinic, with age of onset ranging from 5.6 to 17.5 years and mean onset of 10.7 years. Onset occurred between 10 and 14 for about 65% of the cases. The ratio of boys to girls was about 60 to 40%, and boys had an average onset age of 9.5 compared to 12.6 in girls. Multiple rituals occurred in about half of the cases, with the most frequent ritual being washing. Of the children diagnosed with OCD, 60% had at least one other anxiety disorder, and 20% had a history of at least one prior anxiety disorder. Last, Perrin, Hersen, and Kazdin (1992) reported a lifetime prevalence rate of 14.9% in a clinic sample of 5–18-year-olds who had an anxiety disorder. Thus, it is one of the least common anxiety disorders. There does not appear to be a significant relationship between sex and severity of OCD (Last & Strauss). Valleni-Basille et al. (1994) found that female adolescents reported more compulsions and males reported more obsessions. In a manner consistent with gender ratios of other anxiety disorders, some studies have reported that adolescent girls report more OCD symptoms and greater impairment than do boys (Berg et al., 1989; Maggini et al., 2001).

In summary, the overall data suggest that the prevalence rate is about 2% of the population, is more common in boys, and has earlier onset in boys, with washing being the most common ritual. When children and adolescents reach adulthood, however, the sex difference disappears and the ratio between men and women is equivalent. In older adolescents and adults, age of onset has been shown to be between 14 and 20 in males and between 21 and 22 in females (Bellodi, Sciuto, Diaferia, Ronchi, & Smeraldi, 1992).

Primary Symptoms

- Repetitive and intrusive thoughts or behaviors that significantly impair functioning or cause severe distress
- Obsessions are not about actual life situations or experiences as would be seen in GAD
- Person is aware that thoughts are intrusive and are interfering with functioning
- Person is aware that obsessions and compulsions are causing impairment, although young children may not be aware of these effects
- Compulsions consume an excessive amount of time to perform
- Compulsions tend to be ritualistic and performed in a rigid manner
- Compulsive behaviors include washing, ordering, arranging, classifying, categorizing, or otherwise applying rigid patterns to events or objects
- After objects or behaviors have been ordered, arranged, etc., person checks and rechecks frequently
- High needs for perfectionism on specific tasks or circumstances
- Obsessions almost always are accompanied by compulsions
- Child may engage in secretive behaviors to hide compulsions

Table 5.3 DSM-IV-TR Diagnostic Criteria for OCD

A. Either obsessions or compulsions

Obsessions as defined by (1), (2), (3), and (4):

1. Recurrent and persistent thoughts. Impulses or images that are experienced, at some time during the disturbance, as intrusive and inappropriate and that cause marked anxiety or distress
2. The thoughts, impulses, or images are not simply excessive worries about real-life problems
3. The person attempts to ignore or suppress such thoughts, impulses, or images or to neutralize them with other thought or action
4. The person recognizes that the obsessional thoughts, impulses, or images are a product of his or her own mind (not imposed from without as in thought insertions)

Compulsions as defined by (1) and (2):

1. Repetitive behaviors (e.g., hand washing, ordering, checking) or mental acts (e.g., praying, counting, repeating words silently) that the person feels driven to perform in response to an obsession, or according to rules that must be applied rigidly
2. The behaviors or mental acts are aimed at preventing or reducing distress or preventing some dreaded event or situation; however, these behaviors or mental acts either are not connected in a realistic way with what they are designed to neutralize or prevent or are clearly excessive

B. At some point during the course of the disorder, the person has realized that the obsessions or compulsions are excessive or unreasonable. Note: This does not apply to children

C. The obsessions or compulsions cause marked distress, are time-consuming (take more than 1 h a day), or significantly interfere with the person's normal routine, occupational (or academic) functioning, or usual social activities or relationships

D. If another Axis I disorder is present, the content of the obsessions or compulsions is not restricted to it (e.g., preoccupation with food in the presence of an Eating Disorder, hair pulling in the presence of Trichotillomania, concern with appearance in the presence of Body Dysmorphic Disorder, preoccupation with drugs in the presence of a Substance Use Disorder, preoccupation with a serious illness in the presence of Hypochondriasis, preoccupation with sexual urges or fantasies in the presence of a Paraphilia, or guilty ruminations in the presence of Major Depressive Disorder)

E. The disturbance is not due to the direct physiological effects of a substance (e.g., a drug of abuse, a medication) or a general medical condition

Specify if:

With poor insight: if, for most of the time during the current episode, the person does not recognize that the obsessions or compulsions are excessive or unreasonable

Note: From American Psychiatric Association (2000, pp. 462–463). Copyright 2000 by the American Psychiatric Association. Reprinted with permission

Secondary or Related Features

- Significant effects on overall global functioning in over half of affected children and youth
- Interferes with interpersonal relationships
- May cause embarrassment with peers
- Interferes with emerging independence in adolescence

- Constant fears of compulsions being "found out" by others
- Feelings of helplessness and uncontrollability
- Impairment in ability to spontaneously shift from the ritual behavior
- Does not respond to reasoning to alter or stop the behavior

The most common compulsive ritual is hand washing, reported in up to 85% of cases of OCD (Swedo, Rapoport, Leonard, Lenane, & Cheslow, 1989). Variations of hand washing include ritualistic bathing routines, and similar actions involve washing that must be followed in a particular pattern on a daily basis. If the ritual is interrupted, it must be repeated until done without error based on the child's personal standard of perfection. Other examples of ritualistic behavior include placing objects in precise order or position, frequent recounting although there is no reason to believe that items are missing, retracing steps many times, or following a rigid pattern of preparing to go to bed. In all cases, the behaviors are developmentally inappropriate, time-consuming, and impair social, personal, or academic functioning.

There is a subgroup of children who develop OCD or tic behaviors that are associated with a bacterial infection. Pediatric Autoimmune Neuropsychiatric Disorders Associated with Streptococcal infection (PANDAS) presents with an abrupt onset of OCD or tic symptoms following contracting a Group A β-hemolytic streptococcal infection (GABHS), such as strep throat. The progression of the infection shows acute worsening of symptoms with some periods of improvement or remission (Swedo, 1994; Swedo et al., 1998). The PANDAS subgroup shows five key symptoms: (a) presence of OCD or tic behaviors, (b) prepubescent onset, (c) sudden and intense onset with periods of acute symptom severity, (d) temporal association with GABHS and symptom onset, and (e) neurological abnormalities, such as choreiform (involuntary, rapid, and jerky movements) (Swedo; Swedo et al.). Symptoms resembling ADHD, Tourette's syndrome, and oppositional defiant disorders may be seen. Prompt diagnosis and treatment are essential for the health of the child and also to prevent possible neurological damage. Although PANDAS is a relatively rare condition, the clinician should be alert to its possibility if there is a sudden onset of symptoms or there is a current or recent history of a streptococcal infection. Left undiagnosed, a PANDAS infection might be diagnosed as OCD, a tic disorder, or ADHD and treated with psychotropic medications or psychotherapy. In the meantime, the infection may subside, with the erroneous conclusion that the treatment was effective. If an infection recurs, the symptoms may return, and the process is repeated. Therefore, if there is a suspicion that the behaviors are due to medical causes such as PANDAS, immediate referral to a pediatrician or other medical personnel is indicated.

Comorbidity

Other anxiety disorders and depression and mood disorders are the most common comorbid conditions (Wewetzer et al., 2001), with concurrent mood disorders more common in older children (Geller, Biederman et al., 2001). SAD and GAD tend to be comorbid with OCD, as well (Geller et al.). OCD frequently co-occurs in children and adults with Tourette's syndrome, ranging from 35 to 50%. In children and adults with OCD as a primary diagnosis, the prevalence of Tourette's syndrome is much lower at 5–7% (American Psychiatric Association, 2000; Geller, Biederman et al.). OCD is also comorbid with other Axis I disorders, such as mood and somatoform disorders (Eisen et al., 1999) and with Axis II disorders, for example, Cluster C personality disorders (Steketee, Chambless, & Tran, 2001).

Obsessive–compulsive behaviors often are seen in children with PDD, but they may not meet the criteria for an accompanying diagnosis of OCD. Many children with PDD have a high need for sameness, predictability, and structure and may engage in behaviors that may appear to be compulsive. Although these behaviors may consume time, they are seen as rational to the person, while older children with OCD may see the behaviors as being irrational, but they cannot stop performing them. The child with PDD views the behaviors as being important in and of themselves and not as symptomatic of OCD (D. Meichenbaum, 2006, personal communication). Attempting to alter these behaviors may result in resistance, because the child views them as a part of the behavioral repertoire and not as problematic or impairing.

Differential Diagnosis Considerations

Children often engage in persistent preferences for sameness or have some ritualistic behaviors that are not problematic, such as bedtime rituals or arranging toys or possessions in a constant pattern. These typical rituals have three distinguishing characteristics from OCD: (a) they are not excessive, (b) the rituals are different from those seen in OCD, such as frequent hand washing, and (c) typically disappear by the age of nine (Leonard, Goldberger, Raporport, Cheslow, & Swedo, 1990). With adolescents, "true" ritual behaviors are uncommon, but they may engage in behaviors such as spending an inordinate amount of time in grooming and personal appearance activities. These behaviors are not truly rituals but are more related to concern about how the adolescent appears to others. Obsessions without compulsions in young children are the rule rather than the exception, and the same pattern is generally true for adolescents and adults. The rituals tend to change over time from one to another, for example, washing behavior may give way to counting or ordering rituals. Complexity may increase over time, making it more difficult to conceal from others. As rituals increase in complexity and time consumption, the child or adolescent spends less time with other activities, which can have significant negative effects on social relationships. The child may be embarrassed about the behavior and seek to avoid situations where the behaviors can be seen by others.

The ritualistic compulsive behaviors associated with OCD have some resemblance to perseverative behaviors shown in children with PDD that includes autism. Although the behaviors may appear similar, the distinctions between compulsive and repetitive behaviors are due in part to the goal or intent of the behaviors. In OCD, compulsions must be the result of obsessions that the child is trying to control through the compulsive behavior. Further, compulsive behaviors represent attempts to neutralize anxious symptoms. In contrast, perseverative behavior of children with PDD and autism appears to be more associated with executive functioning deficits in the frontal lobe that impair the child's cognitive flexibility to be able to disengage from the behavior, rather than a direct attempt to neutralize anxiety (Liss et al., 2001).

Criterion D of the DSM-IV diagnostic criteria specifies that Eating Disorder, Trichotillomania, Body Dysmorphic Disorder, Substance Use Disorder, Hypochondriasis, Paraphilia, or a Major Depressive Disorder must be ruled out. The central issue in differential diagnosis from OCD is that the latter may involve obsessive or compulsive behaviors that are the results of these conditions. In true OCD, the ritual is the primary concern and is the source of major impairment. Medical conditions that may mimic OCD, such as PANDAS described above, must also be considered and ruled out if questions about their presence arise.

Psychological Assessment Profiles

In addition to several scales that purport to measure OCD symptoms, established psychological assessment instruments typically show high levels of trait anxiety and generalized distress. Mild to moderate elevations on mood or depression scales may occur. Parent and teacher rating scales may agree if the OCD behavior is pervasive across home and school and is detected as being ritualistic. The behaviors could be infrequent, not recognized as being ritualistic, or the child may be skilled at hiding them, so that parents, teachers, and others may not observe them. If they are observed, they may be considered to be minor issues or as odd, but not as problems requiring intervention. As with other disorders, the degree to which the OCD impairs functioning is the important factor in determining presence and severity.

Social Phobia (Social Anxiety Disorder)

Social phobia is also referred to as Social Anxiety Disorder, and the terms often are used interchangeably. The diagnosis of avoidant disorder (AD) in DSM-III-R was subsumed under social phobia in DSM-IV, because they showed essentially the same characteristics. AD did not require that the fear of social situations or focus on social evaluation, but only on social contact with others. In DSM-IV, the definition and criteria for social phobia were expanded to include fear of situations where the child is exposed to unfamiliar people.

McClure and Pine (2006) suggest that social phobia may describe a disorder where the child is fearful of specific social situations, such as performing in public. Conversely, social anxiety disorder pertains more to high levels of anxiety about a wide range of social situations in which the child feels uncomfortable. The National

Institute of Mental Health (NIMH) uses the term "generalized social phobia" to refer to situations where a person is excessively anxious around anyone other than family members (NIMH, n.d., p. 10). Although the terms may be used interchangeably, there may be different clinical presentations by a child with regard to whether the disorder is manifested in specific or generalized social situations, requiring different approaches to treatment. The "generalized" specifier in the DSM-IV diagnostic criteria for social phobia requiring phobic behavior in most social situations addresses this distinction.

Selective mutism is listed among "Disorders Usually First Diagnosed in Infancy, Childhood, or Adolescence" in the DSM-IV. There has been research over the last several years to suggest that the disorder may be an early form or manifestation of social phobia that develops later in childhood. The behaviors seen in selective mutism of social withdrawal, social anxiety, and lack of social communication are consistent with the general features of a social phobia/social anxiety disorder. Some authors have proposed that selective mutism should not be a separate disorder but be seen as a symptom or subtype of social phobia (Black & Uhde, 1995; Dummit et al., 1997).

Prevalence Rates and Epidemiology

Epidemiological data indicate that social phobia is one of the more common anxiety disorders and is associated with significant impairment. Data from the National Comorbidity Survey indicated a lifetime prevalence rate of 13.1% and a 12-month prevalence rate of 7.9% in adults (Kessler et al., 1994) and is more common in women than men with a 3:2 sex ratio, although clinical studies have not found sex differences (Turner, Beidel, & Cooley-Quille, 1995).

The typical age of onset for social phobia (excluding selective mutism) is about 11–12 years of age, although it can begin in early childhood and shyness and social reticence may be seen as early as 2–3 years of age, often as behavioral inhibition (Kagan, Reznick, & Snidman, 1988). Strauss and Last (1993) compared children with simple phobia to children with social phobia between the ages of 4 and 17. Both groups were referred for treatment about three years after onset, and there was no sex difference in prevalence rates. Children with simple phobia were younger and had earlier age of onset, compared to those with social phobia who showed later onset at postpubertal ages. The data were consistent with other studies that found similar prevalence rates and epidemiological patterns (Essau, Conradt, & Petermann, 2000; Wittchen, Stein, & Kessler, 1999).

Primary Symptoms

- Marked and persistent fear of one or more social or specific situations (specific phobia)
- Marked and persistent fear of nearly all social situations with unfamiliar people (generalized social phobia)

Table 5.4 DSM-IV-TR Diagnostic Criteria for Social Phobia

A. A marked and persistent fear of one or more social or performance situations in which the person is exposed to unfamiliar people or to possible scrutiny by others. The individual fears that he or she will act in a way (or show anxiety symptoms) that will be humiliating or embarrassing. Note: In children, there must be evidence of the capacity for age-appropriate social relationships with familiar people and the anxiety must occur in peer settings, not just in interactions with adults

B. Exposure to the feared social situation almost invariably provokes anxiety, which may take the form of a situationally bound or situationally predisposed panic attack. Note: In children, the anxiety may be expressed by crying, tantrums, freezing, or shrinking from social situations with unfamiliar people

C. The person recognizes that the fear is excessive or unreasonable. Note: In children, this feature may not be present

D. The feared social or performance situations are avoided or else are endured with intense anxiety or distress

E. The avoidance, anxious anticipation, or distress in the feared social situation(s) interferes significantly with the person's normal routine, occupational (academic) functioning, or social activities or relationships, or there is marked distress about having the phobia

F. In individuals under age 18 years, the duration is at least 6 months

G. The fear or avoidance is not due to the direct physiological effects of a substance (e.g., a drug of abuse, a medication) or a general medical condition and is not better accounted for by another mental disorder (e.g., Panic Disorder With or Without Agoraphobia, Separation Anxiety Disorder, Body Dysmorphic Disorder, a Pervasive Developmental Disorder, or Schizoid Personality Disorder)

H. If a general medical condition or another mental disorder is present, the fear in Criterion A is unrelated to it, for example, the fear is not of Stuttering, trembling in Parkinson's disease, or exhibiting abnormal eating behavior in Anorexia Nervosa or Bulimia Nervosa

Specify if:

Generalized: if the fears include most social situations (also consider the additional diagnosis of Avoidant Personality Disorder)

Note: From American Psychiatric Association (2000, pp. 456). Copyright 2000 by the American Psychiatric Association. Reprinted with permission

- Attempts to avoid or escape social situations to reduce anxiety
- Extreme distress if avoidance or escape is not possible
- Extreme shyness or behavioral inhibition in social situations
- "Loner" behavior
- Few friends and active social relationships
- Fear of making public presentations, such as speeches or reports
- Concerns about embarrassment, humiliation, or appearing inept
- Physical symptoms, such as stomachaches, flushing of the skin, or rapid heart rate
- Chronic anticipatory worry about being in social situations

Secondary or Related Features

- Refusal to go to school, which can result in academic underachievement
- Will not answer doorbells or telephones

- Will not volunteer to participate at school or answer questions posed by teachers
- May refuse to eat in a school lunchroom or cafeteria around other children
- May take indirect routes to places to avoid social interactions
- Stays at the back of a large group of children when changing activities
- Avoids attention-seeking
- Resists or refuses to participate in competitive games, especially when changing clothes with others is necessary, such as in physical education activities at school
- Poor leadership skills
- Poor social skills
- Excessive social passivity
- Have a greater tendency to interpret social situations as threatening
- Extreme self-consciousness
- Attention and learning problems at school
- May demonstrate lower levels of empathy and mutual reciprocity with peers and friends
- Increased risk of social exclusion, relational victimization, and bullying
- More pessimistic about future outcomes than peers
- Unpopular with peers

Comorbidity

In the National Comorbidity Survey, social phobia was found to be the most common anxiety disorder and the third most common psychiatric disorder among adults (Kessler et al., 1994). Children with social phobia tend to have higher trait anxiety, general emotional overresponsiveness, and excessive fearfulness (Beidel, Turner, & Morris, 1999), which puts them at higher risk for other anxiety disorders, especially GAD. They also have tendencies toward depressed mood, placing them at greater risk for a mood disorder. Associations with mood disorders, however, are seen more often with older than younger children (Stein et al., 2001). Interestingly, Pine, Cohen, Cohen, and Brook (2000) found a unique association between social anxiety disorder and conduct disorder, noting that the former predicted a relatively benign course for subsequent conduct disorder. Thus, high social anxiety may have a mitigating effect on the development of conduct problems, a pattern not seen in children who have other comorbid anxiety disorders and conduct disorder. In summary, children with social phobia/social anxiety disorder tend to be at risk for other anxiety disorders, mood problems or disorders, social impairments, and frequent periods of distress.

Differential Diagnosis Considerations

As with other anxiety disorders, other diagnoses must be ruled out to confirm the presence of social phobia. A detailed current medical history is needed to determine whether there are medical conditions that may contribute to or explain the behavior, as well as to determine if there are any medications being prescribed. Abuse of licit or illicit drugs must also be ruled out as possible explanations.

PDD may have some behaviors that appear to have social phobia characteristics. However, children with PDD likely will show other characteristics not common to children with social phobia, including global social impairment, stereotypic behaviors, language difficulties, and perseverative behaviors. A child or adolescent with Body Dysmorphic Disorder demonstrates unusual concern or worry about minor or imaginary physical flaws, a characteristic not common to children with Social Phobia. Schizoid personality disorder is very rare in children and adolescents and is characterized by flattened affect, aloofness and detachment, and little or no desire to associate with others, including family members. They do not avoid others to minimize or cope with anxiety, but do so due to lack of interest in others. In contrast, children with Social Phobia often relate well to family members, have some friends, and have some interests in social and interpersonal relationships, despite being uncomfortable. A distinction between Social Phobia and Panic Disorder is that, in the latter, panic attacks can onset suddenly without warning and are not associated with specific feared stimuli. In contrast, most children with Social Phobia typically can be identified as their anxiety resulting from being around others (generalized) or of specific events or circumstances (specific).

Differentiating children with Separation Anxiety Disorder from Social Phobia can be more challenging for the clinician, because the intent of the behavior may be more difficult to determine. There is the possible role of parent reinforcement of separation anxiety behavior that helps to maintain the pattern. Parents of children with social phobia typically do want their children to be socially involved and to have friends and, in fact, may be concerned that their child does not show interest in these activities. A fundamental difference is that children with SAD are not so anxious about being with others but are more anxious about separating from parents. In contrast, chidden with social phobia try to avoid anxiety-producing social situations, although they may show separation behaviors, such as "clinging" if being exposed to social situations appears imminent.

Age of onset for social phobia typically is in the adolescent years, which tends to distinguish it from SAD. Onset can occur at younger ages but is infrequent before about eight years of age. Rates of both normal social fears and social phobia increase over time and tend to peak in adolescence, especially among girls. From adolescence forward, the difference in prevalence rates between boys and girls tends to remain constant (McClure & Pine, 2006). Therefore, adolescent girls appear to be at the greatest risk of developing social phobia at its peak prevalence rate.

Typical Assessment Profiles

Children with social phobia tend to show high levels of general anxiety, social withdrawal, a high level of specific fears, and impaired social skills, which are often reported by adults on rating scales and in interviews. Self-reports tend to confirm general anxiety and withdrawal, but social skills may be reported to be in the average range. Interviews with teachers, parents, and others and direct observations generally will reveal and document the specific conditions where phobic behaviors are seen.

Specific Phobia

Specific phobia represents a class of anxiety disorders where specific, identifiable stimuli or circumstances precipitate an anxiety reaction, perhaps including panic attacks. Unlike other anxiety disorders where symptoms can emerge from cognitive distortions or faulty schemata, specific phobias are associated with reactions to stimuli that both the child and others can identify, such as fear reactions to loud noises or large animals. Although children may have cognitions about fear-producing stimuli, the cognitions are not considered causal in the onset of phobic symptoms. The associated fear may cause the child to attempt to avoid situations that trigger the phobic reactions. They may be precipitated by any of a number of stimuli, which the DSM-IV-TR categorizes as Animal Type, Natural Environment Type, Blood–Injection–Injury Type, Situational Type, or Other Type. Specific phobias show variations as a function of age. For example, fears of large animals tend to occur before age seven but dissipate by adolescence, while phobias of thunderstorms tend to have onset at about 12 years of age.

Prevalence and Epidemiology

Prevalence rates of specific phobia range from about 0.3 to 15.1% with a median rate of 3.5% (Costello, Egger, & Angold, 2004). Like most anxiety disorders, specific phobias appear to occur more often in girls than in boys, and overall prevalence rates tend to remain stable across childhood and adolescence. Unlike other anxiety disorders, such as panic disorder and agoraphobia which tend to increase over the life span, specific phobias tend to decline to occur rarely in adolescence. Frequency of specific phobia occurs more often in clinical vs. community samples. The onset of most specific phobias appears to be about the time that children start school (Costello, Mustillo, Erkanli, Keeler, & Angold, 2003). There is inadequate research to indicate whether specific phobia is related to factors such as SES or culture.

Primary Symptoms

- Marked and persistent fear of specific stimuli or situations
- Avoidance from anxiety-producing situation through crying, hiding, or tantrums

Table 5.5 DSM-IV-TR Diagnostic Criteria for Specific Phobia

A. Marked and persistent fear that is excessive or unreasonable, cued by the presence or anticipation of a specific object or situation (e.g., flying, heights, animals, receiving an injection, seeing blood)

B. Exposure to the phobic stimulus almost invariably precedes an immediate anxiety response, which may take the form of a situationally bound or situationally predisposed panic attack. Note: In children, the anxiety may be expressed by crying, tantrums, freezing, or clinging

C. The person recognizes that the fear is excessive or unreasonable. Note: In children, this feature may be absent

D. The phobic situation(s) is avoided or else is endured with intense anxiety or distress

E. The avoidance, anxious anticipation, or distress in the feared situation(s) interferes significantly with the person's normal routine, occupational (or academic) functioning, or social activities or relationships, or there is marked distress about having the phobia

F. In individuals under age 18 years, the duration is at least 7 months

G. The anxiety, Panic Attacks, or the phobic avoidance associated with the specific object or situation are not better accounted for by another mental disorder, such as Obsessive–Compulsive Disorder (e.g., fear of dirt in someone with an obsession about contamination), Posttraumatic Stress Disorder (avoidance of stimuli associated with a severe stressor), Separation Anxiety Disorder (e.g., avoidance of school), Social Phobia (e.g., avoidance of social situations because of fear of embarrassment), Panic Disorder With Agoraphobia, or Agoraphobia Without History of Panic Disorder

Specify type:

    Animal type

    Natural environment type (e.g., heights, storms, water)

    Blood–injection–injury type

    Situational type (e.g., airplanes, elevators, enclosed places)

    Other type (e.g., phobic avoidance of situations that may lead to choking, vomiting, or contracting an illness in children, avoidance of loud sounds or costumed characters)

Source: American Psychiatric Association (2000, p. 125). Copyright 2000 by the American Psychiatric Association. Reprinted with permission

- Response is excessive to the situation
- Catastrophizing about severe negative outcomes if exposed to the situation
- Escape from situation or clinging and pleading from adults if escape is not possible
- Physiological symptoms of increased heart rate, trembling, and blood pressure

Secondary or Related Features

- Interference with daily functioning
- May interfere with school functioning if the phobia is triggered by stimuli at school
- Ridicule and teasing by peers

Comorbidity

Children with specific phobia are at increased risk for SAD and social phobia/social anxiety disorder. There is evidence that there is comorbidity among the three types of phobias, i.e., social, specific, and agoraphobia (Pine & Grun, 1999). There is no convincing evidence that specific phobia is linked with the development of depression over time or that it is a precursor to other anxiety disorders, such as GAD or OCD.

Differential Diagnosis Considerations

Because the symptoms of Specific Disorder can be similar to behaviors of other anxiety disorders, the clinician should rule out other comorbid disorders that may have specific fearful behaviors, such as OCD, PTSD, Separation Anxiety Disorder, Panic Disorder With or Without Agoraphobia, or Social Phobia. All of these disorders tend to be associated with pervasive impairment, whereas Specific Phobia only symptoms likely will be shown in only specific circumstances and not show pervasive impairment. It is possible that some children with Pervasive Developmental Disorder may show some behaviors that are similar to Specific Phobia, but there will be a history of developmental problems in many areas over several years. It is possible that a child may have one of these disorders in addition to Specific Phobia that may require simultaneous assessment and intervention.

Another differential diagnosis consideration is when children show evidence of school refusal, often referred to as school phobia. It is important to determine if the child's fear of school is based on a fear of specific aspects of school, or if it is related to reluctance to go to school for fear of being bullied or other negative circumstances, parent–child relationship problems, or other issues. If it is determined that the child is experiencing bullying and harassment, attention should be given to altering the school situation, rather than placing all of the responsibility on the child. If it is determined that the reluctance is due to parent–child relationships, then alternative diagnoses and intervention may be considered.

Typical Assessment Profiles

If the child has Specific Phobia only, psychological assessment profiles likely will show no to mild elevations, but likely not in the clinically significant range. Slight elevations in general anxiety and stress may be shown, but any assessment results of significance likely will be shown on specific fear measures, such as the *Fear Survey Schedule for Children-II* (Gullone & King, 1992; Gullone & Lane, 2002).

Posttraumatic Stress Disorder

PTSD is a disorder that emerges following exposure to either acute or chronic events that can occur once or many times. A person can be assaulted or be in a serious accident and develop PTSD or it may develop as a result of repeated exposure to threatening or harmful situations, such as soldiers in war or children exposed to chronic abuse. Its consequences can be severe and cause significant impairment in social, personal, and occupational or academic functioning. PTSD has been known for many years and is comparable to the term "shell shock" and "war neurosis" experienced by soldiers. The significance of PTSD in children and adolescence has become more important with incidents involving school violence, such as shootings at Jonesboro, Arkansas in 1998 and at Columbine High School in 1999. In general, symptoms of trauma are similar in children and adults, although there are some differences, such as children having flashbacks being uncommon.

Prevalence and Epidemiology

Although several studies regarding the epidemiology of PTSD have been conducted on adults, less is known about the disorder in children. Stress reactions have long been recognized in children, but increased interest began after the incident in Chowchilla, California in 1976 when 26 children on a school bus were kidnapped and the bus was buried for 27 hours with the children inside. All of the children escaped, but they were not given any immediate counseling or therapy to address trauma symptoms. Terr (1979) interviewed 23 of the children within about 6–10 months after the event and found that, although their symptoms were similar to those of adults who have experienced trauma, there were some important differences. They did not show hallucinations, flashbacks of reliving the experiences, numbing, or forgetting what had happened. In follow-up interviews four years later, none of the children had forgotten anything about the experience. They relived the experience through talking, storytelling, reenactments, and playing bus-driving or kidnapping games (Terr, 1983). These findings suggest that children process and express trauma differently from adults, which are due, in part, to age and developmental factors.

Research on prevalence rates has shown variation in the percent of children who have patterns similar to PTSD. Fletcher (2003) summarized the results of a meta-analysis of studies in which children and adults had been exposed to traumatic situations. The overall findings of the study indicated that more than 20% of traumatized children showed all DSM-IV symptoms, with the exception of 16% who showed a pessimistic outlook and 12% who could not remember parts of the trauma. Approximately 88% of the children showed at least one of the criterion B symptoms. Seven of the 11 most frequently occurring symptoms were on criterion B:

Reminders were distressing	51%
Reenactment of events	40%
Feeling as if the events were being relived	39%
Intrusive memories of the events	34%
Bad dreams about the events	31%
Trauma-specific fears	31%
Talking excessively about the events	31%

Other frequently occurring symptoms were affective numbing (47%), loss of interest in previously important activities (36%), and avoidance of reminders of the events (32%). The results for children and adolescents were generally similar to those of adults. Approximately 36% of all ages met criteria for PTSD, with age ranges as follows: preschool (39%), school age (33%), adolescents (27%), and adults (24%). These data indicate that children exposed to traumatic situations have a significant risk of developing PTSD symptoms and meet criteria for a mental disorder. Aggressive or antisocial behavior seemed to occur more often in preschool children. Generalized anxiety (39%), guilt (43%), low self-esteem (34%), and dissociative responses (48%) were the most frequent associated symptoms for all ages. The study did not report whether any of the participants received counseling or therapy at any point.

Risks for exposure to traumatic events increases with age. Young children may develop stress disorders from events such as accidents, injury, abuse, and loss of a parent. As children reach adolescence, they are exposed to a greater range of possible stressors, including traffic accidents while driving or being a passenger with a teen driver, death of a parent or close friend, or medical problems. Adolescents are also more likely than adults to be exposed to violence, with boys more likely to be victims of assault and girls to be exposed to dating violence and rape. Kilpatrick, Saunders, Resnick, and Smith (1995) found that 23% of a sample of adolescents had been a witness to violence and were victims of assault and that 20% met lifetime criteria for PTSD. Further, adolescents who have been traumatized have a much greater likelihood of problems with academic achievement, aggressive or delinquent behavior, high-risk sexual behavior, substance abuse, excessive risk-taking, extreme avoidance, depression, and deficits in the development of skills necessary for career preparation, intimate relationships, and general psychosocial adjustment. All of these problems may lead to other disorders in addition to PTSD, such as attachment problems. Traumatic stress is associated with attachment problems in infants, leading to the potential for long-term problems. Cichetti, Toth, and Bush (1988) reported that across studies, 70–80% of maltreated infants developed insecure attachments to caregivers.

Table 5.6 DSM-IV-TR Diagnostic Criteria for PTSD

A. The person has been exposed to a traumatic event in which both of the following were present:
  1. The person experienced, witnessed, or was confronted with an event or events that involved actual or threatened death or serious injury, or a threat to the physical integrity of self or others
  2. The person's response involved intense fear, helplessness, or horror. Note: In children, this may be expressed instead by disorganized or agitated behavior

B. The traumatic event is persistently reexperienced in one (or more) of the following ways:
  1. Recurrent and intrusive distressing recollections of the event, including images, thoughts, or perceptions. Note: In young children, repetitive play may occur in which themes or aspects of the trauma are experienced
  2. Recurrent distressing dreams of the event. Note: In children, there may be frightening dreams without recognizable content
  3. Acting or feeling as if the traumatic event were recurring (includes a sense of reliving the experience, illusions, hallucinations, and dissociative flashback episodes, including those that occur on awakening or when intoxicated)
  4. Intense psychological distress on exposure to internal or external cues that symbolize or resemble an aspect of the traumatic event
  5. Physiological reactivity on exposure to internal or external cues that symbolize or resemble an aspect of the traumatic event

C. Persistent avoidance of stimuli associated with the trauma and numbing of general responsiveness (not present before the trauma), as indicated by three (or more) of the following:
  1. Efforts to avoid thoughts, feelings, or conversations associated with the trauma
  2. Efforts to avoid activities, places, or people that arouse recollections of the trauma
  3. Inability to recall an important aspect of the trauma
  4. Markedly diminished interest or participation in significant activities
  5. Feelings of detachment or estrangement from others
  6. Restricted range of affect (e.g., unable to have loving feelings)
  7. Sense of a foreshortened future (e.g., does not expect to have a career, marriage, children, or a normal life span)

D. Persistent symptoms of increased arousal (not present before the trauma), as indicated by two (or more) of the following:
  1. Difficulty falling or staying asleep
  2. Irritability or outbursts of anger
  3. Difficulty concentrating
  4. Hypervigilance
  5. Exaggerated startle response

E. Duration of the disturbance (symptoms in Criteria B, C, and D) is more than 1 month

F. The disturbance causes clinically significant distress or impairment in social, occupational, or other important areas of functioning

Specify if:
  Acute: if duration of symptoms is less than 3 months
  Chronic: if duration of symptoms is 3 months or more

Specify if:
  With delayed onset: if onset of symptoms is at least 6 months after the stressor

Note: From American Psychiatric Association (2000, pp. 467–468). Copyright 2000 by the American Psychiatric Association. Reprinted with permission

Primary Symptoms

- Reliving or reexperiencing the memories of the event(s)
- Intrusive thoughts
- General fearfulness
- Avoidance of stimuli that could trigger memories
- Excessive distress on the "anniversary" of specific events
- Difficulty talking about the events
- Attempts to suppress memories of the events
- Detachment or withdrawal from familiar people
- Emotional blunting or numbness
- Memory and concentration problems
- Sleeping problems
- Hypervigilance
- Easily startled or exaggerated startle response to stimuli that are related to the events (e.g., loud noises similar to those heard in an automobile accident)
- Pessimism about the future and that the memories will always be present
- Physiological symptoms (muscle tension, aches and pains, etc.)

Secondary or Related Features

- Generalized anxiety
- Depression or mood problems
- Perhaps guilt about having survived the traumatic event(s)
- Aggressiveness
- Irritability
- "Omen formation"—belief in ability to foresee future negative events
- Negative effects on developing close relationships
- General social wariness
- Social skills problems
- Erratic or poor school performance
- Anger toward or fear of perpetrators of traumatic events
- Dissociative reactions
- Lowered self-esteem
- Eating problems

Comorbidity

In the meta-analysis cited above, Fletcher (2003) reported that 13% of the sample met criteria for ADHD and also showed oppositional behavior, although it was not known whether they were a consequence of PTSD or were preexisting patterns. Fletcher notes that it is possible that challenging behaviors associated with these disorders may have placed the children at greater risk for abuse. There is no significant evidence to suggest that merely having ADHD increases the risk for the development of PTSD in children and adolescents. Children with PTSD are at greater risk for developing Panic Disorder, Agoraphobia, Obsessive–Compulsive Disorder, Social Phobia, Specific Phobia, Major Depressive Disorder, Somatization Disorder, and Substance-Related Disorders.

Differential Diagnosis Considerations

In cases of acute onset PTSD, the child will show a rather sudden onset of symptoms, which will help to differentiate it from GAD that tends to have a gradual onset. Although there is the possibility that ADHD is associated with PTSD as noted by Fletcher (2003), sudden onset of symptoms is not associated with ADHD, especially in older children. The child may also show phobic behaviors that are fear reactions associated with reliving the events or the presence of intrusive memories, which are not characteristic of the associated disorders listed in the DSM-IV, including ADHD. It is likely that generalized anxiety will accompany the PTSD along with some mood or depressive symptoms, although they may not meet diagnostic criteria for a mental disorder. When stressed, children may show signs of panic attacks, but most often will be able to discuss the memories that are triggering the behaviors. They may seek to avoid being in new places, which may suggest agoraphobia. Agoraphobia is more associated with being afraid of being in open spaces, while the child with PTSD avoids situations to reduce the possibility of encountering stimuli that might precipitate symptoms. Over time, the child may develop feelings of uncontrollability, helplessness, and hopelessness, which increases the risk for mood disorders. It is likely that anxiety and mood disorders will accompany PTSD and may require simultaneous treatment, as well as monitoring the possibility of suicidal ideation.

Chronic onset PTSD may present more challenges with differential diagnosis, due to its gradual progression as opposed to onset due to a traumatic event. Rather, PTSD becomes part of the child's overall behavior pattern and is more likely to be associated with global impairment, internalizing and externalizing symptoms, and school and occupational problems. Children with chronic onset PTSD are more likely to have comorbid disorders as noted in the DSM-IV than are those experiencing sudden onset. Without accurate diagnosis and treatment, however, sudden onset PTSD may lead to more significant and pervasive impairment, including the development of comorbid disorders. Children with undetected abuse may demonstrate a range of internalizing and externalizing symptoms that suggest PTSD, but extreme caution should be exercised when inferring that abuse is occurring without definitive confirming evidence.

Typical Assessment Profiles

Children with sudden onset PTSD may show extreme and atypical changes in behavior such as withdrawal, irritability, loss of interest in preferred activities, and lowered school performance. They often show highly elevated scores on self-report and multidimensional measures of internalizing problems, especially generalized anxiety and depressive mood. As the stress subsides, these elevations tend to decline and may or may not return to normal levels. Children with chronic onset may show lower, but clinical elevations on these types of scales that are indicative of anxiety, depression, anger, irritability, and dissociation.

Panic Disorder

Panic disorder is characterized by unexpected panic attacks followed by a minimum of one month or longer of (a) persistent fear of having another attack, (b) worry about the implications of the panic attacks, or (c) a significant change in behavior as a function of the attacks (American Psychiatric Association, 2000). The attacks can vary in frequency, duration, intensity, symptoms shown, or their consequences. Over time, the worry about repeated attacks can be almost as debilitating as having the actual attacks and significant impacts on personal, social, and academic or occupational functioning can occur. Panic attacks have sudden onset and reach their peak intensity within 10 minutes. They may be linked to (a) specific situations that always or nearly always precipitate an attack, (b) predispositions for the attacks to occur, although they might not occur on a predictable basis, or (c) lack of identifiable cues that precipitate an attack. Although many anxiety disorders have features of panic attacks, the diagnosis of a panic disorder requires that the attacks not have an identifiable "trigger." The key difference between reactions in other anxiety disorders and panic disorders is that the person having a panic attack perceives dire or catastrophic consequences associated with bodily sensations, such as death from an imagined heart attack or inability to breathe. The autonomic reactions that occur with panic attacks result in awareness of intense bodily symptoms, convincing the person that death is imminent. Over time, the person can develop agoraphobia, which is a pattern of fear and avoidance of situations that are associated with the onset of panic attacks.

Although predicting the onset of panic attacks can be difficult, there is evidence that anxiety sensitivity (AS) is a predictor of occurrence. AS is the tendency to interpret physical symptoms as potentially threatening and the person is hypervigilant about bodily sensations, hence being "anxious about being anxious." With a heightened tendency toward AS, the person is more likely to have panic attacks (Hayward, Killen, Kraemer, & Taylor, 2000, Schmidt & Lerew, 2002; Schmidt, Lerew, & Jackson, 1997). Schmidt, Lerew, and Jackson (1997) found that AS predicted panic symptoms better than did trait anxiety in soldiers in high-stress basic training. AS is considered to be an interpretation bias that predisposes the person to be overly concerned with physical symptoms and creates a tendency to interpret symptoms as warning signs of imminent panic attacks. For example, a nonanxious or non-panic-prone person might have a sudden chest pain that is attributed to gastric distress, but the high AS person would be more likely to interpret it as a sign or "omen" that a heart attack is looming, leading to a panic attack. These research findings suggest that the clinician should consider assessing AS during clinical assessment for persons who have a history of panic attacks. If high levels of AS are present, they may be a focus of treatment to help prevent panic attacks. Assessment of AS in children is discussed in Chap. 8.

Prevalence Data and Epidemiology

There is much less research on the disorder in children and adolescents than in adults. Thus, much of the available information is based on reports and histories of adults with panic disorder. The disorder is two to three times more common in female adults and adolescents than in their male counterparts, and its course tends to be chronic and persistent, even with treatment. Panic disorders in childhood are rare, and onset most often occurs between late adolescence and the mid-30s, with a median onset age of about 24 (Burke, Burke, Reger, & Rae, 1990). Yonkers et al. (1998) reported that only 39% of persons with panic disorder showed remission within five years. Katschnig and Ameing (1994) found that only 31% of patients attained remission within 2–6 years, and Hirschfield (1996) reported that 18% of patients with panic disorder with agoraphobia and 43% without agoraphobia recovered after their first panic episode. These latter data indicate that the presence of agoraphobia predicts a more severe and intractable course that is resistant to change. The DSM-IV states that about one-third to one-half of community-based samples of people who meet criteria for panic disorder also meet criteria for agoraphobia.

In a review of the literature, Ollendick, Mattis, and King (1994) reported that panic attacks occur in 40–60% of adolescents; thus, experiences of panic are common in this age range. Panic attacks and panic disorder occur far less frequently in children and are difficult to assess. Panic disorder is less common than social phobia or specific phobia. In the National Comorbidity Survey, Kessler et al. (1994) reported a lifetime prevalence rate of 3.5% and a 1-year prevalence rate of 2.3% for panic disorder. Kessler et al. also reported higher lifetime prevalence for agoraphobia without a history of panic disorder (5.3%) than for panic disorder with or without agoraphobia (3.5%). Hayward et al. (1992) noted a developmental trend in the development of panic attacks in children with a mean age of 10.3–15.6 years. As the children became older, there was an increase in panic attacks in girls at a higher rate than boys, and age was not a factor in this trend. The reasons for this pattern were not clear but may be related to the often-documented observation of higher rates of anxious symptoms and anxiety disorders in adolescent girls.

Table 5.7 DSM-IV-TR Diagnostic Criteria for Panic Attack

Note: A Panic Attack is not a codable disorder. Code the specific diagnosis in which the Panic Attack occurs (e.g., ...Panic Disorder With Agoraphobia....)

A discrete period of intense fear or discomfort, in which four (or more) of the following symptoms developed abruptly and reached a peak within 10 min:

1. Palpitations, pounding heart, or accelerated heart rate
2. Sweating
3. Trembling or shaking
4. Sensations of shortness of breath or smothering
5. Feeling of choking
6. Chest pain or discomfort
7. Nausea or abdominal distress
8. Feeling dizzy, unsteady, lightheaded, or faint
9. Derealization (feelings of unreality) or depersonalization (being detached from oneself)
10. Fear of losing control or going crazy
11. Fear of dying
12. Chills or hot flashes

Note: From American Psychiatric Association, (2000, p. 432). Copyright 2000 by the American Psychiatric Association. Reprinted with permission

Primary Symptoms

- Physiological symptoms
- Depersonalization
- Feelings of unreality
- High level of state anxiety at the time of a panic attack
- High levels of tension and apprehension

Secondary or Related Symptoms

- Agoraphobia
- Avoidance
- Fear of vomiting
- Fear of impending death
- Fears of having a major psychological episode
- Refusal to eat
- Reluctance or refusal to attend school or participate in school activities
- Reluctance or refusal to participate in out-of-school group and social activities
- Reduced participation in school learning tasks and classroom activities
- Frequent worry about having another panic attack

Table 5.8 DSM-IV-TR Diagnostic Criteria for Panic Disorder Without and With Agoraphobia

Panic Disorder Without Agoraphobia

A. Both (1) and (2)
1. Recurrent unexpected Panic Attacks
2. At least one of the attacks has been followed by 1 month (or more) of the following:
   (a) Persistent concern about having additional attacks
   (b) Worry about the implications of the attack or its consequences (e.g., losing control, having a heart attack, "going crazy")
   (c) A significant change in behavior related to the attacks

B. Absence of agoraphobia…

C. The Panic Attacks are not due to the direct physiological effects of a substance (e.g., a drug of abuse, a medication) or a general medical condition (e.g., hyperthyroidism)

D. The Panic Attacks are not better accounted for by another mental disorder, such as Social Phobia (e.g., occurring on exposure to feared social situations), Specific Phobia (e.g., on exposure to a specific phobic situation), Obsessive–Compulsive Disorder (e.g., on exposure to direct in someone with an obsession about contamination), Posttraumatic Stress Disorder (e.g., in response to stimuli associated with a severe stressor), or Separation Anxiety Disorder (e.g., in response to being away from home or close relatives)

Panic Disorder With Agoraphobia

A. Both (1) and (2)
1. Recurrent unexpected Panic Attacks
2. At least one of the attacks has been followed by 1 month (or more) of one (or more) of the following:
   (a) Persistent concern about having additional attacks
   (b) Worry about the implications of the attack or its consequences (e.g., losing control, having a heart attack, "going crazy")

B. The presence of Agoraphobia…

C. The Panic Attacks are not due to the direct physiological effects of a substance (e.g., a drug of abuse, a medication) or a general medical condition (e.g., hyperthyroidism)

D. The Panic Attacks are not better accounted for by another mental disorder, such as Social Phobia (e.g., occurring on exposure to feared social situations), Specific Phobia (e.g., on exposure to a specific phobic situation), Obsessive–Compulsive Disorder (e.g., on exposure to direct in someone with an obsession about contamination), Posttraumatic Stress Disorder (e.g., in response to stimuli associated with a severe stressor), or Separation Anxiety Disorder (e.g., in response to being away from home or close relatives)

Note: From American Psychiatric Association, (2000, pp. 402–403). Copyright 2000 by the American Psychiatric Association. Reprinted with permission

Comorbidity

Agoraphobia is one of the most common comorbid disorders with panic disorder, and its presence indicates a more difficult trajectory and outcomes. Depression, substance abuse, personality disorders, and other anxiety disorders, especially GAD, are common comorbid problems (Birmaher & Ollendick, 2004; Brown, DiNardo, Lehman, & Campbell, 2001). Specific and social phobia may also occur, which tend to predate panic disorder with onset in adolescence. Whether early developing anxiety disorders serve as precursors to the development of panic disorders is unknown, although a history of high levels of general anxiety may predispose a child to panic attacks. Thus, children who have a history of high trait anxiety, GAD, or pervasive anxiety disorder appear more likely to be at greater risk for the development of panic attacks.

Differential Diagnosis Considerations

The primary symptoms of panic attacks and panic disorder are unique compared to other anxiety disorders. DSM-IV specifies some symptoms for panic attacks but notes that they are not to be coded as disorders. The list is to be reviewed, and if the person shows the appropriate number of symptoms, consideration of panic disorder criteria occurs. The clinician must also consider whether agoraphobia is present, although a history of panic symptoms does not make the development of agoraphobia inevitable and the severity of agoraphobic symptoms varies across individuals (Craske & Barlow, 1988). Although panic disorder has some similar symptoms of other anxiety disorders, the physiological symptoms play a larger role. In GAD, for example, the primary characteristic is generalized worry and the physiological symptoms co-occur. In panic disorder, the emergence of the physiological symptoms that cause fears of impending death, depersonalization, or "going crazy" causes significant anxiety and distress. Depressive symptoms and disorders may emerge as accompanying problems as the person becomes more debilitated with repeated panic attacks. Thus, although depressive disorders may be comorbid with panic disorder, they are not likely to be causal. The symptoms of SAD may also be similar to panic disorder, but the difference is about the focus of the child's fear. In SAD, the primary fear is separation from the primary caregiver. Conversely, the person with panic disorder is afraid of the physiological symptoms and sensations of having another attack. Another distinction between SAD and panic disorder is that SAD typically has a much earlier onset than panic disorder, although the child may have some physiological symptoms. If adolescents are referred for substance abuse, screening for panic symptoms or attacks is recommended due to the high frequency of panic attacks in this age group (Ollendick, Mattis, & King, 1994) and that the substance use may be an attempt to control panic symptoms or anxiety. Most often, panic symptoms or attacks will be documented by observations, history, or interviews.

Typical Assessment Profiles

Children and adolescents with panic disorder are likely to have high scores on measures of generalized anxiety, AS, somatic complaints, and heightened tension. They tend to have specific fears of experiencing sensations that may trigger a panic attack, which is related to AS. On multidimensional measures such as the *MMPI-A*

(Butcher, Williams et al., 1992), adolescents may show generalized distress, depressive symptoms, and signs of hypochondriacal tendencies. Self-report measures of anxiety typically will show elevations, and ratings by parents and teachers may report signs of anxiety, tension, stress, fearfulness, and somatic complaints. Because anxiety and depressive symptoms tend to co-occur, mood problems may be evident, but perhaps not to the level of a diagnosable comorbid disorder. In all cases, the possibility of co-occurring medical problems should be ruled out through history or referral to medical personnel if physical conditions are known or suspected to be related to panic symptoms. The older child or adolescent can also monitor his own physical sensations and maintain a personal log or checklist of panic symptoms, when and where they occur, identification of any precipitating conditions, and psychological and physical reactions. This self-monitoring of symptoms may also help the person to become more aware of precursors to panic attacks, such as physical sensations and circumstances that may cause heightened general anxiety.

A Developmental Psychopathology Perspective on Differential Diagnosis of Anxiety Disorders

Although the DSM-IV addresses developmental issues more effectively than previous versions, it does not provide a comprehensive approach about how developmental factors are implicated in conducting differential diagnosis of anxiety disorders. Taking a developmental psychopathology approach may help to improve the efficiency and accuracy of identifying and documenting anxiety disorders and comorbid conditions in children and youth. Following is a suggested procedure that incorporates principles of developmental psychopathology that will help in differential diagnosis of anxiety disorders.

Distinguish Between Normal and Pathological Anxiety

Because anxiety is a normal human emotion that is experienced frequently by all people, distinguishing it from pathological anxiety can be challenging. Albano, Causey, and Carter (2001) identify three factors that distinguish pathological anxiety from normal levels: (a) it is more intractable, (b) the fear and avoidance is significantly more pervasive, and (c) the degree of interference in the child's daily functioning is much greater. The *degree of intractability* may be manifested in several ways, including (a) resistance to typical methods and levels of intervention that work for most children, (b) resistance to systematic therapeutic efforts, (c) evidence of long-term patterns that worsen or remain at high levels, (d) changing of patterns, or (e) evidence of increasing comorbidity over time. The *pervasiveness of fear and avoidance* can be ascertained by accumulating evidence that anxiety occurs in multiple settings and circumstances through developmental history, observations, interviews, and objective self-report and behavior rating data. Finally, the *degree of interference* can be determined by compiling data about the quality of functioning in social relationships, family functioning, personal care and responsibility, and school performance in both academic and functional areas. Additional data can also be obtained from developmental history, observations, interviews, and objective self-report and behavior ratings. Thus, if the anxiety is determined to be intractable, pervasive, and interfering with daily functioning, it is likely pathological and a formal diagnosis and treatment may be warranted.

Age of Onset

As discussed above, the age of onset varies for each disorder, which can be of help in specifying which anxiety disorders are present. In many cases, children with anxiety disorders will have shown early symptoms of behavioral inhibition, social withdrawal, reticence, shyness, and sensitivity. When considering age of onset, consideration should also be given to the possibility that the anxiety symptoms are secondary to another disorder, for example, PDD, or may be mistaken for another disorder, such as ADHD. By simultaneous consideration of alternative or comorbid diagnoses and age of onset, increased diagnostic accuracy is possible.

Developmental Comparisons

Although age is the most common and reliable index of developmental status and behavioral expectations, it may not be the most accurate indicator in all cases. The clinician should have a thorough understanding of what behaviors and skills are expected at different ages using a broad range of normal as the comparative index. For a child who has coexisting developmental problems, such as language or learning disorders, anxiety is more likely to be present, and behavioral expectations will need to be modified. Many objective measures of behavior and personality may not take these variations into account; therefore, the clinician must use clinical impressions, history, and other information to improve precision in differential diagnosis.

Genetic and Family History Context

Although direct knowledge of genetic predispositions and variations is not likely to be readily known, it may be possible to infer their possible impact by conducting a thorough family history to determine if there is evidence of anxiety disorders or excessive symptoms in immediate family members. Although there is little evidence to suggest that children inherit specific anxiety disorders (Eley, 2001), a positive family history for anxiety disorders increases the likelihood for clinical or subclinical levels of anxiety that may develop into disorders in children and adolescents.

Biological Context

The clinician must make efforts to determine if there are medical or biological reasons for high levels of anxiety. For example, a child may have a chronic illness that causes stress and anxious symptoms, such as asthma or diabetes. The differential diagnosis process should focus on ruling out physical and medical factors (Anxiety Disorder due to General Medical Condition), a Substance-Induced Anxiety Disorder, or coexisting developmental disorders or problems that may be contributory. If these possibilities are not found to be associated with the symptoms, then using available data to determine which anxiety and/or comorbid disorders are present should proceed. Included in consideration of biological factors is temperament characterized by early signs of atypical shyness, behavioral inhibition, social avoidance, and fearfulness. An early positive history of anxious temperament increases the risk for development of a variety of anxiety disorders, especially GAD and social phobia.

Cultural Context

As discussed in Chap. 2, there is relatively little evidence about the similarities and differences among anxiety disorders across cultures. The DSM-IV does include discussion about consideration of cultural factors in conducting differential diagnosis. There is ample evidence to indicate that the internalizing and externalizing dimensions of psychopathology are similar across cultures (Ivanova, Achenbach, Dumenci et al., 2007; Ivanova, Achenbach, Rescorla et al., 2007). In Chap. 2, the cultural context of developmental psychopathology is discussed, including issues of the nature of internalizing patterns and disorders across cultures. That discussion will not be reviewed here, but, when working with suspected internalizing problems of children and youth from minority groups, close attention should be given to the possibility that some symptoms may be due to the effects of cultural practices and degree of acculturation.

Social Context

Although nearly all mental health professionals would agree that behavior is a product of person and environment interactions, the process of differential diagnosis is primarily focused on the symptoms presented by the child. As such, there may be a tendency to overlook or minimize the role of social factors in the development and maintenance of psychopathology. Because children with anxiety disorders typically are not disruptive, do not call attention to themselves, and tend to be socially compliant to minimize anxiety, they may be mistaken as being less capable, unmotivated, or not having difficulties. Consequently, identification and differential diagnosis of anxiety disorders may be undetected or treated as personality differences, rather than a manifestation of psychopathology. Therefore, the clinician should be particularly attentive to conducting a thorough assessment of social factors that may be contributing to the anxiety problems to reduce the possibility of making clinical errors and improve the accuracy of differential diagnosis. These social factors include peer relationships, parent–child interactions, and overall level of social skills.

Family Context

Family context is an important consideration in differential diagnosis of anxiety disorders. In comparison to family of children who have depressive disorders, families of anxious children typically are not highly dysfunctional. The major variable appears to be related to parenting practices, especially with mothers who tend to be intrusive, controlling, overly protective, and reinforcing of anxious behaviors, such as withdrawal, fearfulness, excessive caution, and perfectionism.

School Context

Because children with high levels of anxiety are more likely to try to avoid situations where they are expected to perform, they may underperform academically compared to their level of ability. Over time, their actual levels of achievement may decline, and they may be seen as less capable than their peers. Tasks involving sustained concentration, memory, persistence, and considering multiple elements of information simultaneously become increasingly prevalent and may be affected by high levels of anxiety. As children progress through school, they are expected to assume more responsibility for their learning, and tasks become more difficult, increasing the tendency for high levels of anxiety to occur and to interfere further with performance. Interventions for academic problems associated with anxiety typically involve using strategies such as relaxation training, task analysis, and breaking tasks into smaller components.

Conclusion

The differential diagnosis of anxiety disorders is often a complex task and involves simultaneous consideration of the six contexts discussed above, although information about genetic and biological contexts may be limited or unknown. Thus, consideration of the other four contexts is essential for accurate diagnosis and must include appropriate assessment procedures, which are discussed in Chaps. 7 and 8. Because comorbidity among anxiety disorders in clinical samples and with depression and mood disorders is common, comprehensive assessment is essential across all contexts for accurate differential diagnosis. From a comprehensive assessment that leads to accurate differential diagnosis that is also descriptive, recommendations for intervention can be developed and implemented.

Chapter 6
Differential Diagnosis of Depression and Mood Disorders

Historical Context of Childhood Depression and Mood Disorders

Unlike anxiety that has normal developmental markers and characteristics, depression and mood disorders do not have age-related and predictable courses. Virtually everyone has experiences of being sad or having brief periods of depression associated with a significant distressing event (e.g., loss of a loved one, situational stress), but they do not cause significant or chronic impairment and do not follow a typical developmental course. Although adolescents are often characterized as "moody" or irritable or experience "hassles," their behaviors typically do not meet diagnostic criteria for a depression or a mood disorder and they do not significantly interfere with overall functioning. Like anxiety, however, depression is an internalizing problem that can have negative effects on various spheres of psychological and social functioning. A focus on depression in children and youth is relatively recent, having received increased clinical and research emphasis in the last two to three decades.

Over many years, four perspectives have been presented on whether depression can exist in children and youth, ranging from that it does not occur to being essentially equivalent to adult depression. These perspectives have had significant effects on clinical work and research regarding the nature of childhood depression to the current emphasis on depression as a form of developmental psychopathology. These four perspectives provide an interesting historical context on the development and manifestations of depression in children and adolescents and are discussed by Kaslow and Rehm (1991).

Perspective I: Depression Cannot Exist in Childhood

This perspective is rooted in psychoanalytic theory which assumes that depression cannot exist in children because it is seen as aggression turned toward the self as a function of a harsh, guilt-arousing superego. The psychoanalytic perspective has

T.J. Huberty, *Anxiety and Depression in Children and Adolescents: Assessment, Intervention, and Prevention*, DOI 10.1007/978-1-4614-3110-7_6, © Springer Science+Business Media, LLC 2012 guilt as a central component to depression that is regulated by the superego. According to this perspective, because young children do not have fully developed superegos, they cannot experience guilt; thus, they cannot develop depression. Consequently, from a psychoanalytic view, depression could only emerge in adolescence when the superego is reasonably well-developed and an increased sense of self-awareness is present. This perspective was highly influential for many years in how depression was viewed and prevented it from being considered as a form of child psychopathology.

Perspective II: Depression in Childhood Is Masked

This perspective emphasizes the concept of "depressive equivalents" or that depression is "masked," existing as an internal state of pathology and external behaviors being equivalent to depression. Thus, behaviors such as aggression, hyperactivity, phobias, delinquent behavior, and other behavior problems were considered to be symptoms of depression. Kaslow and Rehm assert that this position cannot be supported, because if every behavior represents depression, it would not be possible to separate depression from other pathologies. Also, these behaviors may have cultural bases, be typical behaviors at certain developmental points, or be attempts to cope with stressful situations. Although this position has found little empirical support and is no longer a major influence on clinical work and research, it is related to the idea that depression can be comorbid with other disorders.

Perspective III: Depression in Childhood Is Transitory

Kaslow and Rehm summarize the work of Lefkowitz and Burton (1978), who proposed three assumptions about childhood depression: (a) if behaviors that are considered indicative of depression occur in all children, they are not pathological and the syndrome does not exist; (b) the commonly accepted symptoms of depression are transitory developmental phenomena and cannot be considered pathological; and (c) if the symptoms dissipate spontaneously, there is no need for intervention. With regard to the first assumption, Kaslow and Rehm point out that, although single symptoms may occur in a population, a depressive syndrome is defined by a constellation of behaviors. Just because a symptom occurs in a large number of people does not make it any less problematic. The second assumption is questionable because developmental stages by nature are transitory, but a child may be attempting to cope with a stressor during that stage. The fact that the behavior may dissipate or others may emerge does not lessen the impact of the behavior at the time. Just because behaviors occur at various developmental points does not mean they are "normal" or should be disregarded. Regarding the third assumption, although a behavior may remit or dissipate over time without intervention, it does not mean that a disorder is not present. Many pathological behaviors dissipate or evolve into other symptoms over time. To say that these changes are merely developmental and are not indicative of a disorder is not consistent with data indicating that depressive symptoms tend to persist over time, recur, and may be precursors to other disorders.

Perspective IV: Depression in Childhood Parallels Depression in Adulthood

This perspective proposes that childhood depression follows the same course and essentially has the same symptoms as depression in adults. The four primary symptom patterns proposed by Beck (1967) for depression in adults are seen in children: (a) affective problems, for example, dysphoria, mood changes, and apathy; (b) cognitive problems, for example, low self-esteem, guilt, and pessimism; (c) motivational problems, for example, avoidance, passiveness, and low levels of energy; and (d) vegetative and psychomotor problems, for example, sleep problems, appetite disturbance, and somatic complaints. Children may show these symptoms as well as other behaviors that are typically developmental (e.g., occasional oppositional behavior), as well as those that are indicative of other internalizing and externalizing problems. That childhood depression is similar to adult depression is the most widely held view and has been supported in clinical research. There may be some child-specific behaviors (e.g., irritability), but the overall constellation of behaviors that characterize a depressive syndrome is essentially the same in children and adults. This chapter adopts this perspective in discussion of the concepts and procedures of differential diagnosis.

DSM Historical Perspectives on Childhood Depression

DSM-I

In DSM-I (American Psychiatric Association, 1952), depression was listed as "Depressive Reaction" under the category of "Psychoneurotic Disorders," which were described as "Disorders of Psychogenic Origin or Without Clearly Defined Tangible Cause or Structural Change" (p. 6). Anxiety was described as being the central characteristic of these disorders, and depression was a "defense mechanism" to control or allay the anxiety. The onset of a "Depressive Reaction" was precipitated by a current event such as a loss and was accompanied by guilt. Thus, depression was not seen as a major diagnostic category but as a subset or reaction of anxiety or neurotic disorders. Manic–depressive reactions were seen as psychotic disorders and were "…characterized by a primary, severe, disorder of mood, with resultant disturbance of thought and behavior, in consonance with the affect" (p. 24). There was no separate category of depressive reactions for children and adolescents.

DSM-II

The DSM-II (American Psychiatric Association, 1968) used a similar nomenclature, renaming "Psychoneurotic Disorders" to "Neuroses" and applying a 300-code designation. "Depressive Neurosis" was used in lieu of "Depressive Reaction" and was described as "...an excessive reaction of depression due to an internal conflict or to an identifiable event such as the loss of a loved one or cherished possession" (p. 40). Depression was given increased recognition as a separate disorder/neurosis, but still focused on anxiety as a central characteristic. It was no longer described as a defense mechanism and was distinguished from "Involutional Melancholia" and "Manic–depression illness," which were major affective and psychotic disorders. "Reactive depressions" or "Depressive reactions" were included under this subcategory (300.4). No distinction was made between adult and child/youth depression.

DSM-III

The publication of the DSM-III (American Psychiatric Association, 1980) represented a fundamental and substantial evolution of formal psychiatric diagnosis with the introduction of the multiaxial system. The broad category of Affective Disorders included three subclassifications: (a) Major Affective Disorders, in which a full affective syndrome was present; (b) Other Specific Affective Disorders, which included a partial affective syndrome with a duration of at least 2 years; and (c) Atypical Affective Disorders, a category of Affective Disorders that could not be classified into one of the other two subcategories. Major Affective Disorders included Bipolar Disorder (formerly Manic–depression) and Major Depression, which were distinguished by whether a manic episode had occurred. Other Specific Affective Disorders included Cyclothymic Disorder (301.13) and Dysthymic Disorder (300.40), the latter being essentially equivalent to Depressive Neurosis in DSM-II. Major Depression was coded as Major Depression, Single Episode (296.2x), and Major Depression, Recurrent (296.3x), with diagnostic criteria of (A) one or more major depressive episodes and (B) a manic episode had never occurred. Bipolar Disorder had three forms: Bipolar Disorder, Mixed (296.6x); Bipolar Disorder, Manic (296.4x); and Bipolar Disorder, Depressed (296.5x). As with previous editions of the DSM, no distinctions were made between adult and child or youth depression.

DSM-III-R

The revised edition of the DSM-III (DSM-III-R; American Psychiatric Association, 1987) made some minor changes to DSM-III regarding depression and mood disorders. "Affective Disorders" became "Mood Disorders," and two major categories were included: Bipolar Disorders that included Bipolar Disorders (Bipolar Disorder,

Cyclothymia, and Bipolar Disorder NOS) and Depressive Disorders (Major Depression, Dysthymia, and Depressive Disorder NOS). The forms of Bipolar Disorder were retained: Bipolar Disorder, Mixed (296.6x); Bipolar Disorder, Manic (296.4x); and Bipolar Disorder, Depressed (296.5x). For Bipolar Disorder, Mixed, criteria included a full symptomatic picture of current or most recent Manic and Major Depressive Episodes and prominent depressive symptoms lasting at least a full day. For Bipolar Disorder, Manic, a current or recent Manic Episode was required. Similarly, for Bipolar Disorder, Depressed, a current or recent Major Depressive Episode was required. Cyclothymia was described as a chronic mood disturbance showing numerous hypomanic episodes and numerous periods of depressed mood or loss of interest or pleasure that were not of sufficient severity or duration to meet criteria for a Major Depressive or Major Manic Episode. The time period for symptoms was 2 years for adults and 1 year for children and adolescents. The criteria for Major Depression were essentially the same as in DSM-III with the addition that the person had never had an "unequivocal Hypomanic Episode." Dysthymia was retained in DSM-III-R, and the possibility of the coexistence of Dysthymia and Major Depression was introduced as "double depression." In all of the mood disorders in DSM-III-R, no specific distinctions were made between adult and child/adolescent occurrences.

DSM-IV/DSM-IV-TR

The fourth edition of the DSM (DSM-IV; American Psychological Association, 1994) and the text revision (DSM-IV-TR; American Psychiatric Association, 2000) maintained the broad category of "Mood Disorders" with those from DSM-III-R and added others that will be discussed below. Increased description of criteria for Mood Episodes was provided to help improve accuracy for making diagnoses. Also included were specifiers for coding the clinical status of the current or most recent episode, for current or recent episodes in partial or full remission, and for describing the course of recurrent episodes. These additions will not be discussed here, and the reader is referred to the DSM-IV-TR for a complete description and discussion. As with the DSM-III and DSM-III-R, no distinctions between adult and child/adolescent mood disorders were made, although some differences in specific behaviors and duration of symptoms were included. Consequently, there continues to be no distinction between adult and child/adolescent depression and mood disorders, which corresponds to the fourth perspective described by Kaslow and Rehm (1991) that adult depression parallels child and youth depression.

DSM-IV Criteria for Depression and Mood Disorders

In the DSM-IV-TR, there are ten Mood Disorders: Major Depressive Disorder (MDD), Dysthymic Disorder, Depressive Disorder Not Otherwise Specified, Bipolar I Disorder, Bipolar II Disorder, Cyclothymic Disorder, Bipolar Disorder

Not Otherwise Specified, Mood Disorder due to a General Medical Condition, Substance-Induced Mood Disorder, and Mood Disorder Not Otherwise Specified. This chapter will focus on Major Depressive Disorder, Dysthymic Disorder, and Bipolar Disorder I and II. Substance-Induced Mood Disorder is a new classification in the DSM and is related to mood disorders that are caused by use of various substances, which are more likely to occur in adolescents than in children. This disorder is the direct physiological result of exposure to a toxin, a drug of abuse, a medication, or another somatic treatment for depression. Due to the relative rarity of this disorder in children and adolescents, it will not be discussed here. However, in conducting clinical assessment for purposes of differential diagnosis, screening for the presence of substance abuse in older children and adolescents should be done, particularly if there is evidence of a mood disorder.

In Chap. 3, Table 3.2 summarizes the typical age of onset, primary symptoms, common comorbid conditions, and developmental trajectories associated with Major Depression, Dysthymia, and Bipolar Disorder. Using a similar format to the discussion of anxiety disorders in Chap. 5, attention is given to prevalence and epidemiology, specific DSM-IV criteria for each disorder, primary and secondary symptoms, comorbidity, differential diagnosis considerations, and typical assessment profiles. The chapter concludes with a discussion of how to use a developmental psychopathology approach to improve efficiency and accuracy when conducting differential diagnosis of depression and mood disorders.

Depressive and Mood Episodes

Unlike anxiety and with the exception of dysthymia, the diagnosis of depression and mood disorders is based in large part upon the presence and recurrence of depressive episodes. To diagnose depression and bipolar disorders accurately, the clinician must consider the essential features of depressed, manic, mixed, and hypomanic episodes. The features of each of these types of episodes should be considered to help improve the accuracy of differential diagnosis (Table 6.1).

These criteria for a depressive mood episode require that the person show either a depressed mood or loss of interest in almost all activities. Typically, these criteria are readily measured through interviews and most self-report measures of depression. Of the nine criteria, they can be grouped into four categories: (a) physical/physiological symptoms (weight loss, sleeping problems, psychomotor agitation or retardation, and fatigue), (b) anhedonia (loss of interest in activities), (c) depressed mood, negative self-evaluation (feelings of worthlessness, excessive or inappropriate guilt), and (d) cognitive symptoms (concentration/memory and suicidal ideation). The criteria require that no signs of mania or hypomania be evident as in a Mixed Episode, are not caused by a substance or medical condition, and significant impairment in typical functioning. In the case of children and adolescents, it is essential that careful and thorough assessment of school functioning be included, rather than relying solely or primarily on parent report or clinical assessment of the child.

Table 6.1 DSM-IV-TR Criteria for Major Depressive Episode

A. Five (or more) of the following symptoms have been present during the same 2-week period and represent a change from previous functioning; at least one of the symptoms is either (1) depressed mood or (2) loss of interest or pleasure

Note: Do not include symptoms that are clearly due to a general medical condition, or mood-congruent delusions or hallucinations

1. Depressed mood most of the day, nearly every day, as indicated by either subjective report (e.g., feels sad or empty) or observations made by others (e.g., appears tearful). *Note:* In children and adolescents, can be irritable mood
2. Markedly diminished interest or pleasure in all, or almost all, activities most of the day, nearly every day (as indicated by either subjective account or observation made by others)
3. Significant weight loss when not dieting or weight gain (e.g., a change of more than 5% of body weight in a month), or decrease or increase in appetite nearly every day. *Note:* In children, consider failure to make expected weight gains
4. Insomnia or hypersomnia nearly every day
5. Psychomotor agitation or retardation nearly every day (observable by others, not merely subjective feelings of restlessness or being slowed down)
6. Fatigue or loss of energy nearly every day
7. Feelings of worthlessness or excessive or inappropriate guilt (which may be delusional) nearly every day (not merely self-reproach or guild about being sick)
8. Diminished ability to think or concentrate, or indecisiveness, nearly every day (either by subjective account or observed by others)
9. Recurrent thoughts of death (not just fear of dying), recurrent suicidal ideation without a specific plan, or a suicide attempt or a specific plan for committing suicide

B. The symptoms do not meet criteria for a Mixed Episode
C. The symptoms cause clinically significant distress or impairment in social, occupational, or other important areas of functioning
D. The symptoms are not due to the direct physiological effects of a substance (e.g., a drug of abuse, a medication) or a general medical condition (e.g., hypothyroidism)
E. The symptoms are not better accounted for by Bereavement, i.e., after the loss of a loved one, the symptoms persist for longer than 2 months or are characterized by marked functional impairment, morbid preoccupation with worthlessness, suicidal ideation, psychotic symptoms, or psychomotor retardation

Source: American Psychiatric Association (2000, p. 356). Copyright 2000 by the American Psychiatric Association. Reprinted with permission

Manic Episode

Manic episodes are characterized by an unusually high level of activity and mood problems that cause impairment in major areas of functioning. Identifying manic episodes in young children can be challenging to differentiate from high levels of activity, distractibility, and impulsivity that may be associated with other problems, such as ADHD. These behaviors are most often associated with bipolar disorder, which remains controversial in children and youth (Table 6.2).

The seven criteria can be grouped into four categories: (a) self-evaluation, which, compared to Major Depressive Episode, is characterized by extreme, inappropriate positive self-evaluation (increased self-esteem and grandiosity); (b) physiological

Table 6.2 DSM-IV-TR Criteria for Manic Episode

A. A distinct period of abnormality and persistently elevated, expansive, or irritable mood, lasting at least 1 week (or any duration if hospitalization if necessary)

B. During the period of mood disturbance, three (or more) of the following symptoms have persisted (four if the mood is only irritable) and have been present to a significant degree:
  1. Inflated self-esteem or grandiosity
  2. Decreased need for sleep (e.g., feels rested after only 3 h of sleep)
  3. More talkative than usual or pressure to keep talking
  4. Flight of ideas or subjective experience that thoughts are racing
  5. Distractibility (i.e., attention too easily drawn to unimportant or irrelevant external stimuli)
  6. Increase in goal-directed activity (either socially, at work or school, or sexually) or psychomotor agitation
  7. Excessive involvement in pleasurable activities that have a high potential for painful consequences (e.g., engaged in unrestrained buying sprees, sexual indiscretions, or foolish business investments)

C. The symptoms do not meet criteria for a Mixed Episode

D. The mood disturbance is sufficiently severe to cause marked impairment in occupational functioning or in usual social activities or relationships with others, or to necessitate hospitalization to prevent harm to self or others, or there are psychotic features

E. The symptoms are not due to the direct physiological effects of a substance (e.g., a drug of abuse, a medication, or other treatment) or a general medical condition (e.g., hyperthyroidism)

Note: Manic-like episodes that are clearly caused by somatic antidepressant treatment (e.g., medication, electroconvulsive therapy, and light therapy) should not count toward a diagnosis of Bipolar I Disorder

Source: American Psychiatric Association (2000, p. 363). Copyright 2000 by the American Psychiatric Association. Reprinted with permission

(decreased need for sleep); (c) behavioral (increased talkativeness, increase in goal-directed activity, and increased social activity or behavior); and (d) cognitive (flight of ideas, distractibility, and inattentiveness). These symptoms are distinguished from Major Depressive Episode, where some symptoms are included in a Mixed Episode, which is an exclusion criterion for Manic Episode. As with other symptoms, manic behaviors cannot be due to use of a substance or a general medical condition and must cause significant impairment in various areas of functioning. In a Manic Episode, there may be psychotic features. The clinician must also consider if any manic symptoms are due to the effects of a somatic antidepressant treatment. If such effects do exist, they cannot be used to meet criteria for Bipolar I Disorder (Table 6.3).

The criteria for a Mixed Episode are straightforward because they combine symptoms from Major Depressive Episode and Manic Episode. Impairment in major areas of functioning is required, and the symptoms cannot be due to use of a substance or a general medical condition. The four categories under Major Depressive Episode and Manic Episode should be considered and described as to their prevalence and contribution to the degree of impairment.

Table 6.3 DSM-IV-TR Criteria for Mixed Episode

A. The criteria are met both for a Manic Episode and for a Major Depressive Episode (except for duration) nearly every day during at least a 1-week period

B. The mood disturbance is sufficiently severe to cause marked impairment in occupational functioning or in usual social activities or relationships with others, or to necessitate hospitalization to prevent harm to self or others, or there are psychotic features

C. The symptoms are not due to the direct physiological effects of a substance (e.g., a drug of abuse, a medication, or other treatment) or a general medical condition (e.g., hyperthyroidism)

Note: Mixed-like episodes that are clearly caused by somatic antidepressant treatment (e.g., medication, electroconvulsive therapy, and light therapy) should not count toward a diagnosis of Bipolar I Disorder

Source: American Psychiatric Association (2000, p. 365). Copyright 2000 by the American Psychiatric Association. Reprinted with permission

Hypomanic Episode

The primary differences between a Manic Episode and Hypomanic Episode are the degree of severity and the extent of impairment. In a Hypomanic Episode, the person must have shown a pattern of nondepressed mood that can be distinguished from an elevated, expansive, or irritable mood. This criterion is different from a Manic Episode that does not require the presence of a nondepressed mood. Both a Manic Episode and a Hypomanic Episode apply the same seven criteria, and three or more must be met or four must be met if the mood is only irritable. In a Hypomanic Episode, the mood disturbance and altered functioning are observable by others, a criterion not required for Manic Episode. A major distinguishing characteristic from Manic Episode is that a Hypomanic Episode does not cause significant impairment in major areas of functioning, hospitalization is not necessary, and there is an absence of psychotic features. Similar to criteria for Manic Episode, the effects of a somatic antidepressant treatment must be considered. If there are such effects, the symptoms cannot be applied to meet criteria for Bipolar II Disorder (Table 6.4).

Major Depressive Disorder

Major Depressive Disorder is the most common mood disorder that children and adolescents experience and that tends to have a progressive course into adulthood. It is the most researched mood disorder, and considerable progress has been made by researchers who have provided data to document the course and trajectory of MDD in children and adolescents. For the most part the symptoms in adolescents and adults are the same, although younger children may not show some of the classic signs of sad mood, anhedonia, and negative self-evaluation. The diagnosis of MDD requires consideration of criteria for Major Depressive Episode and whether there are

Table 6.4 DSM-IV-TR Criteria for Hypomanic Episode

A. A persistently elevated, expansive, or irritable mood, lasting throughout at least 4 days, that is clearly different from the usual nondepressed mood

B. During the period of mood disturbance, three (or more) of the following symptoms have persisted (four if the mood is only irritable) and have been present to a significant degree:
   1. Inflated self-esteem or grandiosity
   2. Decreased need for sleep (e.g., feels rested after only 3 h of sleep)
   3. More talkative than usual or pressure to keep talking
   4. Flight of ideas or subjective experience that thoughts are racing
   5. Distractibility (i.e., attention to easily drawn to unimportant or irrelevant external stimuli)
   6. Increase in goal-directed activity (either socially, at work or school, or sexually) or psychomotor retardation
   7. Excessive involvement in pleasurable activities that have a high potential for painful consequences (e.g., the person engages in unrestrained buying sprees, sexual indiscretions, or foolish business investments)

C. The episode is associated with an unequivocal change in functioning that is uncharacteristic of the person when not symptomatic

D. The disturbance in mood and the change in functioning are observable by others

E. The episode is not severe enough to cause marked impairment in social or occupational functioning, or to necessitate hospitalization, and there are not psychotic features

F. The symptoms are not due to the direct physiological effects of a substance (e.g., a drug of abuse, a medication, or other treatment) or a general medical condition (e.g., hyperthyroidism)

Note: Hypomanic-like episodes that are that are clearly caused by somatic antidepressant treatment (e.g., medication, electroconvulsive therapy, and light therapy) should not count toward a diagnosis of Bipolar II Disorder

Source: American Psychiatric Association (2000, p. 368). Copyright 2000 by the American Psychiatric Association. Reprinted with permission

symptoms of mania and hypomania. The DSM-IV-TR diagnostic criteria are, for the most part, applicable to children, adolescents, and adults (Tables 6.5 and 6.6).

Primary Symptoms

- Anhedonia
- Depressed mood
- Feelings of helplessness
- Feelings of hopelessness
- Psychomotor retardation and vegetative behavior
- Hyposomnia or hypersomnia
- Somatic complaints
- Memory and concentration problems
- Low self-esteem
- Negative affect
- Absence of positive affect

Table 6.5 DSM-IV-TR Criteria for Major Depressive Disorder, Single Episode

A. Presence of a single Major Depressive Episode

B. The Major Depressive Episode is not better accounted for by Schizoaffective Disorder and is not superimposed on Schizophrenia, Schizophreniform Disorder, Delusional Disorder, or Psychotic Disorder Not Otherwise Specified

C. There has never been a Manic Episode, a Mixed Episode, or a Hypomanic Episode

Note: This exclusion does not apply if all the manic-like, mixed-like, or hypomanic-like episodes are substance or treatment induced or are due to the direct physiological effects of a general medical condition

If the full criteria are currently met for a Major Depressive Disorder, *specify* its current status and/or features:

Mild, moderate, and severe without psychotic/severe with psychotic features

Chronic

With catatonic features

With melancholic features

With atypical features

With postpartum onset

If the full criteria are not currently met for a Major Depressive Episode, *specify* the current clinical status of the Major Depressive Disorder or features of the most recent episode:

In partial remission, in full remission

Chronic

With catatonic features

With melancholic features

With atypical features

With postpartum onset

Source: American Psychiatric Association (2000, p. 375). Copyright 2000 by the American Psychiatric Association. Reprinted with permission

- Irritability
- Suicidal ideation
- Flat affect
- Negative attributional style
- Pessimism
- Negative view of the future and the world
- Internal locus of control
- Appetite problems

Secondary or Related Symptoms

- Somatic complaints
- Social withdrawal and passivity
- Difficulties with interpersonal relationships
- Lowered academic achievement
- Low level of initiation

Table 6.6 DSM-IV-TR Criteria for Major Depressive Disorder, Recurrent

---
A. Presence of two or more Major Depressive Episodes

Note: To be considered separate episodes, there must be an interval of at least 2 consecutive months in which criteria are not met for a Major Depressive Disorder

B. The Major Depressive Episodes are not better accounted for by Schizoaffective Disorder and are not superimposed on Schizophrenia, Schizophreniform Disorder, Delusional Disorder, or Psychotic Disorder Not Otherwise Specified

C. There has never been a Manic Episode, a Mixed Episode, or a Hypomanic Episode

Note: This exclusion does not apply if all the manic-like, mixed-like, or hypomanic-like episodes are substance or treatment induced or are due to the direct physiological effects of a general medical condition

If the full criteria are currently met for a Major Depressive Disorder, specify its clinical status and/or features:

Mild, moderate, and severe without psychotic/severe with psychotic features

Chronic

With catatonic features

With melancholic features

With atypical features

With postpartum onset

If the full criteria are not met for a Major Depressive Episode, specify the current clinical of the Major Depressive Disorder or features of the most recent episode:

Mild, moderate, and severe without psychotic/severe with psychotic features

Chronic

With catatonic features

With melancholic features

With atypical features

With postpartum onset

Specify:

Longitudinal course specifiers (with and without interepisode recovery)

With seasonal pattern

Source: American Psychiatric Association (2000, p. 376). Copyright 2000 by the American Psychiatric Association. Reprinted with permission

- Low participation in school-related tasks
- Limited social and recreational interests
- Body image problems, primarily in adolescent girls
- Noncompliance
- Often accompanied by anxious symptoms

Prevalence Data and Epidemiology

Studies of prevalence data for childhood and youth depression have tended to use different approaches, leading to different estimates of the prevalence of depression. Moreover, it is more difficult to obtain some of the more subjective data such as emotional and mood states from younger children. The large study of children aged 9–13 in the United States in the Great Smoky Mountain Study revealed a three-month prevalence rate of 0.03% for major depressive episode plus 1.45% for depression not otherwise specified (Costello et al., 1996). Depression in preschool children is relatively rare, occurring in less than 1% of children (Kashani & Carlson, 1987), although the samples in this age group typically are small. The National Comorbidity Survey consisted of a nationally representative sample that included adolescents aged 15 and older and yielded lifetime prevalence rates of 14% with another 11% reporting minor depression (Kessler & Walters, 1998). Other studies have reported the prevalence estimates of depression in adolescents to range from 4% (Whitaker et al., 1990) to 24% (Lewinshohn, Hops, Roberts, Seely, & Andrews, 1993).

Of concern is that some studies have found that, although children and youth may not meet criteria for a depressive disorder, they may have subsyndromal or subclinical levels of distress. In a sample of 11–16-year-olds, Cooper and Goodyear (1993) found that 20.7% showed significant symptomatology, but did not meet diagnostic criteria for a depressive disorder. When self-report data are considered that do not rely on diagnosis, 10–30% of adolescents may exceed clinical cutoffs for depression (e.g., Garrison, Jackson, Marsteller, McKeown, & Addy, 1990). Of particular concern is that the prevalence of depression in children and youth has shown an increase over the past several years as found in the second National Comorbidity Survey (Kessler, Anenevoli, & Merikangas, 2001). Although the reasons for this increase are not clear, societal changes, family dysfunction, socioeconomic factors, and increased social stress are possible contributors. The prevalence of subsyndromal patterns increases the risk of the development of diagnosable depressive disorders, but also provides the opportunity for early intervention if detected. Taken together, these data suggest that the prevalence of depression or depressive symptoms that reflect significant impairment can range from about 4% to 30%. If 20% is considered as a "middle ground" approximation, the data would indicate that, in a classroom of 30 adolescent students, approximately six would have serious depressive symptoms or disorders and about four of them would be girls, reflecting a 2:1 prevalence rate of girls to boys.

The preponderance of the research evidence indicates that the typical age of onset of major depression is between mid to late adolescence and early adulthood (e.g., Kessler, McGonagle, Swartz, Blazer, & Nelson, 1993). In a nationally representative sample of over 9,000 participants, 25% of adults with depression or dysthymia reported onset to have occurred before becoming young adults and 50% reported onset by age 30 (Kessler, Berglund, Demler, Jin, & Walters, 2005). The developmental course of depression tends to be bimodal, with a rapid increase at age 11 and again after age 15, reaching a plateau from ages 21 to 26 (McGee, Feehan, Williams, & Anderson, 1992; Kim-Cohen et al., 2003; Newman, Moffit, Caspi, & Magdol, 1996).

Numerous studies have shown consistent findings that the prevalence of depression in female adults and adolescents is about twice that of occurrence in males (e.g., Costello, Stouthamer-Loever, & DeRosier, 1993; Kessler et al., 1993). Prior to adolescence, the prevalence rates have been shown to be about equal between boys and girls in diagnosed depression (e.g., Fleming, Offord, & Boyle, 1989; Kashani et al., 1983) or to be slightly higher in boys (e.g., Angold, Costello, & Worthman,

1998; Costello et al., 1988). The preponderance of occurrence of depression in female vs. male adolescents begins at about age 13 (McGee, Feehan, Williams, & Anderson, 1992) and is due in large part to modal increases for girls after age 11 and from the period of age 15–18 (Hankin et al., 1998).

The reasons for the greater prevalence of depression in adolescent and adult females are not clear but may be due in part to social, cultural, and biological factors. Rudolph (2002) and Rudolph and Hammen (1999) suggest that females may have greater social affiliation needs, which gives them more exposure to stressful life events. Compared to males who use active and instrumental coping styles, females tend to cope with stress and depressed mood with a more internalized, ruminative, and passive style (Nolen-Hoeksema, 2000). Angold, Costello, Erkanli, and Worthman (1999b) found a relationship between depressive symptoms and levels of estradiol and testosterone in female adolescents. Thus, the reasons for the higher prevalence of depression in females appear to be due to a complex interaction of biological, social, and cultural factors.

Comorbidity

Depression has high comorbidity with several conditions and disorders in children and youth. Cases of "pure" depression are likely infrequent because they are often accompanied by anxiety, stress, and conduct problems. Depression and anxiety are the most common comorbid conditions, with an approximate median rate of 39% of children with an anxiety disorder also having a depressive disorder and 17% with a depressive disorder also having an anxiety disorder (Angold, Costello, & Erkanli, 1999a). Depression is comorbid with most anxiety disorders, especially GAD, but not with OCD (Costello, Egger, & Angold, 2004). Median comorbidity rates of 27.3% between anxiety and depression and 12.2% between depression and conduct disorders have been reported (Angold et al.). Comorbidity between anxiety and depression is about the same for boys and girls, but the link between depression and substance abuse is higher for boys (Costello, Mustillo, Erkanli, Keeler, & Angold, 2003).

In a review of available studies, Kovacs (1990) found that 30–75% of depressed children also had concurrent anxiety disorders, including separation anxiety disorder, overanxious disorder according to DSM-III-R (now GAD), severe phobias, or obsessive–compulsive disorder. She also suggested that the comorbidity may be a single disorder, which is consistent with Achenbach's (1991) work that did not find a "pure" depressive syndrome and instead found the anxious–depressed syndrome. The mixed syndrome appears to be more common in younger children and separate disorders may be more identifiable in adolescents and adults. In general, anxiety disorders develop before depressive disorders (e.g., Avenevoli, Stolar, Li, Dierker, & Merikangas, 2001; Kovacs, Gastonis, Paulauskas, & Richards, 1989). Depressed girls are more likely to have a comorbid anxiety disorder, while boys are more likely to have conduct and attention deficit problems. Depression usually follows the onset of a conduct disorder, although the reasons are not clear. It may be that they share common genetic predispositions or that depression is the result of the social problems and alienation that result from conduct problems or a combination of multiple factors, including family variables. Thus, comorbidity of depression and other disorders is common and has important implications for assessment and differential diagnosis.

Differential Diagnosis Considerations

Young children with depression are more likely to show general distress and irritability and fewer of the classic signs of depression. Conversely, adolescents are more likely to show depressive behaviors similar to adults. The high comorbidity with anxiety presents particular difficulties in conducting differential diagnosis, due to the frequent overlap of symptoms. A first step in differentiating these patterns is to conduct a thorough developmental history, which may include retrospective reports by parents. Because anxiety most often precedes depression, a developmental history that focuses on anxiety symptoms may provide indicators of early-onset patterns. If anxious symptoms have been present for several months or years prior to the onset of depressive symptoms, differential diagnosis may be particularly difficult and there may be little practical and clinical value in attempting to differentiate them. In these cases, an anxious–depressed syndrome may be the best conclusion, although there may be value in formulating both an anxiety and depressive/mood disorder. The implications for treating the anxious–depressed syndrome are discussed in Chap. 10. Other indicators of anxiety vs. depression are often found by focusing on the presence or absence of positive and negative affect. Children with depression are likely to have high negative affect and the relative absence of positive affect, while the anxious child will have less negative affect and show higher degrees of physiological hyperarousal. Due to the high comorbidity, however, these patterns may not always be clear.

DSM-IV addresses the comorbidity of depression and ADHD, indicating that irritability is seen in both disorders. In ADHD, however, the irritability is not due to sad mood, as is the case with depression. Another strategy is to determine the age of onset of the irritability and mood problems. ADHD typically has onset in the preschool and early school years, while onset of depression typically occurs in mid-adolescence and early adulthood. If the irritability and mood problems can be traced to early onset, there is a greater likelihood that the problem is ADHD rather than depression. It is possible that depression can co-occur with ADHD, but is more likely to be related to consequences of the social difficulties associated with ADHD. Children who have both depression and conduct disorder are less likely to have high levels of generalized anxiety and meet criteria for an anxiety disorder.

Although not common in young children, adolescents who abuse substances, including tobacco and alcohol, are more likely to have depressive symptoms. An adolescent may use substances to "self-medicate" in an attempt to alleviate anxiety or depressed mood. Substance use may also be influenced by peer pressure and the depressed adolescent may engage in these behaviors as a way to be socially accepted. If the use of substances does result in symptom alleviation or social acceptance, the youth is likely to continue the behavior.

Typical Assessment Profiles

Children and youth with Major Depression typically show elevations on self-report depression measures and depression subscales of multidimensional measures. Ratings by parents and teachers tend to be similar to a child's self-report if the depression is moderate to severe, but they may be more discrepant in mild cases. Depressive mood tends to fluctuate, however, and self-reports and ratings show discrepancies over time. The test–rest reliability of self-report measures of depression in children and adolescents tends to decline over extended periods of time, reflecting changes in symptomatology. The degree of profile elevation depends on the severity of symptoms at the time of assessment. Also, if the symptoms are long-standing, they may be reported as less severe than in cases of sudden onset, such as when a trauma occurs and depressive symptoms emerge. In the latter case, high levels of anxiety and agitation are also likely to be present.

Because depression and anxiety are often comorbid, it is common to see elevations on both types of scales, although the elevations are higher on depressive symptomatology. Another reason for elevations on both types of scales is that many of them contain very similar items. If depressive symptoms are significantly higher (e.g., one half to a full standard deviation), depressed mood is likely to be the primary problem. If both depression and anxiety are elevated to about the same level, differential diagnosis is more challenging and suggests either the presence of the anxious–depressed syndrome or relatively distinct anxiety and depressive disorders that may warrant comorbid diagnoses. If the depression is chronic, there may be indications of impaired social skills and low self-esteem. Children and youth with depression also tend to show low motivation, inattentiveness, and passive noncompliance on ratings by parents and teachers.

Dysthymia

Compared to studies on major depression, there are relatively few studies that emphasize dysthymia specifically in children and adolescents. Most often, studies on dysthymia are included in epidemiological surveys on depression and mood disorders. Thus, extensive specific information on dysthymia is lacking in the research literature. Although there are some differences between dysthymia and depression to be discussed below, dysthymia is generally considered to be a milder and more chronic

Table 6.7 DSM-IV-TR Criteria for Dysthymic Disorder

A. Depressed mood for most of the day, for more days than not, as indicated by either subjective account or observation by others, for at least 2 years. *Note*: In children and adolescents, mood can be irritable and duration must be at least 1 year

B. Presence, while depressed, of two (or more) of the following:
   1. Poor appetite or overeating
   2. Insomnia or hypersomnia
   3. Low energy or fatigue
   4. Low self-esteem
   5. Poor concentration of difficulty making decisions
   6. Feelings of hopelessness

C. During the 2-year period (1 year for children and adolescents) of the disturbance, the person has never been without the symptoms in Criteria A and B for more than 2 months at a time

D. No Major Depressive Disorder … has been present during the first 2 years of the disturbance (1 year for children and adolescents), i.e., the disturbance is not better accounted for by chronic Major Depressive Disorder, or Major Depressive Disorder, in Partial Remission

Note: There may have been a previous Major Depressive Episode provided there was a full remission (no significant signs or symptoms for 2 months) before development of the Dysthymic Disorder. In addition, after the initial 2 years (1 year in children and adolescents) of Dysthymic Disorder, there may be superimposed episodes of Major Depressive Disorder, in which case both diagnoses may be given when the criteria are met for a Major Depressive Episode

E. There has never been a Manic Episode, a Mixed Episode, or a Hypomanic Episode, and criteria have never been met for Cyclothymic Disorder

F. The disturbance does not occur exclusively during the course of a chronic Psychotic Disorder, such as Schizophrenia or Delusional Disorder

G. The symptoms are not due to the direct physiological effects of a substance (e.g., a drug of abuse, a medication) or a general medicinal condition (hypothyroidism)

H. The symptoms cause clinically significant distress or impairment in social, occupational, or other important areas of functioning

Specify if:
   Early onset: if onset is before age 21 years
   Late onset: if onset is 21 years or older
Specify (for most recent 2 years of Dysthymic Disorder):
   With atypical features…

Source: American Psychiatric Association (2000, pp. 380–381). Copyright 2000 by the American Psychiatric Association. Reprinted with permission

form of depression. There are some questions, however, regarding whether dysthymia is a unique disorder because it is often difficult to differentiate from depression. In the Methods for the Epidemiology of Child and Adolescent Mental Disorders (MECA) study, for example, few differences were found between child dysthymia and MDD, other than earlier onset for the children diagnosed with dysthymic disorder (Goodman, Schwab-Stone, Lahey, Shaffer, & Jensen, 2000). This lack of meaningful clinical differentiation raises the question of whether dysthymia is a valid diagnosis or is merely a less severe form of depressive disorder (Goodman et al.).

Primary Symptoms

- Generally depressed mood, sometimes at a borderline clinical level
- Flat and relatively invariable affect
- Lack of energy and initiative
- Chronic pessimism and feelings of discouragement
- Sleeping problems (insomnia or hypersomnia)
- Concentration problems
- Indecisiveness

Secondary or Related Symptoms

- Lack of serious suicidal ideation or attempts
- Elevated levels of general anxiety
- Difficulties with occupational or academic responsibilities, but able to function
- Impaired social relationships
- Lack of enjoyment of some activities, but not to the level of anhedonia
- Lack of effort on school-related tasks
- Underachievement

Prevalence Data and Epidemiology

Lifetime prevalence rates of dysthymia with or without MDD are about 6%, and the point prevalence is about 3% (DSM-IV-TR). The onset of dysthymia tends to be early before the age of 21 and can occur in young children. Many children develop "double depression," with an onset of MDD about 2–3 years after the onset of dysthymia (Kovacs et al., 1984). Kovacs et al. indicated that early-onset dysthymia is a risk factor for recurrent or chronic mood disorder and the development of mania. The MECA study (Goodman, Schwab-Stone, Lahey, Shaffer, & Jensen, 2000) indicated that the co-occurrence of dysthymia and MDD is associated with greater impairment than is each disorder by itself. When both disorders are present, referrals to mental health professionals are most often initiated due to the effects of the depressive disorder (DSM-IV-TR). The course of dysthymia tends to be rather chronic and of longer duration than are depressive episodes. Based on a literature review, Birmaher et al. (1996) reported that the mean length of dysthymic episodes is about four years and that about 70% of affected children eventually develop major depression. These data indicate that early detection and intervention for dysthymic disorder may prevent, delay, or mitigate the onset of major depression in children and adolescents.

Comorbidity

The link between dysthymia and depression is well established based on the MECA study and other research. The development of "double depression" with Major Depressive Disorder places children and adolescents at greater risk of developing significant levels of social, personal, occupational, and academic impairment. Although children and adolescents are rarely diagnosed with personality disorders, the DSM-IV-TR suggests that dysthymia may be associated with Borderline, Histrionic, Narcissistic, Avoidant, and Dependent Personality Disorders. Early signs of these patterns may be indicated in adolescence and warrant further assessment and treatment. In children, the DSM-IV-TR suggests that dysthymia may be associated with both Axis I and Axis II disorders, such as ADHD, conduct disorder, anxiety disorders, learning disorders, and mental retardation. Dysthymia most likely develops after the onset of these disorders, particularly those with developmental implications, such as ADHD, learning disorders, and mental retardation. Due to its early onset and chronicity, dysthymia has been called "depressive personality disorder," which predicts a long-term and relatively constant trajectory. Given that the mean length of dysthymic episodes is about 4 years (Birmhaer et al., 1996), the designation of a personality disorder in children should be made with caution (in general, personality disorder diagnoses should not be given to children under the age of 18). When dysthymia occurs simultaneously as a result of a chronic medical condition, eating disorder, substance use, or other problem, the term "secondary dysthymia" is applied.

Finally, dysthymia is associated with short-term and long-term effects of maltreatment. Depressive symptomatology has been found in maltreated vs. nonmaltreated children (e.g., Kim & Cichetti, 2004; Toth & Cichetti, 1996; Toth, Manly, & Cichetti, 1992). Many children who have been maltreated meet diagnostic criteria for dysthymia (Kaufman, 1991). Various explanations have been posited for this relationship, including cognitive style (Gibb, Wheeler, Alloy, & Abramson, 2001), relationship to maternal figures, social support, attributional styles, social competence, and self-esteem (Kaufman; Kim & Cichetti; Toth & Cichetti; Toth, Maughan, Manly, Spagnola, & Cichetti, 2002). In adulthood, men and women who have been physically abused and neglected as children may demonstrate higher prevalence of dysthymia and antisocial personality disorder (Horowitz, Widom, McLaughlin, & White, 2001).

Differential Diagnosis Considerations

The primary differential diagnosis task is to distinguish dysthymia from major depression and anxiety disorders. Although the core difference between dysthymia and major depression is severity of symptoms, there are also some qualitative

Table 6.8 Comparison of Dysthymic Disorder and Major Depressive Disorder

Dysthymic Disorder	Major Depressive Disorder
Depressed mood	Depressed mood
Mild symptoms	Moderate to severe symptoms
Mild to no anhedonia	Moderate to severe anhedonia
Flat affect less observable	Flat affect more severe and observable
Psychosis not present	Psychosis may be present
Symptoms fluctuate	Symptoms present almost every day
Symptoms present daily for 2 weeks	Symptoms present and absent over 1 year
Minimal impairment of functioning	Moderate to severe impairment of functioning
Suicidal ideation less common	Suicidal ideation more common
Suicide attempts rare	Suicide attempts more likely
Mean duration about 4 years	Mean duration of episodes about 7–9 months

differences between them. Table 6.8 summarizes the major differences based on DSM-IV-TR criteria and available research. The similarities and differences are particularly relevant in cases where "double depression" may exist and the clinician is attempting to determine if both dysthymia and major depression are present.

Children and youth with dysthymia are also likely to have some symptoms of anxiety, but they may not meet criteria for an anxiety disorder. If an anxiety disorder is present, it is most likely a mild form of generalized anxiety disorder or social phobia/social anxiety disorder. Whether an anxiety disorder is present depends primarily on whether anxiety symptoms are distinguishable from the dysthymic symptoms and if they contribute to additional impairment or dysfunction.

Typical Assessment Profiles

Children and adolescents with dysthymic disorder typically show slightly elevated or minimally clinically significant scores on self-report measures of depression. Generalized anxiety may also be elevated, but likely at a lower level than depressive symptoms. Ratings by parents may tend to show similar elevations, although teacher ratings may appear to be in the normal range, due to the mild levels shown in the school setting. Irritability, low self-esteem, discouragement, and general distress may also be evident on multidimensional or specific self-report measures. Assessments done at different times are not likely to show significant variations, compared to assessments of major depression, which often show greater variation in symptom severity and comorbidity with other disorders. Distinctions between dysthymia and subsyndromal depressive mood may be difficult.

Bipolar Disorder

Similar to the history of depression and the relatively recent recognition that it can exist in children and adolescents, pediatric bipolar disorder (PBD) has been found to exist within the last 15–20 years. Prior to that time, bipolar disorder was considered to be an adult disorder, although signs of onset could be seen in adolescence. However, PBD remains controversial regarding whether it occurs in preadolescent children and the ways in which it is manifested. The primary difference between Bipolar I Disorder and Bipolar II Disorder is that the former is characterized by mania and the latter by hypomania. Although adolescents tend to show symptoms similar to adults that include mania, this pattern is less common in preadolescents, who rarely show manic symptoms. They are more likely to show hypomanic symptoms, which would suggest that if PBD exists in young children, it is most likely Bipolar II Disorder. Also, depression is more likely to occur before mania or hypomania in young children, and distinguishing hypomanic symptoms from typical variations of mood and behavior or from comorbid disorders is especially challenging. These patterns raise questions as to whether the same criteria for PBD can be applied to children and adolescents. If the criteria cannot be applied, then there is a significant question as to whether it is appropriate to give a diagnosis of bipolar disorder in young children.

Another diagnostic complication is that because depression often onsets first, following the child for a period of time to see if hypomania or mania develops would have to be done. Faedda et al. (1995) reviewed seven studies that followed severely depressed children and adolescents over a 2–4-year period found that about 25% of them became manic. Weissman et al. (1999) contacted a former outpatient sample of adolescents with MDD after 10–15 years. A significant risk for recurrence of depression was noted, but 4.1% had developed Bipolar I Disorder and 1.4% met criteria for Bipolar II Disorder. Overall, there are relatively few data about the diagnostic accuracy of PBD and how to assess and monitor it over time, especially if there are comorbid diagnoses.

The DSM-IV-TR provides criteria for six Bipolar I Disorders (Single Manic Episode, Most Recent Episode Hypomanic, Most Recent Episode Manic, Most Recent Episode Mixed, Most Recent Episode Depressed, and Most Recent Episode Unspecified) and for the one form of Bipolar II Disorder. Due to space considerations, only the criteria for Bipolar I Disorder, Single Manic Episode, and Bipolar II Disorder are provided here. Specific symptoms and their severity will vary depending on whether mania, hypomania, or depression is the primary mood (Tables 6.9 and 6.10).

Primary Symptoms

- Rapid mood shifts
- Irritability
- Aggressiveness

Table 6.9 DSM-IV-TR Diagnostic Criteria for Bipolar I Disorder, Single Manic Episode

A. Presence of only one Manic Episode and no past Major Depressive Episodes

Note: Recurrence is defined as either a change in polarity from depression or an interval of at least 3 months without manic symptoms

B. The Manic Episode is not better accounted for by Schizoaffective Disorder and is not superimposed on Schizophrenia, Schizophreniform Disorder, Delusional Disorder, or Psychotic Disorder Not Otherwise Specified

Specify if:

Mixed: If symptoms meet criteria for a Mixed Episode

If the full criteria are currently met for a Manic, Mixed, or Major Depressive Episode, specify its current clinical status and/or features:

Mild, moderate, and severe without psychotic features/severe with psychotic features

With catatonic features

With postpartum onset

If the full criteria are not currently met for a Manic, Mixed, or Major Depressive Episode, specify the current clinical status of the Bipolar I Disorder or features of the most recent episode:

In partial remission, in full remission

With catatonic features

With postpartum onset

Source: American Psychiatric Association (2000, pp. 388). Copyright 2000 by the American Psychiatric Association. Reprinted with permission

- Rage reactions
- Mood lability
- Dysphoria
- Suicidal ideation
- Hyperactivity
- Restlessness
- Racing thoughts
- Pressed speech
- High level of energy

Secondary or Related Symptoms

- Impaired social relationships
- Oppositional to adult authority
- Social ostracism and isolation
- Difficult to manage and direct
- Destructive
- Poor or variable school performance
- Impatience
- Loud and disruptive
- Difficult to involve in group activities

Table 6.10 DSM-IV-TR Criteria for Bipolar II Disorder

A. Presence (or history) of one or more Major Depressive Episodes

B. Presence (or history) of at least one Hypomanic Episode

C. There has never been a Manic Episode or a Mixed Episode

D. The mood symptoms in Criteria A and B are not better accounted for by Schizoaffective Disorder and are not superimposed on Schizophrenia, Schizophreniform Disorder, Delusional Disorder, or Psychotic Disorder Not Otherwise Specified

E. The symptoms cause clinical significant distress or impairment in social, occupational, or other important areas of functioning

Specify current or most recent episode:

    Hypomanic: if currently (or most recently) in a Hypomanic Episode

    Depressed: if currently (or most recently) in a Major Depressive Episode

If the full criteria are currently met for a Major Depressive Disorder, *specify* its current clinical status and/or features:

  Mild, moderate, and severe without psychotic features/severe with psychotic features

  Chronic

  With catatonic features

  With melancholic features

  With atypical features

  With postpartum onset

If the full criteria are not currently met for a Hypomanic or Major Depressive Episode, *specify* the clinical status of the Bipolar II Disorder and/or features of the most recent Major Depressive Episode (only if it is the most recent type of mood episode):

  In partial remission, in full remission

  Chronic

  With catatonic features

  With melancholic features

  With atypical features

  With postpartum onset

Specify:

  Longitudinal course specifiers (with and without interepisode recovery)

  With seasonal pattern

  With rapid cycling

Source: American Psychiatric Association (2000, p. 397). Copyright 2000 by the American Psychiatric Association. Reprinted with permission

Comorbidity

Comorbidity of PBD is common, with conduct disorder, anxiety disorders, depression, and substance use/abuse being the most frequent diagnoses. A considerable body of research has suggested that ADHD is either comorbid or that bipolar disorder is mistaken for ADHD. Biederman et al. (1996) published a seminal article that provided evidence of comorbidity between juvenile mania and ADHD. A later article by Biederman (1998) asserted more specifically that mania is often mistaken for

ADHD and that clinicians should look at the possibility of misdiagnosis. Severe ADHD shows symptoms similar to juvenile mania, such as excessive talking, press of speech, hyperactivity, restlessness, impulsiveness, and attention problems. It is also possible that the two disorders coexist simultaneously or have common biological or neurological substrates that lead to similar symptomatology. Of concern in misdiagnosis of ADHD for juvenile mania is that treatment for ADHD often involves prescribing stimulant medications. If the syndrome is undetected mania, these medications may increase dysphoric mood and exacerbate mania symptoms.

PBD also tends to be comorbid with conduct disorder in some children, with shared symptoms that include antisocial behavior, noncompliance, aggressiveness, intrusion into the behavior and functioning of others, and social alienation. Biederman, Faraone, Chu, and Wozniak (1999) suggest that there may be a bidirectional relationship between conduct disorder and mania, i.e., that the presence of one is influenced by the other. Thus, if there are symptoms of conduct disorder, they may indicate the presence of mania and the presence of mania may contribute to conduct problems.

Differential Diagnosis Considerations

Distinguishing bipolar disorder from anxiety and MDDs can be difficult because classic mania in young children tends to be rare. Hypomania is more likely, which may appear more like anxiety and depressed mood variations. Although PBD has some symptoms of anxiety and depression, they are likely to be more severe and variable, depending on the dominant mood at the time. Establishing mania and hypomania requires careful taking of developmental history, retrospective reports by parents, and observation and behavior recording over time. Distinguishing manic and hypomanic symptoms from typical developmental variations of mood and behavior can be challenging, as well. If mood problems are present that are readily observable and impairment of functioning is evident, there is a greater likelihood of a mood disorder. Accurate diagnosis of PBD is unlikely to be completed in one assessment or interview session and multiple interactions and data are necessary (Youngstrom, 2010).

An added complication in differential diagnosis is that dysthymic or pure depressive episodes may occur in bipolar disorders that are similar or identical to symptoms of unipolar disorder (Youngstrom, 2009). Also, young children's moods may "oscillate" rather than "rapid cycle" over an ultradian (24 hours) period and resemble a mixed episode and are more common than are rapid cycles seen in adults (Tillman & Geller, 2003; Youngstrom). Thus, rapid cycles seen in adults may not occur in children. Instead, children are more likely to show signs of mixed episodes over brief periods of time.

Differentiating PBD from ADHD may be improved by considering developmental history. PBD typically does not onset in young children, compared to ADHD onset that is often diagnosable at preschool levels. If there is evidence of ADHD at preschool and early school levels, there is a greater likelihood that the problem is not PBD. Of course, it is possible that they are comorbid and that both disorders are present. Another indicator of the difference between the two disorders is that children with ADHD often have coexisting learning problems, often in reading and language skills. Although children with PBD have school problems, there is not a strong body of evidence to suggest that specific learning problems are coexisting problems. The school-related problems of children with PBD are more likely due to not completing work, participating in school tasks, and erratic performance, rather than not being able to read or having specific learning problems.

Typical Assessment Profiles

Children and youth with bipolar disorder demonstrate similar psychological assessment profiles to those with major depression, dysthymia, and anxious symptomatology in self-reports and ratings by parents and teachers. Chronic dysphoric mood is common, and there may be signs of discouragement, hopelessness, low self-esteem, and other symptoms characteristics of depression and dysthymia. Assessment of variability of mood states is best done by charting of the child's moods over a period of time, which should include information about what was happening at the time, potential "triggers," and the reactions of the child and others. Although there are no norms in standardized measures to measure frequency, intensity, and duration of mood variations, a charting procedure may give valuable information about the child's behavior and circumstances surrounding onset of mood variations. These charts may be able to be completed by the child, if she or he is old enough to understand and is willing and able to participate. These charting procedures may also have therapeutic value by helping the child to recognize moods, variations, and factors that precede and follow onset of manic or depressive episodes.

A Developmental Psychopathology Perspective on Differential Diagnosis of Depression and Mood Disorders

Although differentiating pathological levels of anxiety from typical developmental levels of anxiety is important, a similar issue is not seen in children and youth with depression and mood problems. Despite occasionally feeling sad or "blue," children and adolescents do not have typical developmental periods or markers of depression or dysphoric mood. However, the clinician must be aware that children do feel unhappy and also have periods of elation that could be mistaken for dysphoria and mania or hypomania. It is essential to determine if these patterns are normative and if they reflect impairment. The clinician should also be alert to subclinical and subsyndromal patterns that may be precursors to more serious mood problems and also may cause some current impairment.

Age of Onset

Depression and mood disorders typically do not have onset until late childhood or early adolescence and are rare in preschool children. Because there are no developmental markers for depression, onset of symptoms that are not variations of normal mood and cause impairment should not be ignored. Given the recent research on bipolar disorders, it is possible that symptoms of ADHD may be mistaken for manic or hypomanic symptoms, although caution should be exercised and thorough assessment should be conducted. If sudden onset occurs, consideration should be given to the possibility of trauma, effects of ongoing stress, or a medical condition.

Developmental Comparisons

As with all forms of psychopathology, a thorough knowledge of typical developmental patterns and behaviors is essential to understanding depression and mood disorders. Children who have developmental disorders, learning and academic challenges, and social problems are at greater risk of developing depression and mood problems, which may or may not be accompanied by high levels of anxiety. Direct assessment of mood problems in young children is challenging and the clinician must rely on reports from parent and teachers, observations, and clinical history.

Genetic and Family History Context

Research suggests that there is a genetic link between histories of depression in parents and their children, although the transmission appears to be in the form of a general tendency rather than to inherit specific disorders. When conducting differential diagnosis, a family history that is positive for parental depression may suggest that children have a predisposition toward depression that begins early in life. Whether a genetic predisposition contributes to the development of depression or a mood disorder depends on a number of factors, including child vulnerabilities, resilience, and situational circumstances. The absence of a positive family history does not necessarily mean that depression will not develop, but that the risk is reduced.

Biological Context

The clinician should consider and rule out biological factors, such as chronic illness, neurological patterns, medical problems, and substance abuse as possible explanations for depression. Although depression does not appear to be a temperamental variable, such as occurs in anxiety, tendencies toward mood problems could have a biological basis and increase the risk for their development. Unlike genetic factors that are unobservable and unknown if they are factors, many biological factors can be ruled out as possible contributors to the development of depression.

Cultural Context

There is ample evidence to suggest that depression may have cultural correlates regarding SES, with poorer children having greater rates of depression (Offord et al., 1992). When conducting differential diagnosis, cultural factors should be evaluated to determine if they are significant contributors to depressive symptoms. If the child is a member of a cultural group that discourages expression of emotion, the risk for depression may increase. In those cases, the typical diagnostic criteria for depression or a mood disorder may not apply. Although cultural factors may vary in their relative contribution to depressive disorders, there is sufficient evidence to suggest that depression or depressive mood occurs in virtually all cultures.

Social Context

The social environment can have a significant relationship to the development and maintenance of depressive symptoms. Children and adolescents who have depression are more likely to have difficulties with interpersonal relationships, have fewer friends, and function less well in social situations. The clinician will need to try to assess social factors to determine their effects on functioning and how they affect the manifestation of symptoms. Areas to focus on include nature and extent of friendships, participation with peers, social skills, adaptability to social situations, responsiveness to social stressors, and social support. It is important to assess the effects of chronic stress, which, if present, increases the likelihood of the development of depression.

Family Context

The overall structure and functioning of the family are important considerations in differential diagnosis and description of childhood depression. In particular, children with a depressed parent, especially maternal depression, are much more likely to develop depression themselves. Behavior management methods used by parents should also be evaluated because methods that are punitive, arbitrary, inconsistent, or authoritative are likely to cause more stress and mood problems in children and adolescents. Children who are depressed are also at greater risk of feeling mal-treated, which should also be ruled out.

School Context

School is a primary setting where the effects of psychopathology can be shown. Academics and social interactions are highly intertwined, and children who do not do well academically tend to have social problems. Depression can interfere with children's willingness to initiate tasks, concentration, memory, effort, and persis-tence. If the depressed child seems to do well at school, but has more problems at home, then the possibility of dysfunction in family functioning should be explored. Another area to consider is whether the child is the victim of bullying or relational aggression, which is related to a greater risk of depressed mood. In some cases, the bullied child may feel extreme stress and depressed mood, due to not being able to cope with bullying behavior.

Conclusion

As with anxiety, consideration of all six contexts is important to gain a full under-standing of the nature of child psychopathology. Because depressed mood is likely to be exacerbated by social, cultural, family, and school contexts, it is important to consider each one in determining the presence of psychopathology, identifying developmental trajectories, and developing interventions.

Part III
Assessment

Chapter 7
Methods of Assessment

Careful and comprehensive assessment of anxiety and depression is essential to the accurate description and diagnosis that will help to inform and guide interventions. The clinical assessment of children requires a multimethod approach that includes (a) multiple measures, (b) multiple informants, (c) multiple settings, and (d) multiple time periods. Because young children often have not yet developed the cognitive and language ability and personal experiences to accurately self-report their subjective anxious and depressive symptoms, reliance upon observations and information from others, especially parents and teachers, is essential to obtain a thorough clinical picture. Typically, assessment in children using a multimethod approach involves seven components: (a) taking a thorough developmental and family history; (b) direct behavioral observations; (c) interviews with the child, parents, and teachers; (d) completion of behavior rating scales by parents, teachers, and the child; (e) completion of multidimensional personality inventories; (f) completion of self-report measures; and (g) informal methods. These methods provide objective information about the primary symptoms, behaviors, patterns, and their severity. Because anxiety and depression have a significant subjective component, it is necessary to obtain information from as many sources as possible using a multimethod approach. Depending on the developmental level of the child, some self-report methods may not be appropriate due to less developed language and reading skills. Few reliable and valid self-report measures are available for use with children younger than about eight years of age.

Developmental and Family History

A thorough developmental and family history is the cornerstone of psychological assessment and serves to inform and complement other assessment components. From a developmental psychopathology perspective, information should be obtained about the various contexts, i.e., genetic, biological, social, cultural, family, and

T.J. Huberty, *Anxiety and Depression in Children and Adolescents:*
Assessment, Intervention, and Prevention, DOI 10.1007/978-1-4614-3110-7_7,
© Springer Science+Business Media, LLC 2012

school-related factors. Information about genetic factors is not typically available and may be inferred based upon developmental history. Similarly, information about biological factors, such as neurotransmitter dysfunction, is not often available to the clinician. The best information, albeit indirect, about genetic and biological factors will be obtained from records and parent report. In a few cases, information from medical professionals, such as the family pediatrician, child neurologist, or other professionals, may be available and offer valuable information about these two contexts. Although this information may not be readily available or able to be confirmed, a positive family history for genetic and biological factors can be helpful in establishing developmental trajectories, identifying causal and contributing factors, confirming age of onset, and clarifying parents' perceptions of their role in the development of problems. Appendix A provides a developmental history form that can be used to gather comprehensive information as the cornerstone of a clinical assessment.

Behavioral Observations

There are three general methods of behavioral observation: (a) direct observation in one or more natural settings and recording of objective or narrative data, (b) analogue observation, where situations are created to approximate actual circumstances and observational data are obtained, or (c) self-monitoring, where children are taught how to observe and record their own behavior. Direct observation involves observing and recording frequency, duration, or intensity of behavior, perhaps using a coding system or other objective method. The advantages of direct observation include obtaining information about what behaviors are shown, antecedents and consequences of antecedents, how a child interacts with others, and the child's coping abilities in various situations. Direct observations are useful in situations where the child can be observed, and behavior is compared to that of other children or to local or national norms. Observations are particularly useful in school settings, where there are several opportunities to observe in structured and unstructured activities across different time periods and settings.

Analogue methods, while useful, often are only feasible in a clinical situation and involve careful planning, monitoring, and recording of data. Under these conditions, it is unknown if the behaviors seen in a contrived situation are equivalent to a natural setting. Analogue observations can be useful when assessing the interactions between a child and parent. For example, a task could be established where collaborative work between a parent and child is expected that approximates an actual interaction, and observations can reveal the degree to which the parent shows specific behaviors, such as being overcontrolling or intrusive. When observing interactions between a parent and an anxious child, attention might be given to observing whether the parent is collaborative or domineering. In cases of childhood depression, observations of parent–child interactions in analogue settings may reveal parental patterns such as impatience, emotional distancing, or excessive criticism.

Although these observations may not be accurate depictions of actual interactions in natural settings, they may provide information that lead to clinical hypotheses about parent–child dynamics and also inform intervention approaches.

Self-monitoring observations usually are rather straightforward to establish and require teaching a child how to observe and record individual behaviors. For self-monitoring assessment to be effective, the child must be motivated to participate and be able to record the data according to a predetermined plan. One advantage of self-monitoring is that the child may develop increased knowledge and awareness of behavior, which can have therapeutic value. Typically, older children can be taught to self-monitor rather easily, but young children can also record their own data with some modifications for developmental level.

When observing and recording behavior, there are four types of data to collect: (a) frequency counts, where the number of times a behavior occurs in a period of time is recorded, (b) duration recording, where the length of time a behavior persists is recorded, (c) interval recording, where behavior is observed for specific periods of time on a schedule, and (d) latency recording, where the time between a stimulus, such as a direction, and a response is documented. It is a common practice to combine some of these methods, such as determining how long a behavior persists (duration) during one or more periods of time (interval). For example, an anxious child might be taught how to record the number of times feelings of anxiety occurs during the day using a rating scale of intensity.

Obtaining observational data of the behavior of anxious and depressed children often will require duration recording because they may not exhibit behaviors that lend themselves to frequency counting. However, the choice of which methods to use will depend on the behaviors of interest. For example, an anxious child may not show many instances of initiating social interactions or volunteering in the classroom. Consequently, an observer might not only record the few number of times initiation is shown but also record the duration or number of times the child engages in off-task or withdrawn behavior. Latency recording may be useful because anxious children tend to show withdrawal and reluctance to interact or initiate.

There are several coding and observational systems available or observers create them for specific purposes, but they will not be discussed here. All of these systems have common elements, including focusing on specific behaviors, a measurement method (e.g., frequency counting, interaction coding), a basis for comparison (e.g., prior data, norms, or peer normative comparisons), and provisions for observing across settings. Examples of formal coding systems include the *Direct Observation Form of the Child Behavior Checklist* (Achenbach & Rescorla, 2001), the *Behavior Coding System* (Harris & Reid, 1981), and the *Student Observation System of the Behavior Assessment System for Children-II* (Reynolds & Kamphaus, 2004). Although observations are useful and relatively easy to use, there are several threats to their validity: (a) poorly defined observational domains, (b) unreliability of observers, (c) lack of social comparison data, (d) observer reactivity, (e) situational specificity of behavior, (f) inappropriate recording techniques, and (g) biased expectations of the observer (Merrell, 2003). There are several ways to reduce threats to validity and the reader is referred to Merrell (2003) for an excellent discussion of these methods.

Clinical Observations

During the course of assessing anxious and depressed children, it is important to observe their behavior during interviews with and without parents present and during evaluation sessions. Observations of how anxious children and their parents interact may offer some clues to their relationship, contributory and maintaining factors to anxiety, and how the child responds to parental behavior. Examples of behaviors to observe during clinical interviews and assessments include

- Psychomotor movements
- Attention to task
- Task persistence
- Eye contact
- Initiation of interactions
- Responsiveness to questions and directions
- Speech quality, speed, tone, rate, and volume
- Physiological symptoms, such as flushing of the skin
- Need for repetition of instructions
- Perfectionism (e.g., frequent erasures, slow and deliberate actions, frustration at making mistakes)
- Time interval between when a question is asked or a task is presented and when the child responds

Interviews

There are three general types of interviews: unstructured, semistructured, and structured diagnostic methods. *Unstructured interviews* are open ended and permit interviewees to "tell their story" of the situation in a rather conversational manner. There is an agenda, and the interviewer seeks answers to more general questions, but the information is obtained in a more informal format. *Semistructured interviews* are more similar to clinical interviews and have a format, typically are focused on problems and referral questions, and have specific objectives for obtaining information, such as developmental history, family constellation, parenting styles, and behavior. *Structured diagnostic interviews* have specific questions arranged in a predetermined order that is followed. The answers to some questions determine whether other questions are asked. Most often, the goal of these interviews is to determine if there are symptoms that meet diagnostic criteria and to make an initial clinical diagnosis. Some structured interviews are designed to detect various forms of psychopathology, while others are oriented toward specific problem areas. Unstructured interviews will not be discussed here due to their lack of format and focus on specific problem areas.

Semistructured Interviews

Semistructured interviews are characterized by predetermined areas for discussion, such as the behaviors of concern, friendships, and social functioning. Sattler and Hoge (2008) provide an excellent outline for a semistructured interview with parents of a child referred for a behavioral, emotional, or educational problem. The areas covered within this outline include

- Parent perception of the problem
- Home environment
- Neighborhood
- Sibling relations
- Peer relations
- Child's relations with parents and other adults
- Child's interests and hobbies
- Child's daily routine
- Child's cognitive functioning
- Child's academic functioning
- Child's behavior
- Child's affective life
- Child's motor skills
- Child's health history
- Family characteristics or problems
- Parental expectations of the child
- Additional questions

Sattler and Hoge (2008) also include an outline for a semistructured interview with a child, which contains similar items from the child's perspective:

- Information about the problem
- School issues
- Attention and concentration at school
- Home
- Interests
- Friends
- Mood/feelings
- Fears/worries
- Self-concept
- Somatic concerns
- Obsessions and compulsions
- Thought disorder
- Memories/fantasy
- Additional questions

Sattler and Hogue offer suggested questions in each of these areas, which could be modified to specific circumstances. This format is an excellent example of a nonstandardized, semistructured clinical interview approach that provides comprehensive information about the referral problems and possible associated factors.

Standardized, semistructured interviews typically focus more on diagnosis and classification. The *Kiddie-SADS* (K-SADS; Puig-Antich & Chambers, 1978) is the *Schedule for Affective Disorders and Schizophrenia* for children aged 6–17 years. Although the title suggests that it addresses affective disorders and schizophrenia, it covers a wider range of emotional and behavioral symptoms. The K-SADS has been found to have good psychometric properties and has undergone revision since 1978. It is difficult to use, however, and should be administered only by experienced interviewers. It does permit skipping items that are not relevant for a specific case and also has open-ended questions, consistent with the concept of semistructured interview formats. It may be most useful when DSM-IV diagnostic criteria are being considered.

The *Semistructured Clinical Interview for Children and Adolescents* (SCICA; McConaughey & Achenbach, 2001) is a part of the *Achenbach System of Empirically Based Assessment* (ASEBA; Achenbach & Rescorla, 2001). The SCICA is used during interviews, and the clinician rates his/her observations and a child's self-reports with separate norms for ages 6–11 and 12–18 on the Observation Form and Self-Report Form. Mean test–retest reliability across all forms is 0.78, which is acceptable and quite good for a scale of this type. The forms provide open-ended questions that address several areas:

- Children's activities and school performance
- Peer relations
- Family relations
- Self-perceptions
- Feelings
- Parent/teacher-reported problems

The SCICA has two major components: Empirically Based Syndromes and DSM-Oriented Scales, which have subscales listed below:

Empirically Based Syndromes

- Anxious[1]
- Withdrawn/Depressed[1]
- Language/Motor Problems[1]
- Attention Problems[1]
- Self-Control Problems[1]
- Anxious/Depressed[2]
- Aggressive/Rule Breaking[2]
- Somatic Complaints[2]

---

[1] Based on interviewer's observations.

[2] Based on child's self-reports.

DSM-IV-Oriented Scales

- Affective Problems
- Anxiety Problems
- Attention Deficit/Hyperactivity Problems (Inattention and Hyperactivity–Impulsivity Subscales)
- Oppositional Defiant Problems
- Conduct Problems

Structured Diagnostic Interviews

Structured diagnostic interviews are characterized by having a predetermined set of questions that are to be asked verbatim by the interviewer or by a computer program. Depending on the answers given, subsequent questions are asked so that not all items are presented. A primary goal of this approach is to ask questions that narrow the range of primary symptoms that will lead to a clinical diagnosis. These types of interviews, in contrast to semistructured interviews, (a) provide a higher level of quantifiable and objective data, (b) cover a comprehensive range of disorders, and (c) provide greater specificity with regard to symptoms (Costello, Egger, & Angold, 2005; Shaffer, Lucas, & Richters, 1999).

The *Diagnostic Interview for Children and Adolescents-Fourth Edition* (DICA-IV; Reich, Welner, & Herjanic, 1997) contains two interview schedules for use with children aged 6–12, adolescents aged 13–17, and parents of children aged 6–17. The schedules can be used separately, although the authors recommend using both forms. The DICA-IV is a computer program only and has over 1,600 possible questions in 28 categories that are oriented toward DSM-IV Axis I categories. Not all questions are answered, as subsequent questions are selected by the computer program based on answers to previous questions. The time required to complete the DICA-IV is about 60–90 minutes and, because it is computer-administered, requires little direct contact with the child or parent. Psychometric data for the DICA-IV are limited, and evidence from prior versions has shown questionable reliability and validity, especially for differentiation and classification of internalizing disorders. Therefore, the DICA-IV should be used cautiously when attempting to differentiate and classify anxiety and mood disorders.

Diagnostic Interview Schedule for Children-IV

The *Diagnostic Interview Schedule for Children-IV* (DISC-IV; Shaffer, Fisher, Lucas, Dulcan, & Schwab-Stone, 2000) is a highly structured diagnostic interview for children that was developed under the auspices of the National Institute for Mental Health. It covers more than 30 possible child and adolescent disorders and can be administered by nonprofessionals who are properly trained, which can be done rather easily. It is longer than the 1992 version and compares well psychometrically and diagnostically with the earlier version. Due to its high degree of structure, it is most suited to conducting differential diagnosis of child and adolescent disorders rather than a clinical interview that focuses on referral problems and questions. It can be a useful tool for differentiating among anxiety and depressive disorders, as well as across disorders that may reflect comorbidity.

The Initial Clinical Interview

The initial clinical interview has several purposes:

- Clarification of the referral questions
- Obtain developmental and family history
- Gather information about genetic, biological, cultural, social, family, and school factors that may be related to the referral questions
- Perspectives of parents and the child regarding the referral questions
- Observations of clinical behaviors of the child and interactions between the child and the parents to the extent possible
- Formulate initial diagnostic impressions or clinical hypotheses
- Determine what assessment procedures are needed
- Develop a plan to gather additional information
- Obtain parental consent for assessment, treatment, or acquisition of records

Mental Status Examinations

The concept of mental status examinations (MSEs) was developed by Adolph Meyer in 1902 as a procedure similar to the medical examination where all bodily systems are evaluated, such as respiratory, circulatory, neurological, and sensory functions. The MSE is patterned after that model by evaluating cognitive, personality, and affective systems that may be related to psychological functioning. Much of the evaluation is conducted by observation of the client during interviews, although specific questions or tasks may be presented to assess functions such as abstract reasoning, memory, orientation, and judgment. Various methods of the MSE have been developed, and there are often slight variations across methods and measures, but, in general, the areas that are assessed include the following:

- *Appearance*—assesses areas such as dress, hygiene, grooming
- *Attitude*—assesses area such as compliance, cooperation, hostility
- *Behavior*—assesses areas such as psychomotor speed and distractibility
- *Speech*—assesses rate, tone, volume, and pressure of speech

- *Affect*—assesses affect presented by the client to the interviewer and includes reactivity, congruence, lability, range, and quality
- *Mood*—assess mood states reported by the client, such as anxious, labile, depressed, and irritable
- *Thought Processes*—assesses areas such as goal directedness, tangential thinking, organization, abstraction, fund of information, cognitive ability, and amount
- *Thought Content*—assesses presence of suicidal and homicidal ideation, delusions, obsessions, compulsions
- *Perception/Sensation*—assesses for hallucinations and disturbed sensory processes
- *Orientation*—assesses orientation to time, place, and person
- *Memory/Concentration*—assesses short-term and long-term memory, concentration, attention span
- *Insight/Judgment*—assesses degree and quality of insight into problems and adequacy of judgment

A form for conducting an MSE is included in Appendix B that includes consideration of these 12 areas. It is not designed to be exhaustive but will assist the clinician in conducting an MSE with children and adolescents. Care should be taken when conducting an MSE with children and youth, however, due to developmental differences in areas such as insight, judgment, affect, and mood compared to adults.

Although the MSE was developed initially for adults, it can be used for children and youth; however, they may not show some of the severe symptoms such as delusions and hallucinations seen in adults. These phenomena are uncommon in children and, in young children, can be difficult to evaluate and separate from fantasy and developmental variations. Nevertheless, they do occur and should not be ignored when evaluating children and youth. With regard to items such as appearance and self-care, the degree of parental caregiving and supervision should be evaluated if the child is younger and is not as responsible for these areas on a daily basis. Questions posed to children and adolescents must be adapted to their cognitive and language levels. Typically, the MSE is not scored or based on norms but is based on observations, conversations, and perhaps asking questions about abstraction abilities (e.g., analogies) or memory (e.g., serial 7s, counting backward).

Perhaps the most well-known formal approach to evaluating mental status is the *Folstein Mini-Mental State Examination-2* (MMSE-2; Folsetin, Folstein, White, & Messer, 2010). The MMSE-2 is not designed to be a complete mental status evaluation but has standardized items, tasks, and a scoring system to facilitate assessment of mental status. It includes five areas using specific tasks to assess: (a) orientation, (b) immediate recall, (c) attention and calculation (counting and spelling backward), (d) recall, and (e) language (naming, repetition, three-stage commands, reading, writing, and copying). There is a maximum of 30 points, with higher scores indicating better mental status. The norms are applicable from ages 18 through adult, thus is less useful for conducting an MSE with children and adolescents.

Although it may not be necessary or possible to conduct a complete or formal MSE in children and adolescents, the typical areas of assessment should nevertheless be observed and evaluated informally. In some cases, knowledge about areas such as cognitive ability, affect, mood, level of anxiety, and memory and concentration may be obtained from standardized intelligence tests, personality measures, and behavior ratings. An assessment of mental status areas can be useful in evaluating children and adolescents, if it is done carefully and appropriately with regard to current developmental levels.

Behavior Rating Scales

Behavior rating scales are used extensively in the assessment of child psychopathology and often are the major sources of objective information about emotional and behavioral functioning in school-based assessment. They have become increasingly prominent in the last two decades as a result of improvements in psychometric qualities and extensive research in child disorders. The typical format is a list of items or questions, and the informant is asked to indicate the frequency or intensity of behaviors on an ordinal scale, such as "never," "sometimes," "often," or "very often." Each of these descriptors is assigned a number, such as ranging from "1" to "4," and then the item scores are summed to create syndrome or scale scores. There are two important characteristics of behavior rating scales: (a) they reflect the perspective of the informants that may or may not be accurate representations of behavior, and (b) behavior ratings essentially are composites or indexes of ongoing observations of the informant but may not correlate well with actual behavior observation data.

Behavior rating scales have several advantages in child and adolescent assessment: (a) they are objective and are based on empirical concepts;(b) they are relatively easy to administer; (c) they are relatively inexpensive; (d) most of them can be completed in 15–20 minutes; (e) they can elicit information from multiple informants, most often parents, teachers, and the child; (f) diagnostic profiles can be generated; and (g) less clinical inference is required for interpretation. Most behavior rating scales measure multiple aspects of behavior simultaneously and include both internalizing and externalizing items and scales. Lack of informant agreement on behavior rating scales is common and reflects different perceptions and experiences with the child. In their often-cited study of informant agreement on the *Child Behavior Checklist*, Achenbach, McConaughey, and Howell (1987) found low to modest correlations across raters and settings. Interinformant agreement problems tend to be greater with anxiety and mood problems due to the subjective nature of some symptoms. The two primary behavior rating scales currently in use are described below.

The *Achenbach System of Empirically Based Assessment* (ASEBA; Achenbach & Rescorla, 2001) is a frequently used behavior rating system composed of the *Child Behavior Checklist for Ages 6–18* (CBCL/6–18), the *Teacher Report Form* for Age 6–18 (TRF), and the *Youth Self Report* (YSR) for Ages 11–18. There are also versions for ages 1.5–5 and a Caregiver–Teacher form (Achenbach & Rescorla, 2001). The ASEBA is one of the earliest, most well-constructed dimensional behavior rating scale system and has been used in numerous studies of child psychopathology. Like most behavior rating scales, it is empirically derived, created by identifying behaviors that characterize child psychopathology and subjecting them to statistical analysis. Consistent with the majority of research studies, two primary *broad band* dimensions were derived: *internalizing* and *externalizing*. The internalizing dimension characterizes behaviors associated with anxiety, depression, somatization, and withdrawal, while the externalizing dimension is characterized by behaviors such as aggression, noncompliance, and attention problems. Internalizing and externalizing are sometimes referred to as "overcontrolled" and "undercontrolled," respectively. Each of the dimensions is comprised of *narrow band syndromes* where specific behaviors tend to cluster together and are correlated with other syndromes within each broad band dimension. Separate narrow band scores are obtained, and total Internalizing and Externalizing scores for the broad band dimensions are comprised of items in the respective narrow band dimensions.

The CBCL, TRF, and YSR contain the same subscales that are based on factor analysis and are consistent across the forms. The broad band internalizing dimension is comprised of three narrow band scales: (a) Anxious/depressed, (b) Withdrawn/depressed, and (c) Somatic Complaints. Similar to the SCICA, the three forms have:

Empirically Based Syndrome Scales

- Anxious/Depressed
- Withdrawn/Depressed
- Somatic Complaints
- Social Problems
- Thought Problems
- Attention Problems
- Rule-Breaking Behavior
- Aggressive Behavior

DSM-Oriented Scales

- Affective Problems
- Anxiety Problems
- Somatic Problems
- Attention Deficit/Hyperactivity Problems
- Oppositional Defiant Problems
- Conduct Problems

The DSM-Oriented Scales were constructed by having psychologists and psychiatrists from 16 cultures evaluate the items with regard to DSM-IV categories and consistency with cultural patterns. The scales correspond to the internalizing dimension of behavior (Affective Problems, Anxiety Problems, and Somatic Problems) and to the externalizing dimension (Attention Deficit/hyperactivity problems, oppositional defiant problems, and conduct problems). The additions to the ASEBA in 2007 include *Obsessive-Compulsive Problems and Posttraumatic Stress Problems* scales. The CBCL and TRF also include a *Sluggish Cognitive Tempo* scale that is not included on the YSR. The YSR includes a *Positive Outcomes* scale that is not present on the CBCL and TRF.

The informant rates 112 items on each of the CBCL, TRF, and YSR using a three-point rating scale. The item scores are summed by subscale, and the results are presented in standard *T*-scores that permit comparisons across forms. The various forms have been shown to have good concurrent and discriminative validity by comparisons to other behavior rating scales. The scales do not have validity scales to detect response styles or inappropriate responding. Reliability data for the CBCL and YSR forms are quite good, with internal consistency, test–retest, and interrater values generally being 0.90 or greater. Reliability values for the TRF are modest, however, ranging from 0.55 to 0.60. Content, criterion-related, and construct validity are satisfactory based on comparison to factor analysis, companions to other behavioral measures, and standard diagnostic systems (Sattler & Hoge, 2008).

The *Behavior Assessment System for Children-Second Edition* (BASC-2; Reynolds & Kamphaus, 2004) is a well-established behavior rating system that has Parent Rating Scales (PRS), Teacher Rating Scales (TRS), and Self-Report of Personality (SRP) forms. The SRP has three forms: child (8–11 years), adolescent (12–21 years), and young adults (18–25 years attending a postsecondary school). The complete system covers ages 2–25, depending on the specific subscales. For example, the age range for "adaptability" is from 2 to 21, while the age range for "alcohol abuse" is 18–25. In addition to the primary informant scales, there are content scales and composite scales for each form. The BASC-2 includes internalizing, externalizing, social, and school-related scales that provide a comprehensive system of assessing symptoms of psychopathology from multiple informants. Table 7.1 provides a summary of the BASC-2 Primary Scales, Content Scales, and Composites by form and age, and Table 7.2 summarizes the scales of the Self-Report of Personality.

Reporting of results is accomplished through three main scores: primary scales, content scales, and composite scores. For the PRS and TRS, informants respond on a four-point rating scale for each item, while a combination of four-point ratings and true–false are used for the SRP. Unlike the ASEBA, the BASC-2 contains scales to detect response sets and response bias. The PRS, TRS, and SRP have a "faking bad" scale index to detect the tendency of informants to overreport negative behaviors that are normatively atypical. The SRP also has a "faking good" index as well as an index that detects responses to items that are highly unlikely or illogical. The computer scoring program for all three forms has a Consistency index that indicates how often responses to similar items occur and a Response Pattern Index that indicates the number of times a response is different from previous items. These indexes

Table 7.1 BASC-2 Primary Scales, Content Scales, and Composites by Form and Age

Scale	Teacher Rating Scales			Parent Rating Scales		
	Preschool 2–5	Child 6–11	Adolescent 12–21	Preschool 2–5	Child 6–11	Adolescent 12–21
Activities of Daily Living				X	X	X
Adaptability	X	X	X	X	X	X
Aggression	X	X	X	X	X	X
Anxiety	X	X	X	X	X	X
Attention Problems	X	X	X	X	X	X
Atypicality	X	X	X	X	X	X
Conduct Problems		X	X		X	X
Depression	X	X	X	X	X	X
Functional Communication	X	X	X	X	X	X
Hyperactivity	X	X	X	X	X	X
Leadership		X	X		X	X
Learning Problems		X	X			
Social Skills	X	X	X	X	X	X
Somatization	X	X	X	X	X	X
Study Skills		X	X			
Withdrawal	X	X	X	X	X	X

Table 7.2 BASC-2 Self-Report of Personality Clinical and Adaptive Scales

Scale	Interview	Child	Adolescent	College
Alcohol Abuse				X
Anxiety	X	X	X	X
Attention Problems		X	X	X
Attitude to School	X	X	X	
Attitude to Teachers	X	X	X	
Atypicality	X	X	X	X
Depression	X	X	X	X
Hyperactivity		X	X	X
Interpersonal Relations	X	X	X	X
Locus of Control		X	X	X
Relations with Parents		X	X	X
School Maladjustment				X
Self-Esteem		X	X	X
Self-Reliance		X	X	X
Sensation Seeking			X	X
Sense of Inadequacy		X	X	X
Social Stress	X	X	X	X
Somatization			X	X

provide valuable information about the clinical validity of profiles and the degree to which the clinician can place confidence in the ratings of each informant. Profiles that show questionable validity on these indexes should be interpreted with extreme caution, and the clinician should investigate the reasons for the response patterns. Although the BASC-2 does not have specific DSM-IV-oriented scales similar to the ASEBA report forms, the various scales do address several symptoms that are useful in differential diagnosis. The non-diagnostically oriented scales, such as Functional Communication, Leadership, and School-Related scores, offer additional information that is useful in providing a more extensive description of the child's functioning and skills.

Interpretation of Behavior Rating Scales

When one considers the profiles generated from behavior rating scales, they may appear easy to interpret by consideration of various elevations above or below cutoff scores, such as one standard deviation above the mean. However, interpretation that leads to accurate conclusions and recommendations from behavioral rating scales is more complex than merely identifying profile patterns. There is a series of steps to consider when interpreting these measures that will not only improve accuracy but provide additional information about the child and the informants. It is to be noted that some behavior rating scales have specific instructions about how to interpret them and to address questionable responding:

1. If the behavior rating scale has validity scales, determine if the results can be considered valid and should be interpreted. If the results are questionable, the clinician should (a) review the individual responses in an attempt to determine if response biases or response sets are evident and (b) review the results with the informant to determine if they understood the items and task, marked the responses correctly, or perhaps had a response bias based on factors such as prior experiences or perceptions of the child. If the clinician determines that the informants have biases that may not be consistent with other data, then attempts should be made to determine their specific nature though follow-up interviews.
2. If the rating scale is determined to be valid using available psychometric indices or if there are no validity scales, the clinician should conduct a visual inspection of the responses. A high number of extreme ratings on scales having three or more choices suggest response bias, lack of familiarity with the child, or incorrect marking of answers, and caution should be used in interpretation. If the scale appears to be valid, tentative general clinical hypotheses can be formulated that must be compared and validated with information from other informants or developmental and behavioral history. Attention should also be given to items that may have been omitted, either by mistake or intentionally. If items were omitted, the informant can be asked if it was intentional or an oversight. If the omissions were an oversight, the informant can be asked to complete the

omitted items. If the items were intentionally omitted, the clinician should ask the informant for the reasons. Most often, intentionally omitted items occur because the informant does not feel able to answer it accurately. Omission of items can affect whether the complete scale can be completed and scored. Some scales have directions for how to address omitted items, such as by adjusting or prorating scores or scoring them in the least significant direction. If response sets, such as extreme responding, are present, it is useful to conduct a follow-up interview with the informants to discuss some of the items to determine the basis for the responses.

3. After a visual inspection of the responses, the next step is to determine if there are elevated scales above specified or suggested "cutoff" scores, such as one standard deviation above the mean, which is a common lower limit to consider the possibility of clinical significance. Lower cutoff criteria increase the possibility of making "false positive" conclusions about the presence of psychopathological symptoms, although fewer false negative conclusions are likely. The highest elevations above clinical cutoffs should be considered to represent the primary symptom pattern that may indicate the presence of a disorder. Other scales may be elevated as well and may or may not be closely correlated with the primary elevations. For example, it is not uncommon for elevations to occur on both internalizing and externalizing scales, such as depression and aggressive behavior.

4. If the profiles are considered valid and there is no evidence of response bias or inaccurate data, each profile should be compared with other informants' profiles to determine the degree of consistency among them. Discrepancies in ratings among informants are common, and it should not be assumed that one set of ratings is invalid. There are several reasons why ratings can be discrepant among raters: (a) exposure and interaction of the informants may vary, (b) the child's typical behavior varies across settings or persons, (c) the setting creates different conditions for the development and maintenance of behaviors, (d) multiple measures from different developers/publishers may not measure the same behaviors in similar ways, (e) biases or response sets of one or more informants, and (f) conditions or stressors perceived at the time of the ratings. Many computer scoring programs provide interinformant analyses that can be useful for comparing profiles.

5. Until shown otherwise, the clinician should initially accept all ratings as valid reports by the informants, who likely have different perspectives of the child's behavior. The clinician should remember that behavior ratings reflect the perspective of the informants, which may or may not be consistent with each other. With regard to anxiety and depression in children and youth, many of the characteristics are subjective and difficult for observers to report accurately, such as feelings of worthlessness, helplessness, perfectionism, and self-esteem. To the extent possible, corroboration of some of these symptoms must be obtained directly from the child through self-report measures and interviews. It is common for informants to show significant discrepancies in ratings for children who have anxiety or depression.

Personality Inventories

Personality inventories have a long history in clinical assessment and are multidimensional by assessing multiple aspects of psychopathology simultaneously. Most often, these measures are completed in a self-report format and contain items reflective of psychopathology across a wide range of symptomatology. Typically, the items have been empirically derived with few theoretical underpinnings. The items are keyed to specific subscales, which are generated into profiles using standard scores, most often *T*-scores with a mean of 50 and standard deviation of 10. Interpretation of these measures is accomplished through analysis of individual scale elevations and combinations of scales.

Minnesota Multiphasic Personality Inventory

Undoubtedly, the *Minnesota Multiphasic Personality Inventory* (MMPI), developed by Hathaway and McKinley in the 1940s, is the most well-known measure of this type and has been a measure of psychopathology in thousands of research studies since its inception. The current version, the *Minnesota Multiphasic Personality Inventory-2* (Butcher, Graham et al.) was published in 1992. The original version was developed and standardized on adults; however, a version for adolescents, the *Minnesota Multiphasic Personality Inventory-Adolescent* (MMPI-A), was not published until the early 1990s (Butcher, Williams et al., 1992). Prior to the MMPI-A, separate norms for adolescents were used, although there continued to be controversy regarding their appropriateness and accuracy. The MMPI-A is normed for youth aged 14–18, with a recommended seventh-grade reading level. It also contains validity scales to detect patterns such as "faking bad," malingering, and inconsistent responding.

The MMPI-A contains the same basic scales as the MMPI-2:

- Hypochondriasis
- Depression
- Hysteria
- Psychopathic Deviate
- Masculinity–Femininity
- Paranoia
- Psychasthenia
- Schizophrenia
- Hypomania
- Social Introversion

The MMPI-A has more specific relevance in clinical assessment through its Content Scales, which are combinations of specific items and are intended to provide a more thorough clinical description of the person. Some of the Content Scales are useful in more clearly describing various patterns, including anxiety and depression and the contexts of developmental psychopathology. The Content Scales are

- Anxiety
- Obsessiveness
- Depression
- Health Concerns
- Alienation
- Bizarre Mentation
- Anger
- Cynicism
- Conduct Problems
- Low Self-Esteem
- Low Aspiration
- Social Discomfort
- Family Problems
- School Problems
- Negative Treatment Indicators

The MMPI-A is often used in clinical settings as a broad assessment of psychopathology of adolescents but cannot be adapted for younger children. It is a highly clinical instrument with an orientation toward diagnostic labels and differential diagnosis. It is not as often used in schools, however, due to its highly clinical nature, complexity, administration time (60–90 minutes), and perceived relevance to educational achievement and performance. It may be useful for educational purposes in clinical settings where a school component is included.

Personality Inventory for Children: Second Edition

The *Personality Inventory for Children-Second Edition* (PIC-2; Lachar & Gruber, 2001) is a multidimensional measure completed by a parent or caregiver for children and youth aged 5–19. The *PIC-2* contains 225 true–false items and a brief form, the *Behavioral Summary* that consists of 96 items. The scale offers the benefit of having an MMPI-A type of format that can be applied to young children. It is also more descriptive and less focused on diagnostic labels and categories. It has three validity scales to detect inconsistent, random, or biased responding. Like the MMPI-A, the PIC-2 does not have composite scores or a total score but has Adjustment Scales. These scales have subscales that provide more precise descriptions of item clusters. Interpretation is accomplished by investigation and comparison of scales and subscales. There is also a version for Spanish-speaking informants (Table 7.3).

The PIC-2 is unique compared to the MMPI-A and similar measures because it provides parent or caregiver perspectives on a child's social, emotional, and academic functioning. It also provides an index of how the parent/caregiver perceives a child's behavior contributes to family dysfunction and parenting practices through

Table 7.3 Clinical scales
of the Personality Inventory
for Children-2

Cognitive Impairment
Family Dysfunction
Psychological Discomfort
Social Withdrawal
Impulsivity and Distractibility
Delinquency
Reality Distortion
Somatic Concern
Social Skills Deficit

the Family Dysfunction Scale, the Conflict Among Members Scale, and the Parent Maladjustment Scale. This is one of the few measures of child psychopathology that gives the clinician information about family dynamics simultaneously with information about child symptoms and how parent maladjustment may contribute to the development and maintenance of problems behaviors. The PIC-2 also provides parent perspectives on school-related matters regarding cognitive impairment (inadequate abilities, poor achievement, and developmental delay). The PIC-2 has acceptable standardization data and psychometric properties of a nonclinical population. There is a referred sample that appears less representative. It does discriminate among various clinical groups. The PIC-2 appears to be a good instrument to assist in assessing anxiety and depression, although some caution should be exercised in interpretation. The Psychological Discomfort Scale reflects symptoms of anxiety and depression together with the subscales of Fear and Worry, Depression, and Sleep Disturbance/Preoccupation with Death, providing more specific symptom patterns.

The *Behavioral Summary* of the PIC-2 has 96 items that may be useful if there are time constraints for using the PIC-2. Composite scores are provided that are comprised of short versions of the PIC-2 Adjustment Scales. In general, short forms of measures tend to have less reliability; therefore, the PIC-2 should be used when possible. Although the PIC-2 does not have composite scores like the *Behavioral Summary*, the scales under each of the composites can be used as a guide for interpretation of the larger version.

Personality Inventory for Youth

The *Personality Inventory for Youth* (PIY; Lachar & Gruber, 1995a, b) is a rather unique personality measure for children because it can be used with children and adolescents in grades 4–12 or about 8–18 years of age. It is a true–false response format with a third-grade reading level, making it one of the best multidimensional self-report personality measures that can be used with young children. Another unique characteristic and advantage of the *PIY* is that it is a complementary

Table 7.4 Clinical scales of
the Personality Inventory for
Youth

Cognitive Impairment
Impulsivity and Distractibility
Delinquency
Family Dysfunction
Reality Distortion
Somatic Concern
Psychological Discomfort
Social Withdrawal
Social Skill Deficit

measure of the PIC-2, with similar scales and interpretative approaches. Reliability and validity are satisfactory to good. It can be used with the PIC-2 that is completed by parents, and both measures can be directly compared across scales and subscales. Like the PIC-2, the *PIY* provides information about a wide range of internalizing and externalizing patterns and has content related to anxiety and depression. It also contains scales to assess the presence of hallucinations and delusions, which, although relatively rare in children and adolescents, are not typically included in most measures of child behavior. Also, the Family Dysfunction scale gives information about the child's perspective on family problems, another scale not seen in most other measures of child psychopathology (Table 7.4).

Student Behavior Survey

The *Student Behavior Survey* (SBS; Lachar, Wingenfeld, Kline, & Gruber, 2000) is a rating scale completed by a teacher and is appropriate for children aged 5–18 years of age. It has 102 items and is easily completed in about 15 minutes. The SBS has fourteen scales in three sections: Academic Resources, Adjustment Problems, and Disruptive Behavior that are more descriptive than diagnostic in their format, although there are implications for clinical diagnosis. The SBS uses a four-point scale, ranging from "1" ("never") to "4" ("usually"). High scores on the Academic Resources Scale indicate positive characteristics, while high scores on Adjustment Problems and Disruptive Behavior are indicative of emotional and behavioral difficulties. It contains scales about Academic Habits and Parent Participation, which are not often directly assessed in other rating scales.

The standardization samples included children from general education as well as children who were referred for clinical and educational problems. Standardization data suggest that internal consistency reliability is good and that test–retest reliability is acceptable to good, although the latter data are limited. The SBS is a rating scale that is similar in content to the PIC-2 and PIY and may be useful when these latter two measures are used. There are limited research data on the SBS, however, and caution should be used when using the scale (Sattler & Hoge, 2008).

Adolescent Psychopathology Scale

A final multidimensional personality scale to be discussed is the *Adolescent Psychopathology Scale* (APS; Reynolds, 1998) and the Short Form of the *APS* (*APS-SF*; Reynolds, 2000). The APS is a comprehensive self-report measure for youth aged 12–19. A third-grade reading level is required, and this can be completed in about 45 minutes to one hour. There are 20 clinical scales that are related to DSM-IV categories, 5 personality scales, 11 psychosocial problem content scales, and 4 response style/validity scales. The *APS-SF* has scales for 12 clinical disorders and 2 validity scales that assess defensiveness and an index of response consistency. It also includes Academic Problems and Anger/Violence scales not contained in the larger *APS*. Psychometric properties of reliability and validity are good, including discriminant validity. Like the MMPI-A, the validity scales are useful for detecting response style problems, response bias, and random or inconsistent responding. Overall, the *APS* is a good measure of adolescent psychopathology, and the Academic Problems and Anger/Violence Proneness scales are useful in school settings.

Interpretation of Personality Inventories

Standardized personality inventories produce multiscale profiles that are examined for clinical and nonclinical significance. The technical and administration manuals include directions and discussion for how to determine their validity and interpret the profiles. The general approach to interpreting these measures is similar to interpreting standardized behavior rating scales, including determining validity and examining the scales. Although behavior rating scales typically have forms for parent, teacher, and child, personality inventories are self-report measures that do not have parent or teacher forms (with the exception of the PIC-2). Of the personality inventories discussed above, only the PIC-2 and *PIY* can be considered to be comparable parent and child forms, although they were developed and published at different times. Therefore, caution should be used in making direct comparisons of the various scales, although such comparisons may have utility with regard to developing clinical hypotheses from the parent and child reports.

The general approach to interpreting multidimensional personality inventories is similar to, but somewhat different from, behavior rating scales. The reader is referred to the prior discussion of the interpretation of behavior rating scales as a guide to interpretation of personality inventories. Additional considerations include

1. Virtually all of the major personality inventories have validity scales, so these indices should be examined according to the guidelines provided by the test publisher to make a determination whether the scale is valid and can be interpreted accurately. If the scale is valid, then individual and cross-scale comparisons can be made. If the scale is invalid, the clinician should conduct a visual inspection of the responses or review the computer printout to determine what occurred. If the

reason for invalidity is due to inaccurate responding, such as not understanding how to complete the scale, then the task may be too difficult or exceeds the informant's cognitive or reading ability. If the results appear due to malingering, "faking good," confusion, or inability to complete it accurately, readministration of the scale is not likely to produce a valid profile.

2. As with behavior rating scales, personality inventories produce profiles with multiple scales. In general, scales are considered individually and in comparison to other scales to determine clinical patterns that lead to conclusions. The MMPI-2 and MMPI-A are unique with regard to profile interpretation because some scale combinations have more specific interpretation descriptions called "two-point" and "three-point" codes that are composed of two or three individual scales, respectively. Not all scale combinations are provided, and there are more two-point than three-point codes. The suggested clinical cutoff score for scales of the MMPI-A is a T-score of 65. The PIC-2 and PIY clinical cutoff scores vary across subscales, with the lowest being a T-score of 60. Because most standardized personality inventories do not have multiple forms, comparisons to other measures are done clinically. These scales are developed under varying standardization conditions, including different sample stratifications and sizes. Consequently, discrepancies among instruments are common, and clinical interpretations should focus primarily on profile patterns that will assist in forming clinical and diagnostic conclusions.

Self-Report Measures

Many self-report measures assess relatively specific emotional, behavioral, and personality characteristics and patterns, such as anxiety, depression, and anger, as well as eliciting information about cognitive, behavioral, affective, and physiological symptoms. These measures may be individual instruments, such as the *Revised Children's Manifest Anxiety Scale-2* (Reynolds & Richmond, 2008) or the *Children's Depression Scale-2* (Kovacs, 2010). Some instruments contain several scales of this type, such as the *Beck Youth Inventories-Second Edition* (BYI-II; Beck, Beck, & Jolly, 2005). The BYI-II is composed of the *Depression Inventory, Anxiety Inventory, Anger Inventory, Disruptive Behavior Inventory,* and *Self-Concept Inventory* scales. Each measure has 20 items that address each area for children aged 7–18 and permit cross-scale comparisons. The BYI-II scales have the advantage of being normed on the same populations and can be directly compared to each other to create a more complete profile. Psychometric data on the BYI-II are good (Beck et al., 2005).

Other measures can be used to assess correlates of symptoms and syndromes, such as self-concept. Although they may not directly address diagnostic criteria, they offer more comprehensive information about factors that may contribute to understanding the clinical picture presented by the child or adolescent. These types of measures will be discussed here, while more specific measures relating to anxiety and depression will be presented in Chaps. 8 and 9, respectively.

Self-Esteem/Self-Concept Measures

Self-concept is a well-established theoretical concept that has received much research attention over many years. Self-concept has been conceptualized as being both unidimensional and multidimensional. Unidimensional perspectives view self-concept as being a general characteristic where a person has a broad view of self. Other conceptualizations view self-concept as being multidimensional and that self-concept may vary across domains. For example, a child might have a stronger self-concept about schooling and academics but a less well-developed self-view about social skills. Low self-concept is associated with depression, although the nature of the direction between them is unclear, i.e., whether one precedes or is the cause of the other or only that they occur together as part of a pattern of emotional distress. From a risk perspective, it is possible that low self-esteem is a risk factor for depression or, conversely, that depression is a causal factor for the other. Children with high self-esteem tend to be more resilient because beliefs in their ability help them cope with stressful situations.

When conducting interventions, Seligman (1998) asserts that improving self-esteem without a corresponding increase in positive behavior changes is at best misguided, and, at worst, dangerous to the child. Thus, information about self-concept may help the clinician to understand problems such as lack of self-initiation and self-disparagement often seen in anxiety and depression. However, establishing a child's multidimensional pattern of self-esteem/self-concept may have limited value as a predictor of anxiety or depression or as a specific target for intervention.

Multidimensional Self-Concept Scale

The *Multidimensional Self-Concept Scale* (MSCS; Bracken, 1992) is a self-report measure for children in grades 5–12, using a four-point Likert response scale format ranging from "Strongly Disagree" to "Strongly Agree." The 150 items are arranged into six subscales of 25 items each: Affect, Social, Physical, Competence, Academic, and Family. A Global Self-Concept Index is also provided. The psychometric properties are quite good, including strong stability over time and high subscale reliability. As an adjunct measure when assessing anxiety and depression in children, the MSCS provides a good index of self-concept in children. Scores are reported as standard scores with a mean of 100 and standard deviation of 15.

Self-Perception Profile for Children

The *Self-Perception Profile for Children* (SPPC; Harter, 1985) was developed by Susan Harter, who has conducted extensive research and theory on self-concept in children. The SPCC contains 36 pairs of statements and is unique to other self-concepts scales as children are asked to select which statement of a pair is most like them. After this selection, the child answers whether the statement is "really true" or "sort of true." Each item is rated on a four-point scale, with higher scores indicating greater self-concept.

The 36 items are grouped into six self-concept dimensions: Scholastic Competence, Social Acceptance, Athletic Competence, Physical Appearance, Behavioral Conduct, and Global Self-Worth. The method of asking the child to select an item from a pair and rating its importance offers additional interpretive value to the SPCC. For example, if Athletic Competence is rated as low, but the child does not consider it to be important, then less significance may be attributed to it. Conversely, if Scholastic Competence is rated as low and the child feels it is not important, greater significance may be attached to it by a clinician due to the importance of schooling and learning and the discrepancy from the child's perception. As has been discussed, low academic achievement and motivation is a risk factor for anxiety and mood/affective problems. The SPCC also has a teacher rating scale to compare to the child's report as well as a separate importance rating scale completed by the child. This latter scale is compared to the responses on the SPPC to add information about the importance placed on the various domains. The SPCC is a valuable instrument that has been used in many studies. However, caution should be used in interpretation because the norm group was based only on Colorado children and technical data are limited. Results are reported in raw scores rather than standard scores, making it more difficult to compare to various standardized instruments.

Self-Perception Scale for Adolescents

The *Self-Perception Scale for Adolescents* (SPSA; Harter, 1988) is a companion measure of the SPCC and is similar in item content, structure, format, and scoring. It contains items that are more relevant to adolescents and has nine scales rather than the six scales on the SPPC. In addition to the SPPC, the SPPA contain three scales measuring Job Competence, Close Friendships, and Romantic Appeal. Like the SPPC, the norm sample was limited to Colorado and there are limited technical data. However, the scale has been used in numerous studies and appears to be a good instrument. Nevertheless, caution should be used in interpretation.

Piers–Harris Self-Concept Scale II

The *Piers–Harris Self-Concept Scale-Second Edition* (PHSCS-2; Piers, Harris, & Herzberg, 2002) is the revision of one of the most widely used measures of self-concept in children. The scale is normed for children and adolescents aged 7–18 and has 60 items arranged in six subscales:

- Physical Appearance and Attributes
- Intellectual and School Status

- Happiness and Satisfaction
- Freedom From Anxiety
- Behavioral Adjustment
- Popularity

The scale is written at a second-grade level and uses a "yes" or "no" response format. It provides a total score as well as subscale scores and can be completed in about 10–15 minutes. There are two validity scales to detect response bias or random responding. Psychometric properties are acceptable, and the scale can be used for screening in school settings and clinics.

Conclusion

This chapter has provided an overview and summary of major methods and approaches to child and adolescent personality and behavioral assessment that can be used in assessment of anxiety and depression. The measures described are useful in a multimethod assessment of anxiety, depression, and comorbid conditions. When combined with other measures, such as those described in Chaps. 8 and 9, the clinician will be able to conduct a thorough clinical assessment that will lead to accurate diagnostic formulations and interventions of anxiety and depressive disorders.

Chapter 8
Assessment of Anxiety

In addition to the assessment methods described in Chap. 7, there are specific methods, procedures, and instruments to assess anxiety symptoms and disorders. The assessment of anxiety should also be considered from the contextual approach of developmental psychopathology discussed in Chaps. 1 and 2. In this chapter, discussion of methods specific to anxiety and anxiety disorders will be presented and integrated with developmental psychopathology concepts. A case example will be provided that describes the referral questions, the assessment procedures used, diagnostic conclusions, and potential recommendations.

Developmental and Family History

Information about genetic and biological factors as risk factors for anxiety disorders may be obtained indirectly through conducting developmental and family history in the parent interview. Parents may not have detailed information about anxiety-related disorders in family history and may describe relatives in general terms, such as "nervous," "high strung," "worrier," and other anxious terms. The developmental history form presented in Appendix A provides a framework to obtain this information from parents or other caregivers. Of particular relevance is the degree to which there are maternal or paternal histories of general or specific anxiety disorders.

Interviews

Child Interviews

Using a semistructured interview format, the practitioner should conduct a child clinical interview about the nature of the symptoms and the child's perception of them. During this interview, a mental status examination can be conducted, using the

T.J. Huberty, *Anxiety and Depression in Children and Adolescents:*
Assessment, Intervention, and Prevention, DOI 10.1007/978-1-4614-3110-7_8,
© Springer Science+Business Media, LLC 2012

format described in Chap. 7 and the form in Appendix B. Behaviors characteristic of anxiety and other patterns should be observed, using a checklist and clinical notes of behaviors. The following are some key questions or areas to ask the child regarding symptoms of anxiety, although the wording may need to be altered for the developmental and language level of the child. Additional techniques to facilitate discussion of feelings and perceptions might include asking younger children to draw pictures and talk about them, engage in play activities, and using favorite cartoon or television characters as frames of reference for questions. Often, it is useful to ask the child for an example to be sure that the question is understood and to obtain some information about the degree of self-awareness of symptoms. Many of the questions will be answered in the interview as a function of discussion about the referral concerns.

Cognitive Symptoms

- Do you worry about things a lot? If so, what do you worry about?
- Are you able to pay attention and concentrate on your schoolwork?
- How do you feel about yourself?
- Do you need to be perfect at things?
- When you get into new situations, how do you feel?
- Are you happy most of the time?
- Are you able to remember things you have to do or when you take tests at school?
- Do you think things bother you more than other kids your age?
- When things do not go well, such as on a test at school, do you think it was your fault, bad luck, or the fault of someone else?

Behavioral Symptoms

- Do you get nervous and wiggly a lot?
- When you have to do something new, are you eager to do it or are you likely to hold back?
- Do you volunteer to do things and raise your hand in class?
- When you are around new people, do you like to talk with them or are you do you hold back a lot?
- Do you finish most things that you start?
- When you have to do assignments at school, do you spend a lot of time erasing, correcting, or redoing your work?
- When you have to talk in a group or give a speech, do you talk fast or get nervous?
- Do little things bother you more than most people your age?
- When you have a choice to do something easy or something more difficult, which one would you probably choose?

Physiological Symptoms

- Do you sometimes feel like your heart is beating too fast when you are not playing or running?
- Do your hands get sweaty a lot for no reason?
- Do you sleep o.k.?
- Is your appetite o.k.?
- Do you get stomachaches or headaches a lot?
- When you get nervous, does your face or neck get red sometimes?
- Do you feel sick at your stomach or feel like you might throw up a lot?
- When you get nervous, do your muscles get tense?

Parent Interviews

Following the semistructured interview format, the practitioner should elicit information on parents' perspectives on the symptoms, causes, maintenance factors, and consequences of anxiety on the child's personal, social, and academic functioning. Similar to the child interview, the practitioner should address some of the following areas using similar questions and ask for examples.

Cognitive Symptoms

- Do you think _____ worries a lot more than most children? If so, what kinds of things does he (she) worry about and how intense do you think it is, using a scale from one to ten, with ten being the most intense?
- Is _____ able to pay attention well and concentrate on things at home, such as doing homework, staying with tasks, and following through on things he (she) is asked to do?
- Do you think _____ is more sensitive about things than most children?
- Does _____ expect too much of himself and feel that he (she) must be perfect?

Behavioral Symptoms

- Does _____ start a lot of things and not finish them?
- When _____ is in a new situation, is he (she) likely to want to enter into it or to withdraw?
- When _____ is confronted with a challenging situation, is he (she) more likely to be calm and organized or get upset?

- Would you say that _____ is more restless or "fidgety" than most children?
- Would you say _____ is "high strung" or is rather even-tempered?
- Does _____ talk rapidly when under stress?
- Would you describe _____ as irritable or "cranky" a lot of the time?

Physiological Symptoms

- Describe _____'s sleeping patterns.
- Does _____ complain of headaches or stomachaches although is not sick?
- Does _____'s neck or face get red when he (she) gets nervous or upset?
- Does _____ perspire a lot when not playing, such as sweaty hands?
- Does _____ get nauseous or vomit when extremely anxious?
- How is _____'s appetite?

Teacher Interviews

When interviewing teachers about anxiety symptoms, similar questions are asked, but some are more specific to school academic and social concerns. In addition to asking questions related to symptoms, the practitioner should explore situations that tend to trigger anxious reactions, how the child reacts, and how the teacher responds.

Cognitive Symptoms

- Is _____ able to concentrate well on assignments and tasks?
- Is _____ able to remember directions and follow through on them?
- Is _____ able to remember and recall information on tests and other learning tasks?
- Does _____ seem happy?
- Does _____ seem to have a good self-concept?
- Does _____ seem to be a perfectionist?

Behavioral Symptoms

- Does _____ start and complete things most of the time?
- Does _____ volunteer and participate in class?
- Is _____ likely to select easy or difficult tasks?
- Would you describe _____ as fidgety and restless?

- Would you describe _____ as "high strung" and needing more support than others?
- Does _____ talk rapidly at times?
- Would you describe _____ as cranky or irritable?
- In new situations, is _____ more likely to want to participate or to withdraw?

Physiological Symptoms

- Does _____ get sweaty and perspire when nervous?
- Does _____ complain of headaches and stomachaches for no apparent reason?
- Does _____'s skin get red and flushed when performing or participating in social situations?
- Does _____ show a lot of muscle tension?

Structured Diagnostic Interviews

In addition to the structured diagnostic interviews discussed previously in Chap. 7, the *Anxiety Disorder Interview Schedule-Child Version for DSM-IV* (ADIS-C; Silverman & Albano, 1996a, b) has parent and child forms to differentiate anxiety disorders using DSM-IV criteria. The Child Version begins with an explanation of the purpose for the interview to the child and to emphasize that there are no right or wrong answers. The following areas are assessed with the Child Version:

- Background Information
- School History
- School Refusal Behavior
- Separation Anxiety Disorder
- Interpersonal Relationships
- Social Phobia (Social Anxiety Disorder)
- Specific Phobia
- Panic Disorder
- Agoraphobia (With or Without Panic Disorder)
- Generalized Anxiety Disorder
- Obsessive–Compulsive Disorder
- Posttraumatic Stress Disorder (PTSD)/Acute Stress Disorder
- Affective Disorders: Dysthymia
- Affective Disorders: Major Depression
- Externalizing Disorders (Attention Deficit Hyperactivity Disorder/ADHD)
- Screening Questions for Additional Childhood Disorders

  - Substance Abuse
  - Schizophrenia

- Selective Mutism
- Eating Disorders
- Somatoform Disorders

In each of the disorders assessed, questions about the degree of interference of the symptoms, fear ratings, and extent of attempts at avoidance of situations are asked. As each area is assessed, the clinician rates each item and formulates a DSM-IV diagnosis. The clinician also determines the Clinician's Severity Rating (CSR) on a 9-point scale (0–8), which is derived from the child's interference ratings, total number of symptoms endorsed by the child, and impression of each diagnostic category. Mental status is noted, and an assessment of psychosocial stressors is conducted. Consistent with the DSM-IV format, Principal Diagnoses are determined, as well as Additional Diagnoses, with each accompanied by a CSR.

In the Parent Version, the format is similar, but some areas are assessed differently from the Child Version:

- School History
- School Refusal Behavior
- Separation Anxiety Disorder
- Interpersonal Relationships
- Social Phobia (Social Anxiety Disorder)
- Specific Phobia
- Panic Disorder
- Agoraphobia (With or Without Panic Disorder)
- Generalized Anxiety Disorder
- Obsessive–Compulsive Disorder
- Posttraumatic Stress Disorder (PTSD)/Acute Stress Disorder
- Affective Disorders: Dysthymia
- Affective Disorders: Major Depressive Disorder
- Externalizing Disorders

    - Attention Deficit Hyperactivity Disorder (ADHD)
    - Conduct Disorder
    - Oppositional Defiant Disorder

- Selective Mutism
- Enuresis
- Sleep Terror Disorder
- Screening Questions for Additional Disorders

    - Substance Abuse
    - Schizophrenia
    - Mental Retardation
    - Learning Disorders
    - Pervasive Developmental Disorders
    - Eating Disorders
    - Somatoform Disorders

Ratings for interference, persistence, avoidance, and distress are recorded leading to a determination of Principal Diagnoses and Additional Diagnoses, each with Clinician's Severity Ratings. The Parent Version also provides for recording family history and a family genogram, parent interview behavior including psychosocial stressors, treatment history, and medication history. The parent and child forms of the ADIS-C can be useful when evaluating the presence, severity, and history of symptoms and in formulating differential diagnoses.

Observations

Observations of children with anxiety can be challenging because they often do not show overt symptoms; the symptoms may not be frequent and may be more continuous than episodic. In general, anxious children are not disruptive unless they are experiencing comorbid disorders, such as agitated depression, panic symptoms, or externalizing behaviors. Nevertheless, using the observational techniques described in Chap. 7, the clinician can develop a plan for systematic observation, most often in the school setting or perhaps in clinical interviews. Following is a partial list of anxiety-related behaviors or circumstances that are amenable to systematic observation:

- Number of times child initiates behavior, such as volunteering in class
- Latency of time to respond to cues or questions
- Number of different behaviors seen
- Duration of time on-task or off-task
- Number or duration of "fidgety" behaviors
- Rapid speech
- Physiological reactions, such as flushing of the skin
- Number or duration of social interactions initiated by the child or by others toward the child
- Other idiosyncratic behaviors

Syndrome-Specific Measures

In addition to the general self-report measures described in Chap. 7, there are several measures that should be considered as part of a comprehensive assessment of anxiety. Because anxiety has a significant subjective component, the child's perceptions of symptoms and concerns on self-report measures are an important complement to information from parents and teachers. Of course, younger children have more difficulty with self-reports of anxiety, but these kinds of measures can add valuable information for developing a complete clinical picture.

Revised Children's Manifest Anxiety Scale-Second Edition

The *Revised Children's Manifest Anxiety Scale-2* (RCMAS-2, Reynolds & Richmond, 2008) is an individually administered self-report measure of general trait anxiety that has 49 items using a "yes–no" forced choice format. The scale provides norms for children aged 6–19, and it has four subscales: Physiological Anxiety, Worry, Social Anxiety, and Defensiveness. The scale assesses for academic stress, test anxiety, peer and family conflicts, and drug problems, as well. It also has a short form consisting of the first 10 items. The RCMAS-2 also has an Inconsistent Responding Index (IRI), which a type of validity scale to help determine if the question are answered accurately or if there is a reason to question the results, such as a response bias. The subscale scores are presented as *T*-scores with a mean of 50 and standard deviation of 10. A total anxiety score is obtained that is reported as a standard score with a mean of 100 and standard deviation of 15.

The RCMAS-2 and its predecessor, the *Revised Children's Manifest Anxiety Scale* (RCMAS; Reynolds & Richmond, 1985), have been used in numerous research studies and extensively in clinical practice as a measure of trait anxiety. The manual describes generally adequate psychometric properties, which are supported in the majority of research studies. The reliabilities of the factor scores are less robust and should be used with caution. The normative sample is based on more than 2,300 children in geographic regions in the United States and with ethnically diverse groups and is composed of almost identical numbers of males and females. Norms are provided for three age groups: 6–8 years, 9–14 years, and 15–19 years. By using a "yes" or "no" response format, it is appropriate for younger children. A short form consisting of the first ten items can be completed in fewer than 10 minutes and provides a general index of trait anxiety. An audio presentation format is also available. The authors suggest that the scale can provide valuable clinical information about problems such as stress, test anxiety, school avoidance, peer and family conflicts, and drug use. Reynolds and Richmond also state that the scale can be used to identify and monitor anxiety symptoms over time.

Multidimensional Anxiety Scale for Children

The *Multidimensional Anxiety Scale for Children* (MASC; March, 1997) is a self-report measure of trait anxiety for children aged 8–19 years of age containing 39 items that can be completed in about 15 minutes. It proposes to assess all the major areas of anxiety. It contains the following scales and scores:

- Physical Symptoms Scale

  - Somatic Symptoms Subscale
  - Tense Symptoms Subscale

- Social Anxiety Scale

  - Humiliation Fears Subscale
  - Performance Fears Subscale

- Harm Avoidance Scale
  - Perfectionism Subscale
  - Anxious Coping Subscale
- Separation/Panic Scale
- Anxiety Disorders Index
- Total Anxiety Index
- Inconsistency Index

There is also a ten-item short version that provides only a total anxiety score and can be useful as a screening instrument. The full version of the MASC has been shown to have adequate psychometric properties and can be used as part of a comprehensive assessment battery and is preferred over the short version.

State–Trait Anxiety Inventory for Children

The *State–Trait Anxiety Inventory for Children* (STAIC; Spielberger, 1973) is a well-established measure of anxiety for children aged 6–12 that incorporates a measure of state anxiety. There are separate protocols for state and trait anxiety of 20 items each that can be completed in about 5–10 minutes each. The scales do not have separate factors and state and trait scores are derived. The items are rated on a four-point scale, with some reverse-scored to reduce response bias. Raw score totals for each scale are created and converted to percentiles and *T*-scores with higher scores indicating higher levels of anxiety. Norms are provided by gender and grade level, and the standardization sample includes about 35% African American children. Psychometric properties are good with internal consistency values in the 0.80s range, although there are relatively few validation studies. The norms are also quite dated and geographically limited to the state of Florida. The STAIC is used primarily as a research instrument rather than in clinical assessment, but is a good general measure of trait and state anxiety. The state anxiety scale may be useful in assessing level of anxiety before and after a child encounters a stressful situation and for assessing intervention effects.

Internalizing Symptoms Scale for Children

The *Internalizing Symptoms Scale for Children* (ISSC; Merrell & Walters, 1998) assesses a broad range of internalizing symptoms and positive and negative affect for children aged 8–12. The scale contains 48 items on a four-point scale as "Never True," "Hardly Ever True," "Sometimes True," and "Often True." It can be completed in about 10–15 minutes and provides subscale and total score percentiles and standard deviation equivalent scores. The ISSC has two factors that load on specific symptoms: (a) Negative Affect/General Distress (depression, anxiety, and negative self-evaluation) and (b) Positive Affect (positive affect and self-evaluative statement that are not consistent with symptoms of internalizing disorders). Higher scores indicate higher levels of psychopathology or the absence of positive affect.

The psychometric properties of the ISSC are quite good, based on a representative US sample. Internal consistency for the total scale is 0.91 and 0.90 and 0.86 for the two factors, respectively. Validity data are strong, as well, showing good correlations with other self-report measures of anxiety and depression, including the RCMAS (Reynolds & Richmond, 1985), the *Children's Depression Inventory* (Kovacs, 1992), and social skills instruments. The unique aspects of the ISSC are that it includes measures a broad range of internalizing symptoms and positive and negative affect contained in one instrument. As discussed in Chap. 9, the simultaneous assessment of positive and negative affect with internalizing symptoms is important to help distinguish between anxiety and mood disorders. The ISSC is a useful addition to a battery of instruments and procedures when assessing anxiety and depression.

Childhood Anxiety Sensitivity Index

The *Childhood Anxiety Sensitivity Index* (CASI; Silverman, Flesig, Rabian, & Peterson, 1991) is a self-report scale developed to measure anxiety sensitivity. The concept of anxiety sensitivity and its association with anxiety and anxiety disorders were discussed in Chap. 2. Although measures of generalized anxiety offer important information about the type and degree of anxious symptoms, they provide little information about how children feel about them. The CASI attempts to assess the degree of responsiveness to various anxious symptoms and offer some predictive information that could help to develop preventive strategies. An example of an item might be "I worry that I might die if I get nervous." The CASI has 18 items with three response choices: "none," "some," or "a lot." Recent research has found that the CASI has three factors: Physical Concerns, Social/Control Concerns, and Psychological Concerns in a nonclinical sample (Walsh, Stewart, McLaughlin, & Comeau, 2004). Girls scored higher than boys on the Physical Concerns factors and, to a lesser degree, on the other two scales. Girls tended to show higher overall levels of anxiety sensitivity than boys, who showed a somewhat opposite pattern, i.e. scoring lower than girls on the Physical Concerns subscale and somewhat higher on the Social/Control and Psychological Concerns scale. Most studies have shown that the CASI has acceptable reliability and validity, although it should be used with some caution.

Although the CASI is primarily a research instrument, it may be useful for assessment of anxiety when accompanied by other measures of anxiety. It may be more useful as a clinical than a psychometric instrument to gather information about symptoms predictive of panic reactions.

Positive and Negative Affect Scale for Children

The *Positive and Negative Affect Scale for Children* (PANAS-C; Laurent et al., 1999) is a self-report measure of that can be used to assess positive affect (PA) and negative affect (NA) in children who show both anxious and depressive symptoms. It contains 27 items to assess PA and NA and contains adjectives such as "sad" and asks the child to rate the degree to which the items describes her/him on a five-point scale ranging from "1"—"Very Slightly" to "5"—"Extremely." The scale has good alpha coefficients for NA (0.94 and 0.92) and PA (0.90 and 0.89) and good convergent and discriminant validity of NA with self-reports of depression ($r = 0.60$) and anxiety ($r = 0.68$) and PA correlating negatively with depression ($r = -55$) and with anxiety ($r = -0.30$). Although the PANAS-C has been primarily a research instrument, it could be used in clinical assessment. It offers a relatively "pure" measure of PA and NA with items that are similar to items in self-report measures.

Fear Survey Schedule for Children-II

The *Fear Survey Schedule for Children-II* (FSSC-II; Gullone & Lane, 2002) is a revision of the *Fear Survey Schedule for Children-Revised* (Ollendick, 1983), a self-report measure used to assess the presence of children's fears. The FSSC-II was developed with adolescents aged 11–18 and measures frequency and intensity of fears. The scale has high internal consistency values and correlates well with measures of positive and negative affect.

Screen for Child Anxiety-Related Emotional Disorders

The *Screen for Child Anxiety-Related Emotional Disorders* (SCARED; Birmhaer et al., 1997) contains 38 items as a child or parent report measure and has five factors: Panic/Somatic, Separation Anxiety, Social Phobia, General Anxiety, and School Phobia. The SCARED is appropriate for children aged 9–18, and items are answered on a three-point scale. Psychometric properties are good, including being able to discriminate among specific anxiety disorders.

Assessment of Specific Anxiety Disorders

The measures described above are useful in the overall assessment of anxiety symptoms by providing information about trait anxiety, specific symptoms, and correlates of anxiety, such as anxiety sensitivity. Other available measures may be useful to assess specific disorders when accompanied by the above instruments, observations, and interviews. These measures and procedures not only improve differential diagnosis, but also help to identify specific behaviors and symptoms that will improve diagnostic formulation and facilitate the development of interventions.

Social Phobia (Social Anxiety Disorder)

Interviews

The semistructured interview format is recommended to distinguish between two subtypes of social anxiety disorder: (a) the *specific* type which refers to a restricted range of fear or anxiety, such as giving public performances, eating with others, or using a public restroom, and (b) the *generalized* subtype, where high levels of anxiety occur in most social settings. Additional questions may help to obtain specific information about the nature, specific symptoms, degree of perceived impairment, and what the child does to cope with the symptoms and their perceived effectiveness. For the specific subtype, the following questions should be considered, adjusting the language for the child's level:

- In what situations do you feel anxious?
- Are some situations better or worse than other?
- What are you thinking before you start doing the task?
- What are you thinking about while you are doing the task?
- What do you think when the task is over?
- What behaviors do you notice that you do when performing the task?
- Do you have physical signs, such as sweating and upset stomach while you are doing the task?
- What changes in behavior or physical signs do you notice after the task is done?
- On a scale of 1–10, how would you describe the severity of the anxiety?
- What do you do to try to control the anxiety? On a scale of 1–10, how effective is each one?

When assessing the generalized subtype, the following questions should be considered, again adjusting the language for the child's level:

- What kinds of situations make you anxious?
- Do some situations make you more anxious than others?
- What do you think causes you to feel more anxious in some situations than others?
- Do you try to avoid situations more or less than you used to?
- When you are in a social situation that you cannot avoid, what do you think about?
- When you are in a social situation that you cannot avoid, what behaviors do you do to cope with the anxiety?

- When you are in a social situation that you cannot avoid, do you notice physical reactions, such as an upset stomach, tight muscles, or sweating?
- Do some situations cause more of these reactions? If so, please describe.
- On a scale of 1–10, how would you describe the severity of the anxiety in situations that create a lot of anxiety?
- What do you do to try to control the anxiety? On a scale of 1–10, how effective is each one?

Syndrome-Specific Measures

The *Social Anxiety Scale for Children-Revised* (SASC-R; LaGreca & Stone, 1993) is a 26-item self-report measure of social anxiety normed on children in fourth through sixth grades that has three factors: Fear of Negative Evaluations from Peers, Social Distress and Avoidance Specific to New Situations, and Generalized Social Avoidance and Distress. The internal consistency reliability values for the factors were, respectively, 0.86, 0.78, and 0.69, which are acceptable.

The *Social Phobia and Anxiety Inventory for Children* (SPAI-C; Beidel, Turner, & Fink, 1996) is a 26-item measure for children aged 8–17 that has five factors: Assertiveness, General Conversation, Physical and Cognitive Symptoms, Avoidance, and Public Performance. The SPAI-C has strong reliability and validity properties, including good ability to discriminate between clinical and nonclinical samples.

Generalized Anxiety Disorder

Interviews

Because generalized anxiety disorder (GAD) is characterized by pervasive, "free floating," and excessive anxiety that is not caused by specific events or stimuli, interview questions should include trying to determine associated personality characteristics that contribute to overall social and personal impairment. Additional questions should try to determine if there are specific situations that tend to create more anxiety, such as social settings and evaluation situations. Cognitive–behavioral approaches are especially useful for conducting interviews with children having GAD because the factors that elicit general anxiety often are highly subjective and internal. Because GAD is general and pervasive, many questions are common to several anxiety disorders and the reader is referred to others listed above. However, there are other areas that may be useful to explore in interviews:

- Tell me about all the things you worry about and which ones bother you the most.
- When do you know that you are anxious? What things do you notice?

- Do you have trouble concentrating on lots of things? If so, what are they?
- Do you think you are cranky or irritable more than most people your age?
- Do you think you are more serious than most people your age, or are you about like everyone else?
- Do you think you need more reassurance than most people your age?
- Do you think that you have a tendency to be perfect at the things you do?

Syndrome-Specific Measures

The majority of self-report measures of anxiety assess general characteristics, although they often have subscales, such as the MASC, RCMAS-2, and ISSC. Subscales from self-report behavior rating scales and multidimensional personality inventories give indexes of generalized anxiety, all of which are useful as measures in the assessment of GAD. With young children, it may be difficult to access generalized anxious cognitions through self-report measures and variations of play interviews may be useful.

Obsessive–Compulsive Disorder

Interviews

Conducting clinical interviews of children with obsessive–compulsive disorder (OCD) includes areas common to all anxiety disorders, as well as some mood problems. Questions to ask include:

- Describe these repetitive thoughts and when they occur.
- Which ones seem to occur most often and how often do they occur each day?
- How distressing or bothersome are these repetitive thoughts?
- How do these repetitive thoughts affect your ability to do your homework, be with friends, and other things you need or like to do?
- Do these repetitive thoughts seem reasonable or unreasonable to you?
- Do specific things seem to trigger specific repetitive thoughts? If so, what are they, when do they occur, and how often?
- Are there certain beliefs or attitudes that you have about yourself that seem to be related to these repetitive thoughts? If so, tell me about them.

Areas to address for compulsions include:

- The specific behaviors shown, for example, checking, hoarding, and washing.
- Do these behaviors help you to feel less distress?
- Do these behaviors make sense to you? Why or why not?

Syndrome-Specific Measures

Children's Yale-Brown Obsessive–Compulsive Scale

The *Children's Yale-Brown Obsessive–Compulsive Scale* (CY-BOCS; Goodman, Price, & Rasmussen, 1989a, b) is a clinician-administered rating scale that assesses the severity of obsessive and compulsive symptoms. It has an extensive list of specific thoughts and compulsive rituals, each of which are rated on amount of time per day, degree of distress caused, the child's amount of effort expended to resist the symptoms, the amount of perceived control, and degree of interference with normal functioning. A total severity score is obtained by summing the symptom scores. The CY-BOCS has good psychometric properties and can be a useful addition to an assessment battery.

Leyton Obsessional Inventory-Child Version

The *Leyton Obsessional Inventory-Child Version* (LOI-CV; Berg, Rapoport, & Flament, 1989; Berg, Whitaker, Davies, Flament, & Rapoport, 1988) is a downward extension of the adult version of the scale for use with children and adolescents. The LOI-CV contains a list of 44 OCD symptoms that the respondent rates for presence or absence and degree of impairment of functioning. It has four derived factors that can be used as subscales: General Obsessive, Dirt/Contamination, Numbers/Luck, and School-Related Symptoms. Psychometric properties are adequate and the scale can be used as a method to gather information on specific OCD symptoms. The LOI-CV can be found in March and Mulle (1998).

Posttraumatic Stress Disorder

Interviews

Conducting interviews of children and youth with PTSD requires that emphasis be given to the manifestation of symptoms in their onset, type, severity, and impact on functioning. In general, symptoms are shown in three broad categories: intrusive reexperiencing of the events, avoidance of triggering events, and physiological reactions. Caution must be exercised in what and how questions are asked of children who have experienced trauma, especially if it was acute and they are still experiencing symptoms. Depending on what questions are asked and how they are posed, a child who has experienced trauma may feel increased distress during an interview. Adjusting the questions and approach is essential to gather information and to help the child avoid unnecessary discomfort and stress. The following questions can be used as guides, but the wording and format can be changed to accommodate the child's developmental and situational status.

- Do you have nightmares about what happened?
- Do you have trouble going to sleep or staying asleep?
- Do you have a lot of bad feelings or emotions about what happened that occur? If so, what are they?
- How do you think what happened affects you now?
- Are you "jumpy" or startle easier than you used to?
- Do you get tense a lot, especially when you think about what happened?
- Do thoughts and feelings about what happened affect how well you get things down or plan ahead?
- Do you try to avoid or get away from things that remind you of what happened?
- Do you sometimes feel kind of "numb" or find it hard to feel things?
- Do you like to talk about what happened?
- Do you sometimes feel guilty or ashamed of what happened?
- Do you have periods of feeling angry or upset without a good reason?

Syndrome-Specific Measures

There is no specific, well-standardized posttraumatic stress scale that is consistent with the DSM-IV criteria. The use of three or four-point rating scales for specific symptoms may be useful an informal clinical measures to assess the presence and severity of symptoms. The *Traumatic Symptom Checklist for Children* (TSCC; Briere, 1996) is a 54-item measure of symptoms of trauma seen in children aged 8–16. The TSCC has six clinical subscales: Anxiety, Depression, Anger, Posttraumatic Stress, Dissociation, and Sexual Concerns. The scale contains two validity scales that measure avoidance and denial of symptoms (underresponse) and exaggeration of symptoms (hyperresponse). The TSCC is a useful index of traumatic symptomatology that can assist in identifying symptoms and their effects on social, personal, and academic functioning. It may be useful as a measure of treatment effectiveness, but more research is needed on this point.

The *Child Behavior Checklist* is part of the *Achenbach System of Empirically Based* Assessment (ASEBA; Achenbach & Rescorla, 2001) and has the Posttraumatic Symptoms Scale that may provide information from informants about specific PTSD symptoms that were added to the ASEBA in 2007. These items have been shown to be good indicators of traumatic stress in children and adolescents; thus, the system may be especially useful when assessing posttraumatic stress problems.

Separation Anxiety Disorder

Interviews

As the only anxiety disorder specific to children that may have strong parent–child relationship issues, interview questions should focus on both the symptoms and parent–child relationships.

- How do you feel when you are not near your (major caregivers)?
- When you have to leave your parents or house, how do you feel?
- Do you worry about getting hurt, lost, or being hurt when away from your parents?
- Do you have problems getting to sleep or staying asleep?
- Do you like to stay close to your parents?
- Do you like to sleep alone?
- Do you have bad dreams or nightmares about being away from your parents?
- How do you get along with your parents?
- Do you think your parents pay enough attention to you?
- Do you think your parents keep you from doing a lot of things you would like to do?
- Is there anything you would change about how your parents treat you?

Syndrome-Specific Measures

There are relatively few scales that measure separation anxiety (SA) in children and adolescents. Some scales have been developed from research studies, but few are in common use. Many scales such as the SCARED (Birmhaer et al., 1997) and the MASC (March, 1997) have subscales that address SA which can be used to obtain a better clinical picture. The *Spence Child Anxiety Scale* (SCAS; Spence, 1998) also has a SA scale that could be used during clinical assessment. Psychometric properties for the SCARED, MASC, and SCAS generally are good, suggesting that they can be used for clinical assessment.

Specific Phobia

Interviews

By definition, specific phobias reflect fears of identifiable objects or situation that the child can identify and communicate to the clinician. Therefore, questions about the phobias shown by the children should focus on (a) clearly specifying the feared events or situations, (b) the conditions which trigger distress and anxiety, (c) the frequency and intensity of the reactions, (d) the coping methods the child employs, and (e) the perceived effects of these coping methods.

Syndrome-Specific Measures

Depending on the type of specific phobia, some of the measures discussed previously may be useful in assessment, such as the *Fear Survey Schedule for Children-II* (Gullone & King, 1992). Other informal measures are subjective units of distress (SUDS) scales. SUDS scales are often used in desensitization interventions that are described in Chap. 10. They are simple to construct and involve developing a scale ranging from one to ten or ten to one hundred for each fear. Lower self-ratings on these scales give an index of mild anxiety or fear and higher numbers indicate more distress for each phobia. These scales can be used to assess the degree of distress the child feels prior to treatment and can also be used to measure the effects intervention progress.

Children's Anxious Self-Statement Questionnaire

The *Children's Anxious Self-Statement Questionnaire* (CASSQ; Kendall & Ronan, 1990) is a measure to assess cognitive features of phobic behaviors by asking the child to respond to anxiety-related self-statements. It has two subscales: Negative Self-Focused Attention and Positive Self-Concept and Expectations. Although the CASSQ does not assess specific phobias directly, it may be useful in obtaining information about cognitive content that will contribute to the development of interventions.

Case Example

Name: Andrea
Age: 12
Grade: 7

Reason for Referral

Andrea was referred by her parents for problems associated with stress, anxiety, and unhappiness. The problems have been present since early elementary school to a mild degree, but have become more significant in the last year or so. The parents are seeking information on what is causing the problems and what can be done to alleviate them.

Background Information

Andrea lives with her biological parents and sister aged five and a brother aged nine. The family structure is intact, and there are no significant family problems. The parents agree that the mother worries and "hovers" a lot over Andrea, while the father is more "laid back" and does not show much concern about the situation. Andrea met all developmental milestones and is not taking any medications at present. Maternal family history is positive for anxiety disorders, and the mother describes herself as anxious and a "worrier." She also admits to being overprotective and trying to shield Andrea from stressors and difficult situations. Andrea's father has a history of mild to moderate depressive symptoms and reports nonspecific mental health problems on his side of the family. He admits to not being as involved in the family as he should and leaves the primary discipline responsibilities of the children to the mother. Neither parent has participated in mental health counseling or therapy. The mother describes the other children as being anxious, shy, and withdrawn, although they have some friends. Andrea has shown a withdrawn, anxious, and inhibited temperament since preschool and is described by her parents as still being shy, timid, and self-conscious around other children. She does not have a large circle of friends, but always has had two or three friends with similar behaviors and personalities. She has difficulty initiating and maintaining friendships, but gets along well with peers at school who do not reject, tease, or exclude her from social activities.

Her teachers report behaviors similar to those seen by the parents with regard to shyness and anxiety, but describe Andrea as cooperative, well-organized, works hard, wants to succeed, and is eager to please. She enjoys school and is not disruptive or excessively attention-seeking. Andrea has had some academic difficulties in reading and math, although she is not failing and her performance has improved. She has been referred for evaluation for special education, but was not found eligible for services for academic or social–emotional problems. The evaluation indicated that her overall cognitive ability is in the low average range and that her achievement was consistent with her ability and slightly below grade level at about early sixth grade. Although she does show rather significant withdrawal and anxiety, she was not deemed to need special education services because these symptoms were not interfering with her social and academic performance to a marked degree.

Interview Observations and Information

Andrea was apprehensive about entering the first session, but came willingly and was compliant. Initially, she was uncommunicative and answered direct questions with little elaboration and appeared defensive. She maintained little eye contact, talked in a low volume with a monotone, and was reluctant to initiate conversation. She moved frequently in her seat and picked at her fingers. After several minutes of light conversation about school and related topics, her eye contact improved and the behavioral symptoms decreased significantly. When asked what she had been told about why she was there, she stated that "there is something wrong with me because I get really nervous sometimes around people and I get scared a lot. I've been this way for a long time and I really don't think it will change. No matter what I try, I can't stop worrying. When things happen, I always figure either it's my fault or that I have disappointed my mom and dad or one of my teachers." She reported having a few friends and that she gets along well with family and friends, although she does not have anyone with whom she can talk about feelings and problems. She likes school, her teachers, and most of her classmates, but would like to have more friends and do better with her schoolwork. She has one best friend, Erin, but sees her mostly at school, and they have not stayed overnight at each other's house. When asked to give three words that would describe her, she said "nervous," "worrier," and "dumb." She said that she thinks she is "dumb" and believes that she lacks the ability to make friends, although she would like more friends.

During the assessment sessions, Andrea was cooperative and completed all tasks asked of her, but frequently asked if her answers were correct. She said, "Are you trying to find out what is wrong with me?" The examiner responded that "Your parents and teachers have said that maybe you are not as happy as you would like and that maybe we can find some ways to help you." Andrea became more relaxed at that point and maintained better eye contact and talked more readily. She put forth good effort from that point forward and smiled more, engaged in conversation with the examiner, and completed all assessment tasks presented to her.

Mental Status

Andrea's overall appearance including dress, hygiene, and grooming were age appropriate, and she was dressed in blue jeans and a sweater that were neat and clean. She was calm and compliant, although quite reticent and reserved at the beginning, which improved over the first interview session and into the subsequent two assessment sessions. Her psychomotor speed was normal, although she did show some anxious, "fidgety" behavior that decreased over time. Her rate of speech was normal, but had lower volume and tone that would be expected of her peers, but these patterns improved over the sessions, as well. There was no evidence of pressure of speech. When discussing her typical affect, she reported that she feels anxious a lot of the time, but does not become depressed, although sometimes feeling sad. She reported being disappointed in herself that she does not have more friends, but did not have major concerns about this issue. She described herself as frequently feeling "nervous" and "a worrier," but was not sure how to improve. Her affect during the sessions was within a normal range, and there was no evidence of hypomania or depression, although signs of anxiety and sad mood/dysthymia were noted. Thought processes were intact with no evidence of tangential thinking, disorganization, or impairments in problem solving. She did not report having suicidal thoughts and stated no intent or plans to harm herself. There were no indications of delusions, hallucinations, or problems with orientation as to time, place, or person. She did report sometimes having difficulty concentrating and staying on task, because she often worries about not doing well in school and making mistakes. Her insight into her behavior was appropriate for her age and was considered to be good.

Assessment Results

Behavior Assessment System for Children-Second Edition Standard Scores

	Mother	Teacher
Composites		
Externalizing Problems	58	43
Internalizing Problems	69	87
Behavioral Symptoms Index	47	50
Adaptive Skills	33	43
School Problems	–	58
Clinical Scales		
Hyperactivity	47	42
Aggression	68	47
Conduct Problems	57	43
Anxiety	76	96
Depression	52	73
Somatization	69	72
Atypicality	44	44
Withdrawal	62	55
Attention Problems	60	41
Adaptability	37	37
Social Skills	33	51
Leadership	39	36
Activities of Daily Living	31	–
Functional Communication	38	40
Learning Problems	–	73
Study Skills	–	53

Multidimensional Anxiety Scale for Children

	T-score
Physical Symptoms	
Tense/Restless	68
Somatic/Autonomic	70
Total	71
Harm Avoidance	
Perfectionism	62
Anxious Coping	72
Total	70
Social Anxiety	
Humiliation/Rejection	59
Performance Fears	67
Total	64
Separation/Panic	65
MASC Total	68
Anxiety Disorder Index	68

Beck Youth Inventories

Depression	59
Anxiety	65
Anger	35
Disruptive Behavior	37
Self-Concept	50

Personality Inventory for Youth

Validity Scales	
Validity	65
Inconsistency	54
Dissimulation	49
Defensiveness	60
Clinical Scales and Subscales	
Cognitive Impairment	44
Poor Achievement and Memory	42
Inadequate Abilities	50
Learning Problems	43
Impulsivity and Distractibility	43
Brashness	42
Distractibility and Overactivity	41
Impulsivity	50
Delinquency	41
Antisocial Behavior	46
Dyscontrol	39
Noncompliance	42
Family Dysfunction	39
Parent–Child Conflict	39
Parent Maladjustment	40
Marital Discord	43
Reality Distortion	33
Feelings of Alienation	32
Hallucinations and Delusions	42
Somatic Concern	50
Psychosomatic Syndrome	55
Muscular Tension and Anxiety	48
Preoccupation with Disease	40
Psychological Discomfort	40
Fear and Worry	31
Depression	48
Sleep Disturbance	39
Social Withdrawal	53

(continued)

(continued)	
Social Introversion	60
Isolation	38
Social Skill Deficit	46
Limited Peer Status	50
Conflict with Peers	41

Interpretation of the Data

The information provided from the parent and teacher reports generally are consistent with the developmental history and Andrea's current behaviors. Both informants describe Andrea as having primarily internalizing problems with little evidence of externalizing, acting-out behaviors. The mother endorsed a clinically significant level of aggression, but the behaviors noted were about mild disobedience, irritability, and some noncompliance. It is interesting to note that the teacher reported higher levels of internalizing behavior than did the mother, and they were nearly four standard deviations above the mean. Although the possibility exists that the teacher was overreporting negative symptoms, the validity scales were acceptable for the F, Response Pattern, and Consistency scales. The fact that both mother and teacher reports were consistent with each other offers some support for the pervasiveness of the symptoms across settings, with more symptomatology shown in the school setting. Both informants showed clinically significant levels of anxiety with lower, but significant signs of depression, indicating a highly comorbid pattern consistent with an anxious–depressed syndrome. It is more common for teachers to report accurately the presence of externalizing symptoms. That the teacher reported such a high level of internalizing symptoms indicates that the behaviors were of such frequency, intensity, and duration that they were related to some problems in the school setting. Both informants reported high levels of somatization, endorsing items related to complaints about pain and feeling sick without evidence of a physical problem.

Both informants rated Andrea as being low in adaptive skills of functional communications, adaptability, and leadership. The teacher rated Andrea as having better social skills than did the mother, but the teacher rated her as having more learning problems, which was related to overall classroom performance, primarily in language arts and math. The relatively low level of adaptive skills is consistent with a pattern of social anxiety, withdrawal, and general social discomfort. Although the deficits in adaptability are not severe, they are nevertheless of concern, especially given the fact that Andrea is entering middle school and high school where social relationships become increasingly important.

The pattern of responses given by Andrea on the PIY, MASC, and BYI is interesting in its variability across the measures and in comparison to the parent and teacher ratings. The validity indices on the PIY suggest that Andrea's responses were valid and reflected her perceptions accurately. The elevated Defensiveness

Scale, while valid, does raise the question of whether she may have underreported some of her symptoms. All of the scales and subscales were below clinical significance, although some of the subscales are consistent with other data from the parents, teachers, history, and observations. In particular, she reports a very low T-score of Fear and Anxiety (31), although she self-reported tending to worry about things. The Somatic Concern scale is reported as average (T-score = 50), despite the fact that both parents and teachers reported that Andrea sometimes complains of pains and feeling sick.

Conversely, Andrea's responses to the MASC items revealed variability with the PIY results. She reported clinical levels of Physical Symptoms of anxiety, Perfectionism, Performance Fears, Separation/Panic, and reaching clinical significance on the Anxiety Disorder Index. On the BYI, she reported a clinical level of anxiety (T-score = 65) and a tendency toward depressive symptoms (T-score = 59), again suggesting the presence of anxious symptoms and possible comorbid mood problems.

The reasons for the discrepancies among Andrea's self-reports are not clear, but may be related to the types of questions asked, the response formats of the measures, how Andrea was feeling when completing each measure, the salience and valence of the items to her, variance across measures, and idiosyncratic response styles. The differences between her reports and those of her teachers are noteworthy and suggest that how Andrea perceives herself and her behavior is quite different from those who know her. It is also possible that, on some measures, she was less willing to be forthcoming (e.g. Defensiveness scale on the PIY), creating inconsistency in responding. If this hypothesis were true, it could have implications for how to conduct interventions with her. It is not uncommon for differences to be shown within children's responses on similar measures and also between reports of others, such as parents and teachers. In these situations, it is incumbent on the clinician to conduct further assessment through interviews to try to get a clearer clinical picture of the specific nature of a child's difficulties.

Differential Diagnosis

It is beyond the scope of this chapter to discuss differential diagnosis in detail, but the symptomatology is not consistent with Obsessive–Compulsive Disorder, Simple Phobia, Social Phobia, Posttraumatic Stress Disorder, Panic Disorder, or Separation Anxiety Disorder. Despite the variability among the assessment data, Andrea's symptoms are most consistent with Generalized Anxiety Disorder and the overall pattern indicates that she meets the criteria for GAD. Andrea has had symptoms of anxiety for a long period of time and is causing some difficulties socially and at school (Criterion A), and she has difficulty controlling the worry (Criterion B). She reports physical symptoms on the MASC, as do her mother and teacher on the BASC-2 that includes restlessness (Criterion C1) and muscle tension (Criterion C5). She also gave self-reports of having difficulty concentrating and attending (Criterion C3). Thus, she meets three of the five "C" criteria, and only one criterion is required in children. The symptoms are generalized and are not confined to one of the other Axis I anxiety disorders, such as panic symptoms or disorders, Separation Anxiety Disorder, eating disorder, somatization disorder, serious illness, or PTSD (Criterion D). The symptoms are causing the most problems in social areas and school functioning (Criterion E), and there is no evidence of a psychotic disorder, pervasive developmental disorder, or a mood disorder, substance use, or a medical problem (Criterion F). Andrea does have some comorbid symptoms of mood and depression, which are common in children with GAD, but she does not meet the criteria for Major Depressive Disorder, Dysthymia, Bipolar Disorder, or other mood problems.

Developmental Psychopathology Considerations

Genetic/Biological Context

From a genetic context, it appears likely that there is a familiar genetic pattern that may have predisposed Andrea to the development of an anxiety disorder. With a positive family history of anxiety problems on the maternal side of the family, the mother's self-report of anxiety reports that Andrea's siblings have anxiety and that Andrea has shown these patterns since early age; the chances for a genetic/biological and familial predisposition for anxiety seem likely. Although there is no evidence of biological and neurological anomalies in the family history, the likelihood of some dysfunction in functioning is increased.

Cultural Context

There is no evidence that cultural factors play a major role in Andrea's symptoms, although a detailed analysis of these factors was not undertaken. The primary relevant family context variable is the mother's admission that she worries a lot about Andrea and is a "worrier" herself, which may contribute to an overprotective and "hovering" parenting style. If so, her own anxieties may be communicated to Andrea, who may tend to respond to these behaviors and reinforce them.

Social Context

The social context is quite strong in Andrea's case because, although she reports getting along well with others at school, her own social circle is limited to a small number of friends who are similar to her. Without exposure to a wider range of friends who do not show high levels of anxiety, Andrea is less likely to develop alternative behaviors to her anxious, withdrawn, and inhibited demeanor. As she progresses into her adolescence, social interactions and responsibilities will increase, but may be negatively affected by high levels of anxiety.

Family Context

Although there are no signs of significant family dysfunction present, the fact that the mother reports being overprotective and anxious (is a "worrier") indicates a parenting style where Andrea can emulate her mother's anxious behavior and also establishes and reinforces avoidance behavior. The relative lack of paternal involvement in discipline could create confusion for Andrea and lead to some strained relationships with both parents.

School Context

The school context is a major factor to consider for Andrea because her teacher reported high levels of anxiety that are causing some difficulties with task performance, achievement, and social interactions. Anxious and depressive symptomatology is reported at a high level, which has implications for academic achievement and social interactions that may become more prominent in the school setting.

Finally, the long-term developmental trajectory for Andrea could be an increased risk for social problems, the development of a severe anxiety disorder, comorbid depression, and difficulties into adulthood. A pattern is established that suggests Andrea could continue to develop more severe symptomatology that may contribute to continued problems in social, personal, and academic functioning. Intervention is indicated, which will be discussed in more detail as Andrea's case is revisited from a therapeutic perspective in Chap. 10.

Conclusion

The assessment of anxiety disorders in children and adolescents, if done properly, is a complex process that requires a multimethod approach by gathering information from many sources and using many assessment methods. A thorough developmental history will provide important information about the various contexts associated with anxiety disorders and help to identify those contexts that are important contributors to their development, maintenance, and change over time. Thorough assessment will provide a strong basis for conceptualizing, developing, implementing, and evaluating interventions.

Chapter 9
Assessment of Depression and Mood Disorders

Consistent with the format of Chap. 8, this chapter will emphasize methods and procedures for the assessment of depression and mood disorders. Because there is modest to high comorbidity between anxiety and depression, many interview questions are similar, and the various measures contain comparable, if not virtually identical, items and response formats.

Developmental and Family History

The clinician should conduct interviews with parents or other caretakers to gather information about genetic and biological history that may indicate risk factors for depression and mood disorders. It is likely that parents will have more information about relatives with depressive mood than about genetic or biological factors, especially if there is a history of mental health treatment and medication, which are more common with these disorders. The developmental history form in Appendix A can be used to help elicit this kind of information from maternal and paternal family data.

Interviews

Child Interviews

Using a format similar to that described in Chap. 8 for anxiety, a semistructured interview format focusing on the child's perceptions of the problems, symptoms, and impact on functioning should be completed. A mental status examination should be conducted, using a format similar to the one described in Chap. 7 and the form in Appendix B. Wording of questions may need to be altered to correspond to the

T.J. Huberty, *Anxiety and Depression in Children and Adolescents:*
Assessment, Intervention, and Prevention, DOI 10.1007/978-1-4614-3110-7_9,
© Springer Science+Business Media, LLC 2012

developmental level of the child and his ability to respond. Because young children may show some initial reluctance to participating in interviews, asking them to draw pictures, using favorite cartoon or television characters, and participate in play activities may help to facilitate the interview. Asking for examples of feelings or behaviors will help to assess self-awareness of the child's symptoms, for example, "What makes you sad?" or "How do you know you are sad?" Combining questions that are more typical of anxiety should be considered as part of a standard procedure when interviewing about depression and mood problems. As with all semistructured interviews, questions that are answered during the course of the conversation may not need to be asked directly, unless follow-up or clarification is needed. The questions suggested in the cognitive section are intended to help elicit information about cognitive biases and distortions, negative attributions, illogical reasoning, and thinking impairments that are associated with depressed affect and mood. Variations in the format and wording are encouraged to adapt to the level of the child and for preferences of the interviewer, but the goal should remain to gather an informal assessment of type, severity, and degree of impairment. Conclusions, interpretations, or inferences about the answers to questions of the child should consider his/ her developmental level, because younger children or those with cognitive or language delays are less likely to be able to report feelings or recognize the associations among cognitive, behavioral, and physiological symptoms.

Cognitive Symptoms

- Do you tend to think about things in as only being one way or the other or do you look at things at having many possibilities?
- Do you worry that many things will have terrible outcomes?
- Do you have trouble remembering things, such as what you are supposed to do or when taking tests at school?
- Do you have trouble concentrating on things, such as when you have to do school tasks like reading or math?
- Do you find that things distract you more easily than they used to and that it is hard to pay attention?
- Do you think that you have control over what happens?
- Would you say that you have a positive view of yourself?
- When things do not go well, do you tend to blame yourself, other people, or things that happen?
- Would you say that you have a positive view of the world around you?
- Does the future look good for you?
- Do you feel "upbeat" and happy or kind of sad and unhappy most of the time?
- Would you say that you are more likely to see things positively or negatively?
- At times, do you tend to feel that no matter what you do, it doesn't help much?
- Do you think that things will turn out well or that things are not going to change much?
- Do you have a hard time making decisions?

- Do you put things off because you cannot follow through or decide what to do?
- Do you think about hurting yourself? (If there are signs of suicidal ideation, conduct a suicide risk assessment.)

Behavioral Symptoms

- Do you withdraw from others a lot or more than you used to?
- Do you participate in activities about the same or less than you used to?
- Do you find it easy to participate in activities with others?
- Do you find it easy to put forth effort on things, such as work or school?
- Has your work or school performance been o.k. lately?
- Do you cry a lot about things?
- Do you sometimes overreact to situations?
- Do you feel irritable or "cranky" a lot?
- Do you care much what happens to you?
- Do you find it difficult to work or cooperate with others?
- Have you ever tried to harm yourself?

Physiological Symptoms

- Tell me about your sleeping patterns, such as do you get enough sleep, do you get to sleep and stay asleep, or do you have trouble sleeping?
- Is your appetite o.k.?
- Do you have any aches or pains?
- Do you have enough energy to do things?
- Do you feel like you are too "hyper" or too sluggish or just about right most days?

Parent Interview

Cognitive Symptoms

- Does _____ tend to look at things as "black and white"?
- Does _____ tend to "catastrophize" things, that is, expect that even small things will end up disastrous?
- Does _____ have trouble remembering things, such as chores, assignments, or other responsibilities?
- Does _____ have trouble concentrating on things?
- Is _____ easily distracted and have trouble following through on things?
- Is _____ too hard on himself or take on too much blame for things that are not his fault?
- Would you say that _____ has a good self-perception or self-concept?

- Do you think that _____ has a positive view of things?
- Do you think that _____ is hopeful for the future?
- Is _____ happy and "upbeat" or unhappy and sad most of the time?
- Does _____ feel that nothing she does seems to make any difference?
- Does _____ feel that things are bad and there is not much chance they will get better?
- Has _____ ever talked about hurting himself?
- Has _____ ever tried to hurt herself?
- Does _____ have a hard time making decisions?

Behavioral Symptoms

- Does _____ have a lot of friends?
- Does _____ like to participate in groups?
- Does _____ withdraw a lot or more than he used to?
- Does _____ put forth a lot of effort on things?
- How is _____'s work or school performance?
- Does _____ cry a lot?
- Does _____ overreact to small things?
- Is _____ cranky or irritable a lot of the time?
- Has _____ said that he does not care much what happens to him?
- Has _____ done things such as giving away personal possessions?
- Is _____ cooperative with you or others?
- Has _____ tried to hurt himself? (If yes, obtain information to conduct a suicide risk assessment.)

Physiological Symptoms

- Does _____ sleep o.k.?
- Does _____ have problems getting to sleep or staying asleep?
- Does _____ seem to get enough sleep and wake up rested most days?
- How is _____'s appetite?
- Does _____ complain of aches and pains that do not have a physical basis?
- Does _____ have a good level of energy to get things done?
- Is _____ either too "hyper" or too sluggish or just about right most days?

Teacher Interviews

Cognitive Symptoms

- Does _____tend to look at things as "black and white"?
- Does _____tend to "catastrophize" or think the worst is going to happen over almost everything?

- Does _____ have trouble remembering things, such as directions, assignments, facts, or projects?
- Does _____ have trouble concentrating on tasks that require it, such as math or written assignments?
- Does _____ have trouble paying attention or following through on things?
- Is _____ too hard on herself or take on too much blame for things?
- Do you think that _____ has a good self-concept?
- Would you say that _____ has a positive outlook on things?
- Do you think that _____ is happy most of the time?
- Does _____ have an attitude of feeling helpless and unable to do things?
- Has _____ ever talked about hurting herself?

Behavioral Symptoms

- Does _____ have a lot of friends at school?
- Does _____ like to participate in groups at school?
- Does _____ withdraw a lot from other children or teachers?
- Does _____ put forth an appropriate amount of effort on his schoolwork?
- How is _____'s work or school performance in terms of grades or completion of assignments?
- Does _____ cry at school?
- Does _____ overreact to small things?
- Is _____ cranky or irritable a lot of the time?
- Has _____ said that he does not care much what happens to him?
- Is _____ cooperative with you or others?
- Has _____ tried to hurt herself while at school?

Physiological Symptoms

- Does _____ seem sleepy in class?
- Do you or others notice anything about _____'s eating habits at school?
- Does _____ complain of aches and pains that do not have a physical basis?
- Does _____ have a good level of energy to get things done?
- Is _____ either too "hyper" or too sluggish or about right most days of the week?

Structured Diagnostic Interviews

There are no well-developed structured diagnostic interviews specifically for depression in children and adolescents, but comprehensive interviews such as the K-SADS (Puig-Antich & Chambers, 1978), DICA (Reich, Welner, & Herjanic, 1997), and DISC-IV (Shaffer, Fisher, Lucas, Dulcan, & Schwab-Stone, 2000) may be used to gather diagnostic information about a range of psychopathologies that include items to detect depression and mood problems. Items from the ADIS-P (Silverman & Albano, 1996a) and ADIS-C (Silverman & Albano, 1996b) described in Chap. 7 may be useful to assess depressive symptomatology along with anxiety.

Observations

Many of the behaviors seen in depression are similar to those of anxious children, and observation methods are similar. Consistent with the observation methods described in Chap. 7, there are some depressive-related behaviors that can be systematically observed and recorded in social and school settings. Because depression and anxiety tend to be comorbid, attention also should be given to the presence of anxious behaviors. Of particular note is that some behaviors may be low frequency, but high intensity, such as self-injury. Some of these behaviors include:

- Number of times child initiates behavior, such as volunteering in class
- Latency of time to respond to cues or questions
- Number of different behaviors
- Duration of time on-task or off-task
- Falling asleep, "yawning"
- Picking at skin
- Smoking (primarily in adolescents)
- Self-injurious behavior (cutting, scratching skin with objects, putting self in risky situations)
- Inattention
- Slowed speech
- Pressured speech
- Number or duration of social interactions initiated by the child or by others toward the child
- "Fidgety" behavior
- Giving away possessions
- Irritability, anger outbursts
- Other idiosyncratic behaviors

Self-Report and Clinician Rating Scales

The majority of syndrome-specific measures of depression and mood disorders are self-report scales for children aged eight or older. Many of these measures contain "critical items" that indicate high clinical significance, even though a total score might not be significant. Common critical items are those addressing suicidal ideation, plans, or attempts. Other critical items address symptoms such as helplessness, hopelessness, and loss of interest and pleasure in activities.

Children's Depression Inventory-2

The *Children's Depression Inventory* (CDI-2; Kovacs, 2010) is a self-report measure of cognitive, affective, and behavioral symptoms of depression in children aged 7–17 years of age. The initial version was published as a downward extension of the *Beck Depression Inventory* (Beck, Ward, Mendelson, Mock, & Erbaugh, 1961), which has since been revised as the *Beck Depression Inventory-II* (Beck, Steer, & Brown, 1996). The original version of the CDI has been used widely in clinical practice and research and often included in clinical assessment batteries. The scale has 27 items, each consisting of three statements ranging from no symptomatology to severe symptomatology. The child selects one of the three statements for each item that best describes her/him within the past 2 weeks. Scores are assigned to each item from "0" to "2." In addition to a total score, five factors have been derived to offer more precise descriptions of the nature of the depressive syndrome:

- Negative Mood
- Interpersonal Problems
- Ineffectiveness
- Anhedonia
- Negative Self-Esteem

Prior to 1992, scores on the CDI were presented as raw scores with a mean raw score of approximately ten. Cutoff scores ranging from 13 to 19 were used as to determine a clinical level of significance, with scores above 19 indicating severe depression. Currently, the CDI-2 provides T-scores and percentiles for the subscale and total scores. Individual items, such as item 9 that asks about suicidal ideation, should be considered as critical items of concern, although high subscale or total scores may not occur. It can be administered in groups or individually in about 5–10 min. There are also companion parent and teacher report versions.

Factor analytic studies have supported the factor structure of the CDI, although the Anhedonia scale is less robust. Craighead, Smucker, Craighead, and Hardi (1998) found another factor in an adolescent sample comprised of the loss of appetite, sleep disturbance, and fatigue items that was termed Biological Dysregulation. The authors suggest that this factor may not appear until adolescence. Although this proposed factor does not appear in the norms, it may be useful to calculate and determine if it is part of the clinical picture presented by an adolescent.

The CDI has acceptable psychometric properties, including good internal consistency, moderate test reliability, and construct and criterion validity. It correlates well with measures of self-esteem, depression, and cognitive symptoms but does not discriminate well between children with depression and other clinical groups, especially anxious children (Kovacs, 1992). The CDI was not designed to measure specific symptomatology of the *Diagnostic and Statistical Manual of Mental Disorders-Third Edition-Revised* (DSM-III-R; APA, 1987), the version in effect at the time of publication of the CDI. Consequently, it is not directly relevant to current DSM-IV criteria, either. In fact, Kazdin (1989b) found that only about 31% of children with a major depressive disorder scored at the raw score cutoff of 19 on the CDI. The CDI has many items that are similar to those on measures of anxiety, which may reflect the clinical reality of comorbidity with depression more than it indicates a limitation of the instrument. From a clinical perspective, the CDI may be more of a measure of the anxiety–depression dimension than as a "pure" measure of depression. The CDI and CDI-2 are valuable instruments for assessing depression-related psychological distress, but should be used as part of a battery of measures of depression, and not the sole instrument. Indices of depression on other measures, such as behavior rating scales and multidimensional personality inventories, often contain scales for depression that are useful for comparison.

Reynolds Child Depression Scale-2

The *Reynolds Child Depression Scale* (RCDS-2; Reynolds, 2010) is a 30-item self-report of depression appropriate for children in grades 3–6, which would correspond to an age range of approximately 8–12. The protocol is titled "About Me" rather than including words reflecting that it measures depression. The norms were stratified on a US sample of 1,620 children. Items were designed to correspond with criteria for Dysthymic Disorder and Major Depressive Disorder in the DSM-III-R and are written at a second-grade reading level. Items are to be read to children in grades three and four and may be used in individual or group administration, with an approximate time of about 10 minutes. The first 29 items are scored on a four-point scale ranging from "almost never" to "all the time." The final item is a presentation of five iconic faces showing expressions ranging from very sad to very happy and the child selects one of them to reflect current mood. A total score is derived, and there are no data provided in the manual about subscales or factors. The manual reports reliability coefficients ranging from 0.87 to 0.91, with total alpha reliability of 0.90 and split-half reliability of 0.89.

Reynolds Adolescent Depression Scale-2

The *Reynolds Adolescent Depression Scale-Second Edition* (RADS-2; Reynolds, 2002) is a 30-item self-report measure of depression for adolescents aged 11–20 and is a companion measure to the RCDS-2. The self-report form does not mention "depression" in the title, instead identifying it as "RADS-2." The reading level is at the third grade and can be completed in about 5–10 minutes. The RADS-2 is a revision and restandardization of the *Reynolds Adolescent Depression Scale* (RADS; Reynolds, 1989) and is based on extensive research. Like the RADS and RCDS, each item is rated on a four-point scale ranging from "almost never" to "all the time," and a total score is provided. There are also six critical items that may indicate high risk despite a nonelevated total score and an empirically derived cutoff score for clinical depression. The RADS-2 has four factors that add more clinical information:

- Dysphoric Mood
- Anhedonia/Negative Affect
- Negative Self-Evaluation
- Somatic Complaints

Interpretation of the four scales is based upon *T*-scores, percentiles, and item content. The RADS-2 was normed on a stratified sample of 3,300 children based on US Census Data and included some subjects from Canada. The norms also included data from 297 children in a clinically referred sample based on DSM-III-R and DSM-IV criteria. The manual contains extensive evidence of construct validity, and the subscales correlate well with other measures of depression.

Multiscore Depression Inventory for Children

The *Multiscore Depression Inventory for Children* (MDI-C; Berndt & Kaiser, 1996) is one of the more comprehensive and unique measures of child and adolescent depression, containing more items and several subscales. It is a downward extension of the adult version and is normed for children aged 8–17, with 79 items written at a second-grade level in a true–false response format. The unique aspect of the MDI-C is that the items were developed by children themselves, written in their own words. During scale development, children aged 8–13 reviewed potential items, and then items were revised, reworded, or added based on those comments. Consequently, the items are easy to read, are understandable, and are meaningful to the child. The MDI-C can be completed in about 15–20 minutes and yields a total score and eight subscales:

- Anxiety
- Self-Esteem
- Social Introversion
- Instrumental Helplessness
- Sad Mood
- Pessimism
- Low Energy
- Defiance

The scale also includes an Infrequency Index that serves as a validity check for careless, erratic, or inconsistent responding. One item also serves as a Suicide Risk indicator. Results are provided as raw scores, T-scores, and percentiles, based on a standardization sample of more than 1,400 normal children and adolescents. The MDI-C purports to measure various aspects of depression separately that are helpful with treatment planning and monitoring. The scale is described as measuring relatively stable mood states but is less sensitive to more transient fluctuations in mood.

Children's Attributional Style Questionnaire-Revised

The *Children's Attributional Style Questionnaire-Revised* (CASQ-R; Thompson, Kaslow, Weiss, & Nolen-Hoeksema, 1998) is a 24-item measure of attributional biases based on learned helplessness theory that are presumed to be related to the development of depression. The items describe several positive and negative events, and the child chooses one of two possible causes for each, presumably reflecting attributional style. The causes presented correspond to learned helplessness and attributional style theory and literature: internal–external, global–specific, and stable–unstable. Two composites are provided (Positive and Negative), as well as a Depressive Attribution Score (Positive Minus negative). The scale also provides six subscales:

- Good Internality
- Good Stability
- Good Globality
- Bad Internality
- Bad Stability
- Bad Globality

The CASQ-R is an interesting and intriguing instrument but is more useful as a research instrument and has been used primarily in this way. It may be useful in treatment planning using cognitive–behavioral therapy approaches, which typically focus on attributional styles and belief systems as targets for intervention.

Hopelessness Scale for Children

The *Hopelessness Scale for Children* (HSC; Kazdin, Rodgers, & Colbus, 1986) is a 17-item self-report measure of hopelessness for children aged 6–13 using a true–false response format. The HSC does not assess depression directly but shows two related factors: Negative Expectations/Giving up and Unhappiness/Negative Expectations that have been well established as prominent correlates of depression. The HSC measures hopelessness and future expectations, which are cognitive symptoms of depression and relate to Beck's (1987) cognitive model of depression. Higher scores on the HSC reflect greater feelings of hopelessness and are associated with poor school performance, poor social skills, suicidal ideation, low self-esteem, depression, and high CDI scores (Kazdin, 1989a, b).

Beck Hopelessness Scale

The *Beck Hopelessness Scale* (Beck, 1993) is a measure of hopelessness that similar in concept to the *Hopelessness Scale for Children* (Kazdin et al., 1986) described above and is normed for ages 17–80. It is described as a strong predictor of suicidal ideation, intent, and depression. It contains 20 items that are answered in a "yes" or "no" format and may be useful as an indicator of hopelessness, depressive mood, and suicidal ideation when conducting a clinical assessment on older adolescents.

Children's Depression Rating Scale-Revised

The *Children's Depression Rating Scale-Revised* (CDRS-R; Poznanski & Mokros, 1996) is a clinician-administered rating scale of depression for children aged 6–12. It contains 17 items that the clinician completes, based on reports from parent and child interviews and observation. The scale measures 17 symptoms, most of which are scored on a seven-point rating scale, and provides a single summary *T*-score based on a nonclinical, nonrepresentative normative sample. The seven-point scale is described as being able to detect subtle, but notable changes in symptoms over time. The symptoms assessed are

- Impaired Schoolwork
- Difficulty Having Fun
- Social Withdrawal
- Appetite Disturbance
- Sleep Disturbance
- Excessive Fatigue
- Physical Complaints
- Irritability
- Excessive Guilt
- Low Self-Esteem
- Depressed Feelings
- Morbid Ideation
- Suicidal Ideation
- Excessive Weeping
- Depressed Facial Affect
- Listless Speech
- Hypoactivity

The scale also includes suggested interview prompts, guidelines for integrating information from multiple informants, interpretive guidelines for parent interviews, and comparisons of ratings based on informant, as appropriate. Although the CDRS-R has not received much research attention, it may be useful as an adjunctive measure for a clinician's interviews with the child and parent.

Assessing Suicidality

It is beyond the scope of this chapter to discuss suicidality in significant depth, but it is an issue for all clinicians working with depressed children and adolescents. Certainly, a major concern regarding children with depression is the increased risk for suicidal ideation and possible suicide attempts. Not all children who are depressed will attempt suicide, however, and not all children who attempt suicide meet diagnostic criteria for depression. Because not all children and adolescents who contemplate suicide will attempt it and because it is a low frequency occurrence, predicting who will make an attempt is difficult. Conducting a lethality assessment is an important step and should be done as indicated earlier. Responses to critical items on measures such as the CDI-2 (Kovacs, 2010) and RADS-2 (Reynolds, 2002) are important indicators, and further exploration is essential. The following measures may offer important information when assessing suicidality but should not be the only methods used.

Suicide Ideation Questionnaire

The *Suicide Ideation Questionnaire* (SIQ; Reynolds, 1988) is a self-report measure for high school-aged students, and there is a version for middle school students, the *Suicide Ideation Questionnaire-JR* (SIQ-JR; Reynolds, 1987). Both scales assess the frequency and intensity of suicidal ideation over the prior month using the questionnaire and a second phase called the Suicide Potential Interview. There is a total score used as a cutoff, and no subscales are presented. The scales were developed to facilitate school-based prevention programs and may be less applicable for clinical samples. The scales have good reliability and discriminate well between suicide attempters and the normative group. Items are rated on a seven-point scale, and the scale can be completed in less than 10 minutes. Reliability coefficients for the high school version are 0.97 and 0.93–0.94 for the SIQ-JR.

The SIQ-JR has been found to be a valuable measure cross-culturally, showing higher scores among Mexican American youth (Hovey & King, 1996) and highly predicting suicide attempts in Native Indian youth, a particularly vulnerable group (Keane, Dick, Bechtold, & Manson, 1996). It also has been shown to be useful with inner city children and adolescents (Reynolds & Mazza, 1999). Although there is relatively little evidence regarding the scale's sensitivity and specificity, it is one of the best suicidal ideation scales available for adolescents and can be a valuable addition in assessment of suicide risk.

Kronenberger and Meyer (2001) provide a list of areas to consider and assess with regard to child and adolescent suicide risk:

1. Suicidal ideation
2. Precipitating events
3. Peer coping skills
4. Maladaptive family environment
5. Previous attempts
6. Threats
7. Cognitive constriction
8. Emotional turmoil

9. Cognitive desperation
10. Sudden behavioral changes
11. Preoccupation with death
12. Lack of perceived support
13. Conduct problems/antisocial behavior
14. Use of drugs and/or alcohol
15. Psychomotor agitation/poor impulse control

When assessing suicidality, the clinician must determine if an active plan exists that the child or adolescent has formed. An active plan is characterized by definite thoughts of making an attempt, having developed a clear plan, and taken steps toward implementing it, such as gaining access to a weapon. Other signs include whether the child has shown behaviors such as giving away possessions, completing unfinished tasks, and making comments to peers and others about no longer being around, saying "goodbye," and similar statements indicating final steps.

Assessment of Specific Syndromes

Major Depression and Dysthymia

To a great extent, the assessment of major depression and dysthymia follows the same pattern, with major depressive disorder most often seen as being more severe than dysthymia. Also, dysthymia lasts longer than major depression and more than one year in children and adolescents. The methods discussed to this point are designed to assess both the presence and severity of depressive symptoms and are useful in differential diagnosis. Because anxiety and depression tend to be comorbid, specific assessment of anxiety symptoms should be conducted simultaneously while assessing for depressive patterns. Given the discussion by Goodman, Schwab-Stone, Lahey, Shaffer, and Jensen (2000) questioning whether dysthymia is a distinct disorder, the emphasis should be on describing the type and degree of symptom severity. The possibility of subsyndromal depressive symptoms should not be overlooked, which may be reflected in scores on rating scales and under measures being slightly above the norm and that are consistent with indicators of impaired performance, depressive statements from the child or others, or other relevant information.

Recommended Assessment Procedures/Batteries for Depression and Dysthymia

- Systematic observation across multiple settings
- Semistructured clinical interview with child, as appropriate for age and developmental level

- Parent interview
- Teacher interview
- Completion of CBCL or BASC-2 with multiple informants
- Completion of PIY (or MMPI-A)
- Parent completion of PIC-2
- RCDS-2/RADS-2, *Multiscore Depression Inventory for Children*, or CDI-2
- *Multidimensional Anxiety Scale for Children* (MASC) or *Revised Children's Manifest Anxiety Scale-2* (RCMAS-2)
- *Suicide Ideation Questionnaire* if evidence of suicidal ideation or behavior
- Sleep pattern assessment
- *Children's Depression Rating Scale-Revised* (clinician rating)
- K-SADS or the SCICA if a semistructured clinical interview is desired
- DISC-IV if a structured diagnostic interview is indicated
- Optional: cognitive, neuropsychological, and achievement assessment, as indicated
- Others, as indicated (e.g., CASQ-R, PANAS-C, HSC), especially for treatment planning, monitoring, and evaluation

Bipolar Disorder

Bipolar disorder in childhood and adolescence is one of the most controversial disorders of childhood and adolescence. Differential diagnosis and the appropriate instrumentation is challenging due to the lack of specific and unique criteria for bipolar disorder in children. The features of bipolar disorder discussed in Chap. 6 often are comorbid or mistaken for other disorders, such as ADHD. Thus, many of the measures and procedures used to assess mood disorders, such as those listed above, are useful in assessing bipolar disorder. Obtaining a behavioral history of the symptoms is essential to obtaining an accurate diagnosis. Mania or hypomania is a central characteristic in bipolar disorder, but if either of these exists, they most likely will need to be viewed and followed over time. Therefore, in addition, to the instruments and procedures listed above for assessing depression, dysthymia, and other mood disorders, a detailed history obtained through documentation and interviews to determine the presence of mania or hypomania is necessary. A common error may be attributing bipolar symptoms as severe ADHD. In general, bipolar disorder in young children is considered relatively rare, which would increase the likelihood of an ADHD diagnosis. Further, if bipolar disorder in children does occur, it most likely will have an onset in late childhood, rather than in the primary school years. Because children do not often show "classic" manic episodes but are more likely to show hypomania, there is a greater likelihood of Bipolar II disorder. The symptoms of ADHD that include hyperactivity and other externalizing behaviors typically have an onset before the age of five. The two disorders may be comorbid, but if symptoms have emerged prior to school entry, there is an increased probability of

ADHD versus bipolar disorder. There are many checklists available from mental health professionals or the Internet that purport to identify pediatric bipolar disorder, although many of these forms are not standardized. The *Child Behavior Checklist-Pediatric Bipolar Disorder* (CBCL-PBD; Achenbach & Rescorla, 2001) was developed to assess the likelihood of the development of PBD in children over time and has been shown to identify children who later developed bipolar disorder. Biederman et al. (2009) derived data from two identically developed longitudinal family studies of boys and girls aged 6–18 who had been diagnosed with ADHD according to DSM-III-R criteria that were collected over a 15-year period. At an average follow-up period of about 7 years, the CBCL-PBD predicted subsequent diagnosis of bipolar disorder, major depressive disorder, and conduct disorder, as well as impaired functioning and a higher likelihood of psychiatric hospitalization. Thus, the CBCL-PBD may be useful when questions regarding childhood bipolar disorder occur.

A useful acronym for assessing bipolar symptomatology in children, adolescents, and adults termed "GRAPES" is provided by Youngstrom (2010):

G—Grandiosity: child demonstrates beliefs and behaviors of grandiosity, such as being the best basketball player in the world or being able to create a spaceship to fly to other planets. This level of grandiosity may not be a true delusional pattern, but rather reflects significant overestimation of one's abilities or rational possibilities for accomplishments. In children or immature adolescents, the clinician must distinguish between grandiosity and overactive imagination or fantasy. The primary distinction is that the child will acknowledge an overactive imagination or fantasy, while the child with bipolar disorder will not recognize the grandiosity and unrealistic nature of his beliefs and self-estimations.

R—Racing thoughts: demonstrates racing thoughts by conversation and self-report, which are characterized by rapidly changing thoughts and sentences, often without apparent connections among them. The person may not see the patterns as problems, but as signs of creativity or ability.

A—Activity: demonstrates episodes of high goal-directed activity and can accomplish many tasks during these episodes. At other times, the level of goal-directed activity may be considerably lower.

P—Pressured speech: demonstrates rapid and pressured speech, as if feeling that there is much to communicate and must do it quickly. The tone may be variable, and the volume may increase and decrease in an atypical manner.

E—Elated: shows an expansive, euphoric mood and appears happy during this phase of bipolar disorder that is in contrast to depressive episodes.

S—Sleep: demonstrates a limited need for sleep and can function rather well on a few hours of sleep per night. The person may report not needing a great amount of sleep, in contrast to someone who is depressed and wants to sleep but is unable to attain or maintain a normal sleep cycle. The depressed person who has disturbed sleep is more likely to have impaired functioning.

Case Example

Name: Adam
Age: 11
Grade: 5

Reason for Referral

Adam was referred by his teacher because he has been demonstrating defiant and aggressive behavior at school, including noncompliance, fights and confrontations with other students, call others names, low academic performance, and disinterest in school. Recently, he has been talking about guns and how they can be used to hurt people, but he has not made threats toward anyone, brought a weapon to school, or otherwise caused concerns about directly harming anyone.

Background Information

Adam lives with his biological parents, an older brother aged 13 and a younger sister aged 8. The family is of a lower SES background, which contributes to financial stress, and Adam has made comments that he wishes his father made more money so that he could buy more video games. There is a family history of domestic conflict, and divorce has been discussed frequently over the past several years. There is no evidence that Adam or his sisters have been physically harmed, but his mother describes the home environment as being "tense" and "stressful" at times with frequent arguments. She describes Adam's father as being "emotionally distant" from the family and that he has a history of depression, as well as in his immediate family. She describes herself as being chronically depressed and has been taking antidepressants for several years. She admits that parenting is inconsistent, but that she tries to do the best she can, and feels she gets too impatient with the children. At times, Adam shows aggressive and defiant behavior at home, but has not harmed his siblings although they argue frequently. She reported that Adam has been diagnosed with ADHD since the second grade, which is approximately when his aggressive behavior seemed to become evident. However, the diagnosis coincides with an increase in family conflicts. He is taking dexmethylphenidate for ADHD, which has moderated his inattention, impulsiveness, and distractibility.

An interview with Adam's teacher revealed that he is an average student and gets mostly "C" and "D" grades, primarily because he does not complete his work, turn in assignments, or participate much in class. He was referred for an educational evaluation in the third grade and was found to have average to high average ability with achievement in the average range, but was not determined to be eligible for special education services. Although Adam does show aggressive behavior at times in unstructured settings, such as during recess and lunch, his typical pattern is to be quiet and withdrawn in the classroom. He does not have many friends and rarely initiates interactions with others, often spending time by himself. Adam is described as being angered easily about situations that are rather typical during the school day, such as being bumped accidentally in a line for the cafeteria. In these situations, he often accuses the other student of bumping into him intentionally.

Interview Observations and Information

Adam was reluctant to participate in the assessment sessions and asked the examiner if he was "…trying to find out if there is something wrong with me." He maintained little eye contact with the examiner and was slow in his responses to questions. He did not want to talk about his problems at school, only stating that school is "boring," "dull," and "dumb." He dislikes homework and does not care about his grades. When asked about his relationships with his siblings, he said that they get along well most of the time, but that they do argue at times. He said that he is somewhat afraid of his father who gets angry sometimes, but denied being physically abused by either parent. Concerns about his mother were evident in his comments about her "always being sad" and that it "…must be hard dealing with me and my problems. I have ADHD, you know." As the initial interview progressed, Adam became less resistant and engaged in conversation more easily. When asked about social relationships, he said that he does not have many friends, but admitted that he would like to have more friends. He reported that he does not have anyone to talk with when he feels stressed or sad. Although he tries to talk with his mother, he feels like he is adding to her problems; therefore, he keeps his feelings to himself.

Mental Status

Adam's hygiene, dress, and grooming were appropriate for his age. His attitude was somewhat passively hostile, although not aggressive and he showed some signs of minor agitation. His psychomotor speed varied from normal to slowed, although it improved during the evaluation sessions. His speech rate and tone were in the normal range, and there was no pressure of speech. He tended to speak in a low volume at the beginning of the sessions, but there was improvement. His mood and affect were flat, and he reported that he feels "down" most of the time and unhappy at home and at school. Overall mood in the evaluation sessions was depressed with little variability. Thought processes were intact, and there was no evidence of disorganization or tangential thinking. He denied any suicidal or homicidal ideation, and there were no signs of hallucinations, delusions, or disturbances in orientation. Short- and long-term memory processes were intact, although Adam's insight into his own behavior was considered to be mildly to moderately impaired.

Assessment Results

Behavior Assessment System for Children-Second Edition Standard Scores

	Parent	Teacher
Composites		
Externalizing Problems	80	67
Internalizing Problems	70	50
Behavioral Symptoms Index	80	72
Adaptive Skills	31	33
School Problems	–	57
Clinical Scales		
Hyperactivity	74	64
Aggression	75	78
Conduct Problems	81	57
Anxiety	54	45
Depression	78	58
Somatization	67	47
Atypicality	57	82
Withdrawal	87	60
Attention Problems	69	64
Adaptability	23	27
Social Skills	31	33
Leadership	40	42
Activities of Daily Living	34	–
Learning Problems	–	54
Study Skills	–	34

BASC-2 Self-Report of Personality

School Problems	76
Attitude to School	72
Attitude to Teachers	74
Internalizing Problems	69
Atypicality	51
Locus of Control	78
Social Stress	75
Anxiety	47
Depression	78
Sense of Inadequacy	68
Emotional Symptoms Index	68
Attention Problems	67
Hyperactivity	49
Inattention/Hyperactivity	59

(continued)

(continued)

Personal Adjustment	28
Relations with Parents	31
Interpersonal Relations	17
Self-Esteem	41
Self-Reliance	45

Personality Inventory for Youth

Validity Scales	
Validity	63
Inconsistency	54
Dissimulation	51
Defensiveness	64
Clinical Scales and Subscales	
Cognitive Impairment	69
Poor Achievement and Memory	68
Inadequate Abilities	61
Learning Problems	64
Impulsivity and Distractibility	59
Brashness	49
Distractibility and Overactivity	50
Impulsivity	72
Delinquency	64
Antisocial Behavior	54
Dyscontrol	62
Noncompliance	71
Family Dysfunction	58
Parent–Child Conflict	64
Parent Maladjustment	52
Marital Discord	52
Reality Distortion	53
Feelings of Alienation	53
Hallucinations and Delusions	52
Somatic Concern	52
Psychosomatic Syndrome	52
Muscular Tension and Anxiety	53
Preoccupation with Disease	52
Psychological Discomfort	55
Fear and Worry	50
Depression	66
Sleep Disturbance	44
Social Withdrawal	53
Social Introversion	53
Isolation	51
Social Skill Deficit	65
Limited Peer Status	53
Conflict with Peers	77

Revised Children's Manifest Anxiety Scale Standard Scores

	Standard Score
Total Anxiety	48
Physiological Anxiety	8
Worry/Oversensitivity	7
Social Concerns	13

Children's Depression Inventory Standard Scores

Total Score	63
Negative Mood	49
Interpersonal Problems	57
Ineffectiveness	54
Anhedonia	71
Negative Self-Esteem	62

Interpretation of the Data

Examination of the assessment results indicates both internalizing and externalizing patterns across all informants, although the severity of symptoms varies. Adam's mother and teacher rated him as high on externalizing symptoms and behavioral symptoms, and his mother rated him as clinically significant for internalizing problems. His mother rated him high on depression, but the teacher did not. It is possible that Adam does not show the classic signs of depression in the classroom, and the externalizing and withdrawn behaviors are seen more often. Both informants reported high levels of aggression and hyperactivity. The teacher's high rating on Atypicality suggests that he sees some unusual behaviors at school that are not seen in typical students, such as thought problems or severe inattention. It is interesting to note, however, that the high score on internalizing symptoms is due primarily to high scores on depression.

There are no elevations on the anxiety subscales or on the RCMAS, suggesting that Adam is showing a high degree of depressive symptomatology that is not accompanied by anxiety, although it is seen more at home than at school. The CDI shows a slight elevation in the Total Score ($T=63$), which is due primarily to the high score on Anhedonia ($T=72$). Adam also reports a high locus of control, social stress, depression, and sense of inadequacy on the BASC-2 Self-Report, providing more evidence of depressive mood and symptomatology. Inattention problems that are characteristic of ADHD are reported, although it is possible that some of these symptoms are related to depressed mood. The high level of anhedonia is likely related to Adam's disinterest in school and lack of friendships, because he derives little enjoyment from events and people in his environment. He has low self-esteem, which is also related to depression and feelings of discouragement. Adam is irritable and "cranky," which are symptoms of depression in children.

Adam also reports perceptions of cognitive and learning problems on the PIY, indicating that he believes he is not a good student, which likely is related to his negative attitude toward school and his teachers. On the PIY, he endorsed items associated with Dyscontrol, Noncompliance, Family Conflict, Depression, and Social Skills Deficits that are primarily due to Conflicts with Peers, indicating that Adam has some awareness of problems in his life. He has a negative attributional bias that is associated with depression.

Differential Diagnosis

The data indicate that Adam has both internalizing and externalizing symptoms, primarily depressed mood, some conduct problems, inattention, hyperactivity, and withdrawal. The depressed mood appears to have been present for more than two years, but there is no evidence of specific depressive episodes that would meet criteria for Major Depressive Disorder. His behavior pattern appears most similar to Dysthymic Disorder, Early Onset (300.4), with the pattern being present for at least a year in children (Criterion A), and he has low energy, low self-esteem, and concentration difficulties (Criterion B). Although a detailed history of the pattern is not available, the mother and Adam report that the symptoms have been present for more than a year (Criterion C); there has not been a Depressive Episode (Criterion D); no Manic Episode (Criterion E); there is no evidence of psychosis (Criterion F); there is no indication of substance use, drug abuse, or medical problems (Criterion G); and there is distress and impairment at home and at school (Criterion H). He is considered to be "cranky" and "irritable," which is a symptom of Dysthymia in children (DSM-IV-TR, p. 378). Although an Adjustment Disorder is a consideration, the symptoms and history are not consistent with criteria for an ongoing adjustment problem. He is at greater risk for the development of Major Depressive Disorder as shown in up to 75% of cases in clinical settings (DSM-IV-TR). Dysthymia is associated with a higher incidence of ADHD and conduct disorder (DSM-IV-TR, p. 378). Although Adam does not meet criteria for conduct disorder, the current diagnosis of ADHD and the presence of ADHD symptoms suggest that it is a comorbid condition.

Developmental Psychopathology Considerations

Genetic/Biological Context

There is no direct evidence that Adam's problems are associated directly with genetic or biological factors, although the mother's history of depression may suggest a predisposition that is transmitted. There is no history of significant health problems, head injury, or developmental disorder that has a genetic or biological basis.

Cultural Context

There are no racial or ethnic factors that play a role in Adam's behavior. The family is having financial struggles, which adds a socioeconomic variable that may increase family and individual stress. Added stress may contribute to more severe symptoms for Adam and other family members, which, in turn, will affect family functioning and interactions. Thus, the cultural context is one of external factors increasing risk for personal and family dysfunction.

Social Context

Adam's social relationships and interactions are impaired, and he gets little reinforcement and positive feedback from the home or school environment. Having impaired social relationships and skills likely will continue to lead to isolation, withdrawal, and unhappiness and increase the risk that Adam will develop Major Depressive Disorder within a few years, especially without treatment. As he becomes more unhappy and depressed, he will likely show more social dysfunction and less ability to cope with stressors. Further, the social environment provides many opportunities for children to learn how to regulate their emotions, but Adam is not able to learn and practice strategies to develop these skills. Rather, he expresses emotion in a more depressive manner and ability to appraise situations, express and suppress appropriately, and control his impulses is lacking. As he continues to have social difficulties, his self-esteem is likely to become lower, leading to increased feelings of lack of self-efficacy and competence.

Adam's social situation is cyclic, that is, as he becomes more isolated, withdrawn, and depressed, his social relationships become more marginalized, leading to less inclusion and fewer opportunities to develop social skills. Without social skills, his ability to develop social skills becomes more difficult that may lead to greater depressive mood. If sufficient social skills are not developed, he is likely to have more difficulties in adolescence and beyond, when greater demands for social skills, acumen, and competence are necessary.

Family Context

Adam's family situation is a major factor in the exacerbation and maintenance of his depressive and aggressive symptoms and can be viewed from two perspectives: (a) family dynamics and functioning and (b) parenting relationships. With regard to family dynamics and functioning, the stresses among family members create tension, apprehension, and a perception of lack of control over events. Adam may feel helpless to change the family situation and that there is little hope of significant change, which helps to maintain his depressive symptoms. The relative absence of positive affect by his parents may impair his ability to learn proper social behaviors and emotion regulation skills.

Parenting behaviors may become a source of added stress and depressive mood for Adam. Because his mother is also depressed, there is a greater likelihood of the presence of negative parenting behaviors, including (a) withdrawal, lack of engagement, flat affect, and unresponsiveness (Field, Healy, Goldstein, & Guthertz, 1990) and (b) hostility and intrusiveness (Cohn, Matias, Tronick, Connell, & Lyons-Ruth, 1986), which may be associated with an increase in Adam's depressive mood. His mother is also more likely to demonstrate less communication, engagement, and positive behaviors in her interactions with him and his siblings. His mother may also be more punitive, emotionally detached, and negative and less affectionate and comforting (Blatt & Homman, 1992), which may lead to impairment in Adam's problem-solving skills, mood, and learning of appropriate social behaviors.

School Context

Currently, Adam is showing behavioral and academic performance problems at school, much of which appears due to his depressed mood. His depression is contributing to irritability, social withdrawal, and ineffective social relationships. Although schools are primarily oriented toward developing academic skills, they also are a major source of social learning and competence. Adam's behavior that is associated with his depressed mood is causing social problems, as well as his unwillingness to engage actively in school-related tasks.

Conclusion

Adam's case is complicated from an intervention perspective due to the complexity of his family situation and the contributions of family stressors and parental psychopathology to the development and maintenance of his depressive symptoms. His case is consistent with research literature and clinical practice findings that children who are depressed have a much greater likelihood of family dysfunction. Consequently, interventions likely will involve working with the family, Adam, and in the school setting. Family therapy is indicated as one approach to reducing the effects of the dysfunction on Adam, which will involve discussing the role of the family problems on Adam's depression. Adam likely will also need some direct intervention, using CBT approaches, which will be discussed in Chap. 11 as his case is considered from a therapeutic perspective. He would also benefit from school-based interventions to help improve both his social relationships and academic performance, which are highly interrelated. These interventions should include consultation with the classroom teachers and school psychologist to focus on emotional and behavioral concerns as well as his academic performance. Improvement within any of these spheres should have a positive effect on other areas.

Part IV
Intervention and Prevention

Chapter 10
Interventions for Anxiety Disorders

A number of psychological therapies and interventions have been developed over many decades that are considered forms of psychotherapy, counseling, and other conceptualizations of treatment approaches. Although many types of models and approaches exist, this chapter will focus on those approaches that have shown evidence of effectiveness. Cognitive–behavioral, behavioral, and pharmacotherapy methods have been found to show likely efficacy in treating children and adolescents with anxiety disorders. Research on the efficacy of these methods for children is relatively recent, and fewer studies exist than for adults. The vast majority of pharmacotherapy research for anxiety disorders has been with adults, but there is sufficient evidence of effects with children that warrant its consideration in some cases.

When considering interventions for anxiety problems for children and youth, the clinician should remember that most anxiety interventions that have been studied have focused on ages 7–14 with a mean age of about 10.6 years (Barrett, Rapee, Dadds, & Ryan 1996; Kendall, 1994; Kendall et al., 1997). Often, studies use different ages of participants and variable treatments and have other differences, making it difficult to generalize results. Older children might not respond the same way to a manualized treatment as would a younger child. Differences in language ability, experience with therapy, motivation, degree of family involvement, social factors, and cultural variations are but a few possible factors to consider when developing and implementing anxiety treatments. Developmental differences within and across age ranges as factors in anxiety interventions have not been systematically studied, especially with older adolescents. Therefore, the clinician should have a thorough understanding of current research on anxiety intervention effectiveness with children and adolescents and be prepared to adapt current approaches to the unique circumstances of the case. This chapter will focus primarily on cognitive–behavioral therapy (CBT) and, to a lesser extent, the medications commonly used to treat anxiety disorders.

T.J. Huberty, *Anxiety and Depression in Children and Adolescents:*
Assessment, Intervention, and Prevention, DOI 10.1007/978-1-4614-3110-7_10,
© Springer Science+Business Media, LLC 2012

Foundations of Cognitive–Behavioral Therapy

The basic concepts and tenets of CBT rest in the overall premise that how people think, feel, and behave are fundamental to the development and maintenance of mental disorders. CBT techniques are particularly suitable for disorders such as anxiety, depression, and anger because many of the symptoms are based upon the child's beliefs and perceptions of circumstances. Because these three conditions tend to be highly comorbid, there is some overlap among them that has implications for designing and implementing CBT interventions. The interaction among affect/feelings, behavior, and cognition components is bidirectional, i.e., each component affects and is affected by the other components. Figure 10.1 shows the relationship and bidirectionality among the components.

Whereas some therapies focus on alleviation of specific symptoms, CBT takes both a therapeutic and educational approach, helping the child to understand the three components and how each interacts with and influences the others. For example, a child who is highly anxious may perceive a situation as threatening (cognitive), feels fearful (affective), and attempts to avoid or escape the situation to reduce the negative thoughts, feelings, and physical discomfort (behavioral). The child may not understand all of these components and how each contributes to and maintains the others, leading to a continued pattern of avoidance, escape, or other ineffective coping methods. The goals of CBT include helping the client understand these components, their emergence, effects, and interactive nature and to develop methods for altering cognitions, beliefs, and behaviors that lead to impairment.

In cognitive–behavioral theory, the integration and balance among these components is of central importance to the emotional functioning of the child or adolescent in an interpersonal context. Therefore, how children and adolescents interpret their experiences has significant determining effects on what they believe, how they feel, and how they react to situations. In the CBT perspective, people are considered to be active participants in their environment, being affected by and affecting those around them, in contrast to a "passive" perspective where things are presumed to happen to them. For example, children who have been severely abused certainly have experienced events and circumstances that were done to them, but how they perceive, interpret, and react to these stressors are major determinants of their psychological and interpersonal outcomes.

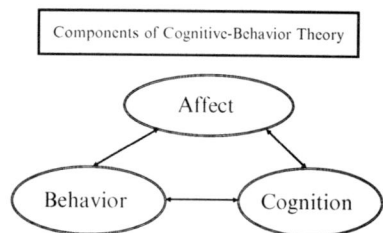

Fig. 10.1 Components of cognitive–behavior theory

The Development of Cognitive Schemata

As experiences develop and accumulate over time, cognitive schemata are formed, which are templates for action that contain cognitive products, operations, and structures. This content can be accurate or inaccurate based on how information is processed through the schemata, which are primary determinants of the child's behavior. Schemata are relatively situation specific and are activated during times of stress, mood variations, or other circumstances that cause the automatic thoughts to be activated. Schemata are not directly accessible and are theoretical constructs, but they do serve to provide a framework to help a child or adolescent understand their dysfunctional beliefs and how they affect their perceptions, feelings, and actions. Schemata reflect the child's basic beliefs about self, others, the world, the future, and potential outcomes.

The automatic thoughts that are part of the content of schemata are a central focus of therapy and can be identified through Socratic questioning, self-reports, and various forms of assessment. Schemata have a developmental characteristic because they begin to form early in life and are built upon and reinforced over time. Schemata prepare one for action and can be positive as well, but negative schemata can contribute to difficulties. Young (1999) considers negative schemata to be a risk factor for the development of emotional distress in children and adolescents. Even in the young, preverbal child, negative schemata develop about how the world is perceived, such as might occur in child abuse and neglect. Although childhood schemata are not as well formed and crystallized as those of adults, they become more so with the passage of time through being reinforced and additional learning (Young). An important concept in CBT is the *content specificity hypothesis*, which suggests that different emotional states are characterized by rather specific cognitions, for example, cognitions for anxiety, depression, and anger. There is a direct link between automatic thoughts and schemata in CBT, where emphasis is placed on altering these thoughts, which, in turn, alter the well-formed schemata.

Cognitive–Behavior Therapy with Children and Adolescents

CBT was originally developed with adults in the 1950s and 1960s, and its application to children is more recent within the last 15–20 years, showing a significant increase in research and practice. The basic concepts and principles of CBT apply to children, adolescents, and adults. These similarities include:

- A collaborative, problem-solving approach between client and therapist.
- The therapist acts as a coach, diagnostician, and educator.
- The therapist is not presented as an "expert" or major impetus of change.
- The client is an active participant in the therapy process.
- CBT requires the commitment, participation, and permission of the client.
- CBT utilizes homework that includes learning new skills to address dysfunctional schemata, false beliefs, and automatic thoughts that impair functioning.

- CBT provides opportunities for rehearsed, supervised, or in vivo practice under the guidance of the therapist.
- CBT is problem-focused, active, and goal-oriented.
- CBT provides mechanisms to evaluate progress and to provide ongoing feedback to the client about progress.
- Techniques used are, for the most part, evidence-based.
- Methods are established for formative and summative evaluation of the effects of treatment on outcomes.

There are some important differences, however, between children and adults when applying CBT principles and techniques. Apart from obvious developmental differences, a major distinction between children and adults is that children rarely refer themselves for psychological treatment. They are viewed by adult caretakers, usually parents, as having difficulties that require intervention. Younger children are less likely to see a need for treatment, and although adolescents may have sufficient self-awareness and insight to realize they are having difficulties, they nevertheless do not often refer themselves. Conversely, adults are much more likely to be self-referred, except in cases where they are court-ordered or encouraged to seek services, such as part of an employee assistance program. Further, children typically do not have a choice whether to go for therapy, whom they will see, or understand the mode of treatment or orientation of the therapist. They also may not have a choice about how many sessions will occur and when they will terminate.

Consequently, the therapist's initial task of establishing rapport, conducting diagnostic formulations, engaging the child in the process, and building a collaborative relationship may be more difficult than with adults. Adults are also more likely to have a basic understanding of psychotherapy and what to expect, while a child typically has little or no knowledge of the process. Therefore, the therapist must work with the child to educate him or her about what to expect and that it is a collaborative endeavor. This approach is especially important for children who are likely to have at least a moderate amount of anxiety because the situation is unfamiliar and they are working with adult strangers. Children are most likely to view adults as authorities, believe that they have little control over the situation, and may be inclined to accept what they perceive the therapist wants. Because CBT is a collaborative process, the therapist must work to develop the relationship and communicate that not only is the child in control to a great extent but that the outcomes of the process will depend substantially on the child's efforts and participation. Through the course of treatment, the child will develop a greater sense of control, a factor that is often lacking in children who experience anxiety and depression.

The Initial Interview with the Anxious Child

Although the majority of children entering therapy for the first time may be apprehensive, anxious children are more likely to show higher levels of worry, fear, and discomfort than adults. They may show high levels of anxious symptoms and have more difficulty expressing themselves at the outset. Because anxious children are unusually sensitive to others' opinions and expectations of them, they may try to meet perceived expectations, be acquiescent, and try to appear confident and capable. They also tend to have a threat attributional style and to have fears of evaluation; therefore, they may be reluctant to say or do things that they believe would make them appear incompetent. Therefore, it is important to lay some initial groundwork for establishing a working relationship by addressing the following.

Initial Discussion with the Child About the Referral

Although children should be given some initial information and explanation of why they are seeing a therapist, often they do not understand what will happen or are told little or nothing by parents or others. An initial question should be "What have you been told about why you are coming here?" If the child does not respond or does not seem to have an understanding of why she is there, a response such as the following could be offered:

"Your parents tell me that you have been worried about some things (difficulties at school, problems with sleeping, etc.), and I wanted to talk with you about that. Is that o.k.?" Most often, the child will assent because they believe they are expected to comply with adults. If, however, the child appears hesitant, unwilling, or otherwise reluctant to engage in conversation, the therapist should engage in rapport-building activities and alternative conversation before pursuing dialogue about the reason for referral. Anxious children may give assent to talking due to tendencies to want to please others, but nevertheless feel uncomfortable. Therefore, the therapist may need to proceed slowly to build rapport and reduce the child's discomfort to a level that permits discussion.

At the point that the clinician determines that the child is willing to engage in some initial discussion of the referral issues and the therapist has gained explicit assent to proceed, the interviewer should again pose a question such as "What have you been told about coming here or why do you think you are here?" If the child does not seem to know, a statement such as "Your mom and dad tell me that you seem to worry a lot and that you are not as happy about things as you used to be. What do you think about that?" can start a conversation. Although it is important to use wording with all children that they are not being blamed for the problems, anxious children are more likely to believe that they are the reason for difficulties. Therefore, care should be taken not to make statements that the child might interpret as being blamed for the problems. As the interview progresses, the therapist should use language and dialogue to communicate that his or her role is to understand the problems, work with the child to develop solutions to the problems, and serve as a coach or educator to develop skills to address them.

Conceptualizing Clinical Problems from a CBT Perspective

Friedberg and McClure (2002) provide a framework for conceptualizing therapy from a CBT perspective that serves as an excellent guide for developing a plan for interventions. Their approach has six steps:

- *Presenting problems*—In this phase, a clinical picture of the referral problems and primary symptoms is developed with clear descriptions of cognitive, behavioral, physiological, and other patterns.
- *Test data*—Formal and informal psychological assessment measures may be used, such as self-report measures of anxiety or depression.
- *Cultural context variables*—In this step, factors such as socioeconomic status, cultural values and beliefs, and family variables are considered with regard to developing the treatment plan.
- *History and developmental milestones*—A careful developmental history is taken to assess factors such as the length of time the problems have existed, family constellation, when developmental milestones were accomplished, personal interests, school success, and interpersonal relationships.
- *Cognitive variables*—Attention is focused on identifying beliefs, distortions, expectations, biases, and other cognitive processes that may contribute to the development and maintenance of the problems.
- *Behavioral antecedents and consequences*—In this phase, factors that tend to trigger behaviors, such as fear or depressed mood, are identified. Also, factors that maintain or exacerbate the symptoms are identified, including parental behaviors or expectations.

From this case conceptualization approach, three products emerge:

1. *Provisional formulation*—The first phase is a clinical picture of the child or adolescent's current circumstances and internal perspective. This phase is not a clinical diagnosis from a DSM-IV perspective but considers the presenting problems, assessment data, cultural context, history and developmental information, behaviors, and cognitive variables that are analyzed and integrated into the clinical picture.
2. *Anticipated treatment plan*—After the provisional formulation is completed, a tentative treatment plan is developed to guide the work between the therapist and the child. Consideration must be given to unique circumstances of the child and the presenting problems, such as the anxious child who might need relaxation training that would not be appropriate for a nonanxious child. The formulation will help to determine which CBT methods are indicated and what modifications might be needed.
3. *Expected obstacles*—In this phase, the therapist tries to anticipate problems that might develop so that the treatment plan can be adapted to address possible barriers.

Cognitive–Behavioral Therapy for Anxiety Disorders

Because anxiety is a basic human emotion, it is not feasible to eliminate it as a symptom of an anxiety disorder. It is associated with normal developmental changes and with reactions to fears and apprehensions of everyday living. Rather, the primary goals of interventions for anxiety using a CBT approach are fivefold: (a) reduce anxiety to manageable levels, rather than complete elimination of symptoms, (b) educate the child about the cognitive, behavioral, affective, and physiological symptoms of anxiety and how they interact and affect functioning, (c) learn new coping and management strategies, (d) practice and implement the learned skills under therapist guidance and coaching, and (e) develop the child's ability to implement these strategies successfully following the formal termination of treatment.

Research Evidence on Cognitive–Behavior Therapy for Anxiety

There is substantial evidence that using CBT to treat anxiety in children has positive outcomes (e.g., Barrett et al., 1996; Kendall et al., 1997) and is considered "probably efficacious" (Ollendick, King, & Chorpita, 2006), indicating that the treatment shows promise of efficacy but that more research is needed. Some studies have used randomized clinical trials, showing medium to large effect sizes comparing clinical groups to wait-list control groups (Barnish & Kendall, 2005; Compton et al., 2004). In a review of treatments using CBT, Cartwright-Hatton, Roberts, Chitsabesan, Fothergill, and Harrington (2004) reported that 56% of treated anxious youth no longer met criteria for their anxiety disorder, and 63% remained without disorder at 6- and 12-month follow-up. One of the advantages of structured or manualized treatment is the control of treatment conditions while being able to adapt and adjust the protocol for individual children. Thus, CBT as an individual, evidence-based intervention for anxiety disorders has sufficient empirical support to judge it to be "probably efficacious," but more research is needed.

Anxious children engage in excessive negative "self-talk" and internal dialogue that exacerbates and perpetuates a cycle of worry, apprehension, anticipation of threat, and negative outcomes. Because cognitions and beliefs are viewed as "behaviors" in cognitive–behavioral theory, they are the targets for intervention. At first impression, adding and developing more positive self-talk might appear to be the primary strategy, under the assumption that positive talk would overshadow or replace negative self-talk. Kendall (1984), however, suggested that the treatment goal should be to reduce negative self-talk and that the therapeutic benefit comes from the development of nonnegative thinking. Treadwell and Kendall (1996) found that changing anxious children's negative self-talk, rather than adding positive self-talk, was the mediator of anxiety reduction. The decrease in negative self-talk is the result of increased problem-solving and coping skills. Table 10.1 presents some examples of changes in cognitions as a result of application of CBT techniques.

Table 10.1 Examples of pretreatment and posttreatment anxious cognitions

Pretreatment cognition	Treatment goal	Posttreatment cognition
"I must be perfect in everything I do"	Reduce negative self-talk that the only acceptable personal standard is perfection	"I don't have to be perfect to be successful and happy in what I do"
"If I don't do well on this test, I will not get into a good college"	Reduce negative self-talk that one possible negative outcome has catastrophic consequences	"Even if I don't do well, I will have many opportunities to do well on other tests and I will be able to go to a good college"
"I do not deserve rewards unless I achieve at a high level"	Reduce negative self-talk that only high achievement is worthy of rewards and to learn how to self-reward	"It is o.k. to reward myself for less than perfect achievement and for putting forth my best effort"
"If I try to become a part of the group, I know I will not be accepted because I'm sure they will not like me"	Reduce negative self-talk that preconceived beliefs are accurate and will lead to negative outcomes	"I do not know if all kids in the group will like me, but I have to try if I want to make friends. I can't expect that everyone will like me and that's o.k."
"I am afraid that if I try to do this, I will fail and everyone will laugh at me, so I am not going to try"	Reduce negative self-talk that failure in inevitable and that social humiliation will occur	"I don't know for sure that I will fail, but if I do not try, I know I cannot succeed. As long as I try my best, what some others may think does not matter that much"

These examples reflect that the therapist works with the child by identifying irrational beliefs and negative self-talk, developing goals to change them, and producing rational, realistic, and productive self-talk. The therapist uses instruction and coaching techniques and materials to control anxiety and reduce negative self-talk. As skills are learned, practiced, and applied, the quality and quantity of negative cognitions are changed, reducing their impact on functioning. This phase of CBT is the educational component where children learn skills, practice them in the safety of the therapeutic environment, make necessary changes, and prepare to apply them in actual settings.

The case of Emily and her need for perfection and high achievement demonstrates how a therapist can obtain information from a client to begin formulating a treatment program.

Therapist: You have said that you feel you have to be perfect in everything you do. Can you tell me more about that?

Emily: I just feel that being perfect or nearly perfect is the only way to be sure I can succeed.

Therapist: Can you give me an example of something where you work to be perfect?

Emily: When I am preparing for a test at school, I will study for hours and hours and go over things many times. It takes me a long time to prepare for things like that. Straight "A's" and being at the top of the class are important to me and I worry about not being able to do that all the time.

Therapist: So, would it be correct to say that you have very high expectations of yourself and being the best and being perfect is very important to you?

Emily: I would say it is more than just very important because I seem to spend most of my time worrying about doing everything perfectly. Whenever I have to take a test, I start thinking about how I need to get a perfect score. It does bother me sometimes and I know I don't have to be perfect to get good grades, but I still do it. Sometimes, I even think it's silly, but I still feel I need to be perfect.

Therapist: Does this working and worrying interfere with other parts of your life?

Emily: It does, because I don't have many outside interests and don't spend as much time with my friends as I would like.

Therapist: On a scale of 1 to 10, how much does this worrying and perfectionism bother you?

Emily: I'd say it would be at least a "9."

Therapist: Would you like to change so that you don't worry about this as much and it doesn't interfere with other things?

Emily: I would like to but I don't want to take a chance on not doing my best. I also worry a lot about letting my parents down if I don't do my best. Maybe I shouldn't feel this way, but I do.

Therapist: Do you know other people who do about as well as you do who are not as perfectionistic?

Emily: My best friend, Susan, is a very good student and does not feel the way I do. She also has a lot more time for hobbies and friends than I do.

Therapist: So, you know at least one person who does well, but does not think the way you do?

Emily: Yes, and I probably should be more like her, but I can't seem to do that.

Therapist: If you were to try to make some changes, what would they be?

Emily: I still want to achieve well, but I would like to feel that I don't have to do everything perfectly. I realize that working to be perfect is making me tense and upset sometimes, but right now, I can't seem to separate them.

Therapist: But you said your friend Susan can do that, so it seems that it is possible. What makes you think you can't?

Emily: I don't really know, but, now that you mention it, maybe I can be successful but not be so perfectionistic.

Therapist: Is that something you think you would like to work on?

Emily: Yes, I would, but it seems like it's going to be hard to do.
Therapist: Change can be hard at times, and I am here to help you accomplish your goal, and we can work together. Perhaps we can discover some new ways of thinking and behaving that may help you be more effective in dealing with these thoughts. Would that be o.k. with you?
Emily: Yes, I would like to give it a try.

Analysis of the Dialogue

In this dialogue, the therapist does several things. The questions asked are designed to gather information on Emily's perspective on her thoughts and beliefs, rather than clarifying symptoms from a diagnostic perspective. The dialogue is problem-focused, and the therapist does not spend time searching for the causes of the problem or suggesting that it is a personality deficit that must be corrected. The therapist does not state or imply that any of Emily's beliefs are irrational, incorrect, or otherwise judged to be inappropriate. However, Emily did state that she realized she does not have to get perfect scores on tests to do well or get "As," and she has some awareness that it may be irrational (i.e., "silly" and "Maybe I shouldn't feel this way") to think this way. A key component of CBT treatment for anxiety is helping the client to become aware that some thinking is irrational and is contributing to the problems. Questions are asked that elicit information from Emily directly to develop an initial assessment of her cognitions about perfectionism and how it affects her. The therapist begins to challenge her thinking by pointing out that not everyone who is highly achievement motivated has a high level of perfectionism. However, the therapist avoids looking for the causes of the dysfunctional beliefs and does not "interpret" them to Emily. As therapy proceeds, focus remains on the dysfunctional beliefs and developing skills to help her change her negative thinking. Emily shows the typical attribution of the perception of threat that most children do not experience, who enjoy going to school and do not experience it as anxiety-producing. In this dialogue, Emily's threat attribution is that if she is not perfect, she will fail.

Emily's automatic thoughts are contained in her schemata that she must be perfect, which are activated to a high level when she must perform. She has some awareness that her thoughts are irrational and illogical but is uncertain if she can modify them enough to reduce the impact on her functioning. She maintains some uncertainty whether she can separate needs for achievement and perfectionism but indicates a desire to go forward. Acknowledgement that the perfectionism bothers her to a significant degree ("at least a 9 on a 10-point scale") suggests that she may become amenable to changing her dysfunctional beliefs and behavior.

Finally, the therapist follows Emily's statement that she would like to work on the problems and seeks her consent to participate and collaborate in therapy. The therapist communicates that therapy is a collaborative process and that her cooperation and commitment are essential. The therapist is not presented as an "expert" who will "fix" her problem. At this point, the nature and process of the therapy would be explained, and Emily and the therapist would continue to develop the collaborative relationship. The degree to which the family would be involved in the treatment process would require further assessment and planning.

Exposure Component

In additional to the focus on the beliefs and beliefs of the client, CBT also uses direct exposure to anxiety-producing stimuli, especially when treating specific problems, such as fears, evaluative situations, and tasks that cannot be avoided. The primary premise is that systematic, graded exposure to the anxiety-producing event improves the ability to develop coping strategies to reduce anxiety. As children develop new skills to cope with their symptoms, they are exposed to more anxiety-producing situations. Exposure to low anxiety-producing situations occurs first where learned skills are practiced, followed by moderate and then higher anxiety-producing stimuli as the child improves the ability to cope with situations. If the progression is too rapid, then the process is slowed and returned to prior levels where anxiety was manageable. At the beginning, the therapist may use imaginal techniques, where the child imagines being in the anxiety-producing situation. After the ability to handle imaginal situations with little or no anxiety is developed, the child is gradually exposed to in vivo situations, where placement in the actual setting is introduced gradually. These in vivo situations are important because the child applies the strategies in actual anxiety-inducing situations.

These exposure activities are developed in collaboration between the child and therapist, and methods are included in the process for feedback and modifications as needed. When not in the therapist's office, the child keeps notes of practice sessions at home and elsewhere, feelings and moods between sessions, and evaluation of the effectiveness of practice. This information is reviewed with the therapist during each treatment session. The actual process may be based in preestablished treatment protocols, such as manualized programs, or through programs developed for a child's specific symptoms.

Exposure Hierarchies

Whether exposure to anxiety-producing stimuli is imaginal or in vivo, both methods involve the development of hierarchies linked to the child's initial and progressive levels of anxiety. Through the collaborative process, the therapist and child develop a hierarchy for each specific fear or situation, beginning with an image or action that produces little or no anxiety for the child. Then, a fear or situation that produces a slightly higher level of anxiety is identified and placed next in the hierarchy. The process continues until a hierarchy of several steps is identified that the child agrees is reasonable. As treatment progresses, the hierarchy is subject to change by adding, removing, or rearranging steps, depending on the child's response at each level. The exposure process gradually desensitizes the child to the anxiety-producing stimulus, creating a new schema and reducing the automatic thoughts and tendencies to avoid situations that cause anxiety. For some children, Friedberg and McClure (2002) suggest that perhaps writing the steps down on cards and then having the child arrange them in order of anxiety-producing intensity may be more useful.

Each of the steps in the hierarchy is assigned a number, typically ranging from 1 to 100, that indicates the least to most anxiety-producing step. The child is asked to report this number, known as a *subjective unit of distress*. Used by the client to indicate the level of the anxiety and how it changes over the course of therapy. For children and young adolescents, a smaller range may be better, such as from 1 to 10, because they may not be able make fine discriminations in a 100-point scale.

Systematic Desensitization

Both in vivo and imaginal approaches are forms of *systematic desensitization* that use hierarchies to reduce anxiety. For some problems, each approach is used separately, while both approaches may be used for other problems. Both methods involve the child in practice of skills and gradual exposure to situations that elicit anxiety. The child identifies the event or circumstance that causes anxiety and that is to be overcome. Then, the therapist works with the child to develop the hierarchy that will be followed. In an in vivo approach, actual events or situations are identified that will be the settings where new skills are practiced. An example of an in vivo desensitization is shown in developing a hierarchy for a child who is highly anxious about going to school. In this approach, the child develops strategies and behaviors to improve the ability to be in a school setting. In imaginal approaches, the hierarchy is presented in the therapist's office with another neutral stimulus, such as relaxation, play, or other activities. An example of an imaginal approach is when the therapist and the child develop a hierarchy of steps about fear of going to school and pair the hierarchy with relaxation training. The goal of this approach is to help the child to recognize automatic thinking that contributes to fears of failure or apprehension. In some cases, imaginal and in vivo approaches may be used together to accomplish treatment goals. Following is a dialogue between Michael and a CBT therapist about fear of going to school.

Therapist: So, Michael, I understand that you are going to start at a new school and you are very worried and nervous about it. Do you want to be able to go to this new school?

Michael: Well, I have to go, but I miss my friends at my old school and I do not make new friends that easy.

Therapist: That is very understandable. Leaving friends and starting at a new place can be difficult for lots of people.

Michael:	Yeah, I have done this before and it doesn't seem to get any easier. I know I have to do it, but it's still hard. Do you think there is something wrong with me?
Therapist:	Your feelings are not unusual and it happens to a lot of people when they have to make changes, so it does not mean that there is something wrong with you. I think that if we can work together, we can come up with a plan that will help you to go to this new school more easily. One way to start is to figure out a series of steps that might help us to understand how much anxiety you feel as you think about going to school. Would you like to try that?
Michael:	O.k., what do we have to do?
Therapist:	We would figure out some steps that involve getting ready to go to school all the way to actually being there and find ways to make it easier at each step. The steps would be based completely on what you think and feel. Once we know all of these small steps, then we can begin practicing them and gradually moving from home to your classroom desk.
Michael:	O.k. Let's give it a try.
Therapist:	As you think about going to this new school, what would be the worst part of it that would make you the most anxious?
Michael:	The worst part would be actually going into the classroom and sitting down at a desk.
Therapist:	As you think about what you would have to do to get to this classroom, what would you have to do that would not cause you to worry or be anxious?
Michael:	I would be fine at home having breakfast and getting dressed.
Therapist:	Let's start with something that doesn't bother you too much about going to the new school. After you have breakfast and got dressed, what would go next that might make you just a little bit more anxious?
Michael:	Putting on my coat and backpack would be next.
Therapist:	O.k., so that would be step two. What would be next?
Michael:	Opening the front door and going outside.
Therapist:	Step 3. What would be next and cause a bit more anxiety?
Michael:	Going to the car and opening the car door.
Therapist:	So going to the car and opening the car door would be step 4. What would be next and cause slightly more anxiety?
Michael:	Sitting down in the car and fastening my seat belt.
Therapist:	So that would be step 5. What would be next?
Michael:	I'm not sure, maybe getting to school?
Therapist:	Would there be something in between getting in the car and getting to school that might make you more anxious than sitting down in the car and fastening your seat belt? Is there something that has bothered you in the past about this?
Michael:	Well, when I'm riding to school, I get nervous as I get closer. I can just feel myself getting more uptight and stressed out the closer I get.

	Definitely riding in the car as I get nearer the school would make me anxious.
Therapist:	So, it seems like getting closer to school is a time when you are especially aware of your physical signs of anxiety and how you think and feel about it. Does that sound about right?
Michael:	Absolutely and I hadn't realized it until you said that. If I could learn how to relax and not be as tense as I get closer to school, I think that would help.
Therapist:	This is an example of how your thoughts, feelings, and physical signs occur together when you are anxious. If you can learn how to handle them together, you may feel less anxious in other situations. So, should we add a step about riding in the car here?
Michael:	That makes sense to me. So what step is that?
Therapist:	That would be step 6. What would be next?
Michael:	The next one would be arriving at school.
Therapist:	Step 7. What is next?
Michael:	Opening the car door and getting out.
Therapist:	So opening the car door and getting out would be step 8. What is next?
Michael:	Walking up the sidewalk to the door.
Therapist:	All right, that is Step 9. And what is next?
Michael:	Opening the door and walking in.
Therapist:	Step 10. And next?
Michael:	Walking down the hall and arriving at the classroom door.
Therapist:	That would be step 11. What would be next?
Michael:	Opening the door and going into the room.
Therapist:	Step 12. So now you are in the room and are getting closer to your desk. What would be next?
Michael:	The next step would be sitting down at my desk.
Therapist:	So that is step 13 and you have sat down at your desk, which is what you were most afraid of. Does this seem like a good set of steps to you?
Michael:	Yes, it does, at least for now.
Therapist:	So we have 13 steps. What we will do now is practice each of these steps here until you feel comfortable with them. When you feel comfortable with each one, we will move to the next one and practice them altogether. Eventually, we want to get to the point where you can get up in the morning, have breakfast, get dressed, ride to school, get out and go to your classroom, and sit in your desk and feel comfortable.
Michael:	That sounds like a big accomplishment and I would be very happy if I could pull it off but even thinking about it makes me anxious.
Therapist:	It is very natural and normal to feel anxious about doing new things and many others your age often feel the same way. As we work together, we will find ways to help you deal with situations that make you anxious.

Analysis of the Dialogue

In this example, Michael has done the major work of establishing the hierarchy with the therapist's guidance. As the hierarchy is implemented, the child and therapist may decide that some steps can be added, deleted, consolidated, or rearranged. Eventually, a final hierarchy is established that produces the desired results with continued, gradual exposure leading to minimal anxiety that does not interfere with school. Generally, 8–12 steps in a hierarchy are reasonable, although more or fewer may be needed in some situations. Too few steps may not allow the child to master anxiety sufficiently to move to the next step comfortably, while too many make it difficult for the child to distinguish meaningful differences between steps, wasting time and effort for little benefit.

The same process is used in imaginal desensitization, except that muscle relaxation is introduced simultaneously with principles of counterconditioning. Through deep muscle training and relaxation, the child experiences a highly relaxed state while the hierarchy is presented from the least to most anxious. This approach uses the concept of *reciprocal inhibition*, a method of behavior therapy where one behavior is inhibited by the co-occurrence of another incompatible behavior. In imaginal desensitization, anxiety cannot occur simultaneously with relaxation; thus, it is inhibited from occurring.

It is beyond the scope of this chapter to give detailed instruction in relaxation training, but the general format is to teach the child to go through progressive tension and relaxation of major muscle groups beginning with head and neck muscles and moving through the body to the legs and feet. After the child is in a highly relaxed state, the hierarchy is introduced from the least to most anxious. While relaxed, the child is asked to imagine each of the steps in the hierarchy and indicate when anxiety increases. At that point, the therapist returns to the prior step to reduce anxiety and then moves forward when the child is comfortable. The process continues until the child reaches the top level in the hierarchy and is comfortable imagining being in the situation.

As each step is presented, the child indicates by a simple movement or comments if anxiety becomes too intense. The therapist returns to a prior step in the hierarchy that did not produce anxiety and repeats the process until anxiety is minimized. Then, the next step is presented and the process continues. If treatment is successful, the child eventually will be able to master the last step of the hierarchy with little or no anxiety. As the child becomes more skilled at relaxation, it can be self-induced at home or at school through self-instruction or by playing a recording of the therapeutic session. Often, moving through a hierarchy requires more than one session with the therapist and the relaxation procedure in induced each time prior to presenting the hierarchy. Typically, some steps of the hierarchy are introduced at subsequent sessions to assure that there has been no relapse and that prior steps do not cause anxiety. If anxiety is shown at some prior steps, the process is repeated. Less time likely will be needed to move through previously practiced steps, and then steps not yet addressed are attempted. Imaginal desensitization may be done alone or combined with in vivo desensitization with the same hierarchy.

Muscle Relaxation Training

In deep muscle relaxation, the child is instructed to follow a series of steps for each muscle group: (a) tense the specific muscle, but not to the point of extreme discomfort, (b) maintain the muscle tension for 5–10 seconds while focusing on its unpleasantness, (c) relax the muscle back to its original state, and (d) upon relaxation for about 30 seconds, focus on the difference between the tensed and relaxed state and how pleasant it feels to be relaxed. The process is repeated two to three times for each muscle, which is followed in the same way for the next muscle. The process begins at the head and moves downward to the feet, each time going back to the previous muscle, adding it to the sequence, and progressing forward. The setting for relaxation training should be a quiet room with low illumination and a comfortable chair. The therapist should talk in a low, quite, and somewhat monotone manner to instill and maintain a relaxed state. In most cases, a full training session can be completed in about 15–30 minutes, depending on the number of muscles to be relaxed and the child's responsiveness. An example of a sequence is:

- Closing the eyes firmly
- Clenching of the teeth and mouth
- Tensing of the neck muscles
- Tensing of the shoulders
- Pulling the arms up to the body and then back to a comfortable position
- Clenching of the fists
- Tensing of the stomach muscles
- Tensing of the thigh muscles
- Tensing of the calf muscles
- Tensing of the ankles and feet

Anxiety Intervention Programs

Intervention programs can be established for specific behaviors, such as performance anxiety or specific fears. Many programs use a multiple session format contained in a manual for the therapist to follow, and the child often has a workbook or package of assignments to complete at various points during the treatment. Usually, about half of the sessions are designed to teach anxiety reduction and coping methods, with the remainder designed to practice the learned skills in actual settings. Each session typically includes a "mood check-in" to monitor the child's mood and progress from week to week. At first impression, a manualized approach might seem to be rigid and not individualized for the child. In fact, manualized approaches are flexible and can and should be adapted to the specific needs of the child, rate of progress, specific symptoms, and the amount of training and practice necessary to go to the next step.

One of the most well-known and empirically supported anxiety reduction programs is *Coping Cat* by Kendall and Hedtke (2006). The *Coping Cat* program is a manualized treatment approach to treat generalized anxiety and related symptoms with the goal to enable the child to function without therapy after several sessions of treatment. The program is evidence-based and is composed of a therapist's handbook and a workbook for the child with examples and homework to be completed over several weeks. Specific activities are planned for each session, but flexibility is given to the therapist to make some adjustments in the program. The program is designed to be used with individuals or groups. It is based upon the FEAR acronym:

F = Feeling Frightened (recognition of physical symptoms)
E = Expecting bad things to happen (recognition of anxious self-talk)
A = Attitudes and Actions that are effective (use of behaviors and coping self-talk)
R = Results and Rewards (child self-evaluates and self-rewards for effort)

Feeling Frightened

This part of the *Coping Cat* program focuses on helping the child to recognize and cope with the physiological symptoms of anxiety when they occur. Treatment activities include using materials from the workbook, role playing, modeling, and focusing on helping the child to use muscle relaxation techniques to reduce tension and sensations.

Expecting Bad Things to Happen

This component is consistent with the anxious child's tendency to have an attributional bias toward threat and the associated expectation of negative outcomes. This bias contributes to the child's misinterpretation of events and the development and automatic use of negative self-talk. Working together, the therapist and child develop strategies to replace negative thoughts. Because young children and adolescents often are not accustomed to identifying and talking about feelings and cognitions, the *Coping Cat* workbook contains worksheets using cartoon characters and drawings, and the child might be presented with a task to write down what a character is thinking. Then, the child is asked about his own thoughts prior to beginning to change negative self-talk.

Actions and Attitudes

There are two primary goals in this step: (a) help the child to develop problem-solving strategies to cope with anxiety and (b) encourage the child not to use maladaptive strategies. A five-step problem-solving approach is taught: (a) the child is encouraged to approach the situation as a problem and to set goals, (b) the therapist and child generate possible alternatives with little evaluation or judgment, regardless of how feasible they may or may not be, (c) after generating possible solutions, each is evaluated by the child and therapist to determine if they are likely to be effective, (d) from the viable alternatives, one is selected to be used, and (e) a plan is made to put the chosen alternative into action. The therapist models strategies and behaviors, and the child is asked to observe and practice them. Workbook activities supplement the problem-solving training to prepare the child to use these newly acquired skills in nonclinic settings. By acquiring and practicing new skills that are effective, new attitudes toward anxiety-producing situation will develop simultaneously with a reduction in negative self-talk.

Results and Rewards

The final step of the FEAR plan involves teaching the child to self-monitor behavior and to learn the use of contingency management for successful coping with anxiety. Positive reinforcement is used and may be self-administered, or the therapist may work with the parent to assist the child. Rewards may be given for demonstrating effective coping strategies, changing ineffective cognitions (e.g., reduction of perfectionistic attitudes, reduced catastrophizing), developing new strategies, or effort. The therapist teaches the child how to self-rate and record progress using informal rating methods.

Coping Cat Session Format

The Coping Cat program consists of 16 sessions and two parent sessions that are summarized below:

1. Describe the program and build rapport with the child.
2. Review the goals of treatment; begin helping the child to identify feelings and distinguish anxious, worried feelings from others; encourage the child to use bodily cues to identify different feelings (e.g., facial expression, body position).
3. Review distinguishing anxious, worried feelings from other feelings; child learns more about somatic responses to anxiety and identifying somatic responses.
4. Normalize the experience of anxiety; review goals of treatment and discuss expectations for outcomes; begin to construct a hierarchy of anxiety-eliciting situations.
5. A parent session is conducted at this point to maintain contact and cooperation with the parents and to gather additional information about the child's needs.
6. Begin creating a hierarchy of anxiety-eliciting situations; introduce relaxation training; review of recognizing somatic cues that show tension and anxiety; demonstrate the connection between somatic cues and relaxation exercises.

7. Review relaxation training; introduce the function of personal thoughts and their impact on responses in anxiety-producing situations; help the child to recognize self-talk (expectations, automatic questions, and attributions) in anxious situations and to develop and use less anxiety-producing self-talk.

8. Review the concept of anxious self-talk and reinforce modification of anxious self-talk into coping self-talk; introduce the concept of developing and using strategies to manage anxiety.

9. Review relaxation training; introduce the concept of evaluating or rating one's performance and self-rewards for performance; review other steps in the plan for coping with anxiety.

10. Review all previously introduced skills by formalizing the four-step FEAR plan to use when feeling anxious and practicing its use in nonstressful situations.

   Feeling frightened? (Recognizing the anxiety or fear).
   Expecting bad things to happen. (Recognizing the anxious self-talk).
   Actions and attitudes that will help? (Developing coping strategies).
   Ratings and reward? (Self-evaluation and self-reward).

   Mid-assessment session occurs here to review and summarize skills presented in the first half of the treatment; also work with parents to design in vivo experiences to meet the child's needs.

11. Describe the change in types of activities from the training segment to the practice segment; in group treatment, this session includes a group social event to celebrate the skills learned and to continue to heighten group cohesion and affiliation.

12. Practice the four-step coping plan under low anxiety-provoking conditions, including imaginal and in vivo. (If using a group approach, all children are involved.)

13. Practice applying skills for coping and in vivo situations that produce low to moderate levels of anxiety. (If using a group approach, all children are involved.)

14. Practice applying the skills for coping with anxiety in in vivo situations that produce high levels of anxiety. (If using a group approach, all children are involved.)

15. Practice applying skills for coping with anxiety in in vivo situations that produce low to moderate levels of anxiety; in vivo involves individual children and other group members are observers or participants, depending on the nature of the individual child's fears; each child prepares an in vivo situation that is tailored to his/her unique anxiety and fears; compare self-rating of performance with those of other observers using recorded session as demonstrative aid.

16. Continue practice of applying skills for coping in in vivo situations that produce high levels of anxiety in each child. (This session involves individual children.)

17. Continue practicing applying skills for coping with anxiety in in vivo situations that produce high levels of anxiety. (This session involves individual children.)

18. Continue practicing applying skills for coping with anxiety in in vivo situations that produce high levels of anxiety. (This session involves individual children.)

Postassessment sessions are conducted to review and summarize the treatment program, make plans with the parents to help maintain and generalize skills, and bring closure to the therapeutic relationship.

Camp Cope-a-Lot

Camp Cope-A-Lot (Kendall, 2008) is an interactive computer program consisting of 12 sessions to treat child anxiety. It is based on the *Coping Cat* program and contains high-quality graphics and contest that is engaging for children with anxiety. The reader is referred to www.workbookpublishing.com for more information on the program.

Involvement of Parents

Parents are not involved in the program sessions and do not participate directly in the treatment of the child. Instead, the parents provide important historical, developmental, and diagnostic information and are informed about the nature of the treatment so that they can determine if it is acceptable. They serve as consultants and collaborators and meet with the therapist after sessions four and nine to discuss the treatment plan. The therapist also offers suggestions to parents that they can use to help facilitate treatment activities and effects at home and continues to offer support to the family.

The *Coping Cat* program is not designed to conduct family therapy but to focus on helping the child to develop effective anxiety-reducing strategies. It may be that there is some significant parental or family psychopathology that should be addressed, but the focus of the *Coping Cat* and similar programs is on the child. A thorough assessment of family dynamics and individual psychopathology may be indicated before family treatment is undertaken. If such treatment is indicated, there is a family *Coping Cat* program that uses similar strategies and actively involves parents (Howard, Chu, Krain Marrs-Garcia, & Kendall, 2000).

The FRIENDS Program

Parents most often refer their children for psychological treatment, rather than the children referring themselves. Children may have some implicit understanding that they are feeling distress but are not likely to have familiarity with understanding of psychotherapy or counseling. They are not likely to ask their parents to get help for them, and they may be reluctant, perhaps due to fears of retaliation, feelings of blame, or about admitting there is a problem. Parents are more likely to refer when the perceived problems have reached a high level of intensity where significant disruption in personal, social, family, or academic functioning is occurring. In some cases, working with the family may be indicated, either to assist with treating the child's anxiety or to address parental psychopathology or family dysfunctions that contribute to the problems. This discussion will not focus on parental or family psychopathology per se, but upon involving parents in the treatment of childhood anxiety. The *FRIENDS* program (Barrett, Lowry-Webster, & Turner, 2000a, b, c, d, e, f) focuses on parents as well as anxious children. "FRIENDS" is an acronym for the program that emerged from Kendall's *Coping Cat* program:

Feeling Worried?
Relax and Feel Good
Inner Thoughts
Explore Plans
Don't Forget to Practice
Stay Calm, You Know How to Cope Now

There is a child component in *FRIENDS* that evolved from the Australian version of the *Coping Cat* program, the *Coping Koala* program. The same principles inherent in CBT and the *Coping Cat* program are found in the *FRIENDS* program. Parents are included in the *FRIENDS* program from two perspectives: (a) they can be effective in facilitating new experiences that can give the anxious child more opportunities to practice newly acquired skills and (b) to model adaptive beliefs and cognitive processing on a daily basis. Also, parents may learn how some of their behaviors may have contributed to or helped to maintain child and youth anxiety and learn how to modify or stop those behaviors. As discussed in Chap. 3, parental behavior such as anxiety, overcontrol, and reinforcement of avoidant behavior may contribute to a child's anxiety. High levels of parent anxiety may have a negative or less productive effect on treatment. Cobham, Dadds, and Spence (1998) found that children with one or more parents with an anxiety disorder responded less well to treatment. Comorbidity of anxiety and depression was shown in a study by Southam-Gerow, Kendall, and Weersing (2001), who found that maternal self-reports of higher levels of depressive symptoms were associated with less favorable outcomes of CBT with anxious youth.

The *FRIENDS* program has four main goals: (a) to help children view their body as their friend as it alerts them when they are feeling anxiety or distress, (b) be their own friend and reward themselves for their efforts, (c) make friends to help build social support networks, and (d) talk to their friends when they face difficult or worry situations. The program uses peer learning, experiential learning, and family-directed problem solving, with emphasis on the learning, cognitive, and physiological components. Specific skills are taught in each of these three areas that maintain anxiety. The child is taught specific skills and parents are taught how to help create opportunities to practice these skills in daily life. Similar to the *Coping Cat* program and other anxiety treatments, techniques include teaching problem solving, use of rewards, reduction of negative self-talk, self-reward, and learning relaxation and deep breathing activities. The program consists of ten sessions and two "booster" sessions for children and youth.

The first three sessions focus on building group participations, cohesion, and therapy guidelines and teach about identifications of emotions, the links between thoughts and feelings, and skill development. The next six sessions focus on the various components of the *FRIENDS* program with training in problem-solving skills and exposure included. The last session emphasizes the development of generalization and maintenance of strategies. The two "booster" sessions review the various strategies taught in the program.

The parent component consists of four sessions that include:

1. Explanation of the *FRIENDS* program, learning deep breathing and muscle relaxation, and the physiological, cognitive, and learned aspects of anxiety.
2. Parents work on identifying their own thoughts, their child's thoughts, and learn and practice problem-solving skills.
3. Learning about reinforcement, rewarding their child for effort, evaluating progress, and how they as parents approach situations.
4. Learning skills for developing positive family skills, parents working together to present a common approach to their child's anxiety, and strategies for maintenance, addressing potential difficulties, and continued practice.

Evidence of Efficacy for Family Intervention for Childhood Anxiety Disorders

One of the first studies to involve families in treatment of childhood anxiety was conducted by Howard and Kendall (1996) who worked with six clinically anxious children aged 9–13. The treatment protocol included CBT with the children and parent involvement using a multiple baseline design. They found significant improvement in diagnostic status, improvement in child and parent report measures, and parent and child reports of postintervention coping skills.

Kendall, Hudson, Gosch, Flannery-Schroeder, and Suveg (2008) used a randomized clinical treatment design to assess the effects of child and family modalities in the treatment of anxiety. Individual cognitive–behavioral treatment (ICBT), family cognitive–behavioral therapy (FCBT), and family-based education/support/attention (FESA) active control groups with random assignment to treatment conditions were used with children aged 7–14 who had a principal diagnosis of separation anxiety disorder, social phobia, or generalized anxiety disorder. Children showed improvement in all conditions, although ICBT and FCBT were superior to FESA in reducing the presence and severity of the primary anxiety disorder and ICBT was considered superior to FCBT by teachers' reports of child anxiety. Documented treatment gains were maintained at 1-year follow-up. When both parents had an anxiety disorder, FCBT outperformed ICBT. This study suggests that CBT approaches are effective and that the introduction of family-based treatment can add to positive outcomes. The authors concluded that ICBT and FCBT were comparable in their effects and that including parents is not essential to therapeutic gains in anxiety-disordered children. Parents are involved in ICBT, however, in their role as collaborators; therefore, it would be incorrect to assume that they should not be involved with their child's treatment. For the youth who did not show gains, parental involvement did not account for the lack of benefit. Of particular note is that teachers reported improvement in child anxiety symptoms, although they knew little about the treatment itself or the condition to which each child was assigned. These data provide evidence of external validity for the effects of the cognitive–behavioral treatment, whether it is individual or family-focused.

Having anxious and nonanxious parents in the study was considered from two perspectives: (a) did treatment for child anxiety affect parental anxiety and (b) did parental anxiety moderate child outcomes? The data indicated that about 40% of maternal diagnoses of anxiety were not found at posttreatment, but there was no difference across treatment conditions. There was a moderating effect of mother anxiety on child outcomes, i.e., children of nonanxious mothers were significantly more likely to be free of their principal diagnosis at follow-up compared to children with anxious mothers. The authors concluded that "…the presence or persistence of a parental anxiety disorder seems to detract from treatment of a youth anxiety disorder" (p. 295).

Considerations for Involving Parents in Treatment for Child and Youth Anxiety Disorders

There is no question that parents should be involved in the treatment of anxiety disorders, but the issue of whether they should be involved as collaborators or co-clients is an important clinical consideration. The Kendall et al. (2008) study suggests that direct parental involvement is not necessary to produce positive child outcomes and that parents who have anxiety disorders may have a moderating effect of treatment efficacy. Some considerations regarding the extent of parental involvement include:

- Whether the parents have significant anxiety disorders that might impact treatment
- Whether the parents are committed to positive outcomes for the child
- Whether the parents can serve as effective collaborators in treatment
- Whether there is significant family psychopathology, such as marital distress
- Whether there is significant parental psychopathology that is best addressed in adult treatment

Despite the research evidence on the involvement of parents in the direct treatment of childhood anxiety disorders, however, it is recommended that parents be actively included as collaborators and facilitators in treatment. Their help should be enlisted to create opportunities for the child to practice newly learned skills, such as taking the child to social events, practicing new skills learned in therapy (e.g., speaking in public), and providing rewards and encouragement as treatment progresses.

Parents may also benefit from psychoeducational sessions to learn about anxious symptomatology, how they may be reinforcing the child's behavior, and how they may be imbibing the development of coping skills. If parents feel that they are a part of the treatment process, they are more likely to continue involving the child in therapy and helping to maintain long-term outcomes.

Pharmacotherapy

The use of medications to treat childhood anxiety disorders has increased over the last several years, although there is not a vast amount of research on the types of drugs and their effects on children. Compared to adults, there are fewer studies on whether medications are effective or have long-term side effects in their use with children, especially young children. Consequently, the use of medications to treat pediatric anxiety remains controversial. Nevertheless, medications to treat anxiety disorders in children are prescribed frequently, and the psychologist is in an important position to observe, monitor, and evaluate their effects and to serve as a collaborator with parents and prescribers.

Medications Used to Treat Anxiety in Children and Adolescents

Antidepressants

The primary medications used to treat anxiety symptoms and disorders in children and adolescents include antidepressants in three groups: (a) selective serotonin reuptake inhibitors (SSRIs), (b) tricyclics (TCAs), and (c) monoamine oxidase inhibitors (MAOIs). Although these medications are most often used to treat depression, they are often effective for treating anxiety. SSRIs affect the transmission of serotonin in brain cells, enabling them to better communicate with each other. They represent the newer class of antidepressants and have few side effects.

The TCAs are older drugs to treat depression but can be used to treat anxiety symptoms. TCAs block reabsorption (reuptake) of serotonin and norepinephrine by brain cells and may also inhibit reuptake of dopamine. They also block other cell receptors, which account for some of their side effects, including dry mouth, dizziness, blurred visions, constipation, drowsiness, nausea, increased blood pressure, headaches, weight gain, and disorientation and confusion (Mayo Clinic, 2008).

MAOIs are the oldest of the antidepressants but continue to be used in some cases and can relieve anxiety symptoms. Their actions prevent the enzyme monoamine from oxidizing serotonin, norepinephrine, and dopamine, keeping these neurotransmitters at levels that maintain a high level of mood. Some of the side effects of MAOIs are similar to those of TCAs, although there are more of them and they can be more severe. The side effects include constipation, nausea, diarrhea, stomach upset, fatigue, dry mouth, dizziness, low blood pressure, light-headedness, decreased urine output, decreased sexual function, sleep disturbances, muscle twitching, weight gain, blurred vision, headache, increased appetite, restlessness, shakiness, trembling, weakness, and increased perspiration. Due to these serious side effects and interactions with certain foods, over-the-counter medications, herbal supplements, and SSRIs, they are not recommended unless other medications are ineffective (Mayo Clinic, 2008; National Institutes of Mental Health, n.d.). In rare cases, the simultaneous use of SSRIs and MAOIs can result in a condition called "serotonin syndrome" where serotonin levels become too elevated, which can lead to fluctuations in blood pressure, confusion, nausea and vomiting, restlessness, hallucinations, extreme agitation, increased heart rate, seizures, coma, or death (Mayo Clinic).

Antianxiety Medications

More recently, medications that specifically address anxiety symptoms have been developed. Most of these medications are benzodiazepines that have few side effects. The most common members of this group are clonazepam, lorazepam, and alprazolam. Buspirone, an azapirone, is a more recent drug that treats generalized anxiety disorder (National Institutes of Mental Health, n.d.). Appendix D lists some of the medications commonly used to treat anxiety, primary side effects, and the disorders for which they are often prescribed. It should be noted that more medications are available to treat anxiety, but they may not be approved for use with children, are not commonly prescribed, or there are insufficient data about them.

Evidence of the Efficacy of Medications to Treat Anxiety Disorders in Children and Adolescents

The biology of anxiety disorders is focused on the role of stress and associated responses in the development of anxiety. The primary brain centers involved in stress–response systems are the brainstem arousal centers, the amygdala in the anterior temporal lobe, the septohippocampal system, the orbital-frontal cortex, anterior cingulate gyrus, and the dorsolateral and ventromedial prefrontal cortex. Much of the research on medications that impact these central nervous system structures has yielded important information about the role of these structures in stress–response mechanisms and anxiety disorders (Helm, Owens, Plotsky, & Nemeroff, 1997).

Brain mechanisms that are involved in a child's response to threat are inherent in the central nervous system and contribute to the expression of anxiety in everyday life and, when severe or chronic, increase the likelihood for anxiety disorders. Presumably, medications help to treat anxiety disorders by reregulating neurotransmitters involved in the stress–response system. The combination of medications with psychological therapy reflects the biopsychosocial approach to treatment. Following is a summary of research on the use of medications for treatment of major anxiety disorders.

Separation Anxiety Disorder

Imipramine has been used to treat Separation Anxiety Disorder (SAD), but the results have been mixed (e.g., Bernstein et al., 2000; Gittleman-Klein & Klein, 1971; Klein, Koplewicz, & Kanner, 1992), partially due to treatment design and comorbidity of depression. Although benzodiazepines have been tried in the treatment of SAD, they can cause behavioral disinhibition in children, which can contradict their use. The Research Unit of Pediatric Psychopharmacology (RUPP) Anxiety Group (2001, 2003) found that fluvoxamine produced an improvement rate of 78% in a group of children with SAD, social anxiety disorder, and GAD compared to 29% in a placebo group. These data suggest that the SSRIs may be useful in treating SAD and also have the advantage of few side effects.

Generalized Anxiety Disorder

The RUPP (2001, 2003) studies cited above found that fluvoxamine was better than a placebo, but unlike social anxiety disorder, GAD was not found to be a predictor of nonresponse to the medication. Rynn, Siqueland, and Rickels (2001) found that sertraline was effective compared to a placebo in the treatment of GAD in children and adolescents. There is some evidence that fluoxetine may have benefit for treating child and adolescent overanxious disorder, separation anxiety disorder, and social phobia (Birmaher et al., 1994; Fairbanks et al., 1997). In general, however, the research evidence on medication treatment of GAD in children and adolescents is limited.

Obsessive–Compulsive Disorder

The use of medication to treat OCD in children and adolescents has been studied rather extensively compared to other childhood anxiety disorders. Studies have found that fluoxetine, fluvoxamine, and sertraline were superior to placebo in the treatment of OCD in children and youth (e.g., Geller, Hoag et al., 2001; March et al., 1998; Riddle et al., 2001). The safety of the SSRIs suggests that they may produce good outcomes with relatively little risk of side effects.

Social Phobia/Social Anxiety Disorder

Studies using medications to treat childhood social phobia/social anxiety disorder (SAD) were conducted by the Research Unit of Pediatric Psychopharmacology

(RUPP) Anxiety Group (2001, 2003). Using fluvoxamine to treat anxiety disorders in children and adolescents, the RUPP group found that the medication was superior to a placebo, but a SAD diagnosis was a moderator of treatment outcome, in that those with SAD did not respond as well to the medication as did participants with GAD or separation anxiety.

Specific Phobia

There have been no randomized studies using medications to treat specific phobia in children and adolescents (Ginsburg & Walkup, 2004). The results obtained by Fairbanks et al. (1997) using fluoxetine in a sample of children and youth aged 9–18 with mixed anxiety disorders found that 4 of 6 subjects with specific phobia responded well. No studies were found that combined CBT or other therapies with medications to treat specific phobia. Thus, there is little evidence about the use of medication in children and youth with specific phobia, but the SSRIs appear to have potential value with few side effects.

Posttraumatic Stress Disorder

There is relatively little research on pharmacotherapy of PTSD in children and adolescents, and only one randomized controlled trial (RCT) could be found (Cohen, 2001). In general, strategies to treat PTSD focus on specific symptoms, such as sleeping problems or generalized anxiety. Most of the evidence is based on clinical reports with little or no control of comorbid conditions. Results from studies with adults with PTSD suggest that SSRIs may be helpful in treating the disorder in children and youth, although more RCTs are needed, including those that compare psychotherapies in combination with medication.

Panic Disorder

There is little research on the treatment of panic disorder in children and youth regarding either psychotherapy or medication. A study by Barlow, Gorman, Shear, and Woods (2000) compared the single and combined effects of CBT and imipramine on a sample of 312 patients, although the subject characteristics were not described. Presumably, the subjects were adults who had a diagnosis of panic disorder who were randomly assigned to imipramine only, CBT only, placebo, CBT plus imipramine, or CBT plus placebo groups. Both imipramine and CBT were superior to the placebo in the acute phase (3 months) for the Panic Disorder Severity Scale (PDDS), but not for the Clinical Global Impression (CGI) scale. After six months, both medication and CBT were superior to placebo on both the PDDS and CGI. Combining the treatments had little advantage in the acute phase but showed more substantial effects following maintenance. Each treatment showed significant effects during maintenance and at follow-up. CBT showed continued effects at follow-up. Thus, CBT as a psychotherapeutic intervention and imipramine appear to have promise in the treatment of panic disorder in children and adolescents, but more research is needed.

Considerations in Medications vs. Psychotherapy

As with many other childhood disorders, the research evidence suggests that treatment of anxiety with a combination of medications and psychotherapy is more effective than either by itself. However, the ongoing concerns with medications with children may cause parents and physicians to approach their use with caution. Unless the anxiety symptoms are severe and significantly interfere with the delivery and effectiveness of psychotherapy, it may be advisable to begin with CBT to determine if it is effective. If it is not effective or the child cannot respond well due to the severity of the anxiety symptoms, then medication may be indicated in combination with CBT.

Treatment of Specific Disorders

Although it is beyond the scope of this chapter to provide detailed descriptions of evidence-based treatments for specific anxiety disorders, there are some general goals and strategies that are common and unique to each disorder. As stated earlier, the overall goal of interventions is to reduce symptoms to a manageable level and not to eliminate them, because it is neither desirable nor feasible to eliminate anxiety entirely. Therefore, the clinician should focus on developing techniques to help the client to identify cognitive, behavioral, and physiological symptoms and how they interact to affect functioning. As treatment progresses, the child will develop skills and strategies to reduce the likelihood of anxiety rising to a level of impairment and to view fewer situations as threatening. The selection of specific strategies may be affected by whether the child is taking medication for anxiety or other disorders, such as depression. If medications are used, the clinician should become familiar with (a) the specific medication(s), (b) the dosages, (c) the anticipated optimal treatment effects, (d) common and uncommon side effects, including possible drug interaction effects, (e) duration of medication therapy, (f) information on dosage adjustments over the course of psychological interventions, (g) when optimal effects are expected, and (h) signs of misuse, abuse, or discontinuation without prescriber approval or knowledge. These factors may influence decisions about the nature and course of psychotherapy. For example, if a medication is prescribed that reduces physiological symptoms, the child may be more responsive to the treatment program by being better able to focus on cognitive symptoms and automatic thoughts. If possible, the clinician should develop an ongoing collaborative relationship with the prescriber to monitor and collaborate on the treatment plan. Following are descriptions of general treatment goals and general treatment strategies for the more common anxiety disorders seen in children and adolescents.

Separation Anxiety Disorder

General Treatment Goals

The overall goal in treating SAD is to increase the child's ability to be apart from parents, family members, or others and to reduce the fear and apprehension about being separated from caregivers. The child is likely to have some generalized anxiety symptoms as well as some apprehension about specific situations. The child must also learn how to manage anxiety when separation from familiar people occurs and learn to be comfortable with others.

General Treatment Strategies

Traditional behavior therapy, rather than CBT, appears more likely to be effective in the treatment of separation anxiety disorder. However, behavior therapy strategies should be positively oriented and not include negative or punitive techniques. In general, reinforcement for gradual success in separating from caregivers is suggested, rather than sudden, abrupt separation. Reinforcement for small steps and successes in separation is recommended that includes self-reinforcement strategies.

Generalized Anxiety Disorder

General Treatment Goals

Because GAD is characterized by "free-floating" anxiety that pervades across situations and does not have specific "triggers," establishing treatment goals can be challenging. The clinician should work with the child to identify situations that most often elicit anxiety and cause the greatest amount of impairment. From the list of situations, the therapist and child should develop a list of behaviors and situations that will become the focus of treatment. In general, no more than two to three behaviors or situations should be focused upon because it is difficult to manage and focus on more than this amount at one time.

General Treatment Strategies

A combination of CBT and behavioral approaches has been found to be effective in helping children with GAD to manage their anxious symptoms. Teaching anxious children how to recognize the triggers of anxiety that come from physiological symptoms helps them to employ learned strategies to avoid a severe anxious reaction. At this time, most of the research has been conducted on children aged 7–14; therefore, research on older adolescents needs to be expanded. Whether parents should be involved is unclear, but the available evidence suggests that parental involvement is more likely to have positive effects if the parents do not have significant psychopathology.

Obsessive–Compulsive Disorder

General Treatment Goals

The general treatment goals are to reduce the intrusive obsessions that serve as stimuli for the production of compulsive behaviors. Reduction in faulty cognitions that contribute to the obsessive patterns and reduction in compulsive behaviors are primary foci in treating OCD.

General Treatment Strategies

CBT methods to correct faulty cognitions have been shown to reduce the frequency of obsessions. Exposure to the feared stimulus and response prevention are effective methods to treat obsessions and compulsions, respectively. Techniques used with these methods include in vivo exposure to feared stimuli, imaginal exposure to feared catastrophes, and instructions to refrain from rituals and avoidance have been shown to be effective.

Social Phobia (Social Anxiety Disorder)

General Treatment Goals

Two primary goals in the treatment of social phobia are (a) to reduce avoidance of social situations that create anxiety and (b) to increase the child's frequency of initiating and maintaining social interactions. In both situations, a small amount of anxiety may remain, even if treatment is considered successful. Hopefully, residual anxiety symptoms will not cause impairment.

General Treatment Strategies

Much of the research has suggested that CBT approaches are effective in treating social phobia. Programs such as *Coping Cat* that include cognitive challenging and disputation may be effective. Social skills training, modeling, rehearsed practice, and strategies that encourage social interactions have been found to be effective in treating social phobia. Children with social phobia also tend to have many characteristics of GAD; therefore, CBT approaches for GAD may help to reduce social phobia symptoms.

Specific Phobia

General Treatment Goals

In contrast to Social Phobia, children who have Specific Phobia are afraid of specific object or situations but do better in other circumstances. Thus, the treatment goal is to reduce anxious reactions to these situations and, if possible, reduce the tendency to avoid them, because avoidance may not always be possible. Therefore, the child must learn how to identify and cope with the specific fear-producing stimulus.

General Treatment Strategies

Ollendick and King (2000) reviewed the available literature and concluded that participant modeling and reinforced practice have been shown to be effective in treating social phobia. Other treatments that have not been as well researched but are likely to be helpful are participant modeling, imaginal desensitization, filmed modeling, in vivo desensitization, and verbal instruction. With the exception of verbal instruction, a common element of these strategies is direct or indirect exposure to the social situations that precipitate social anxiety. Gradual exposure to the feared situation may also be appropriate.

Posttraumatic Stress Disorder

General Treatment Goals

The majority of studies of treatment of PTSD have focused on helping children and adolescents to confront their traumatic thoughts, feelings, memories, and physiological reactions. The overall goals are to help the child to reduce the frequency and severity of these symptoms and to replace them with positive thoughts and feelings and to reduce the physiological reactions that are precipitated by memories or other stimuli that tend to trigger reliving of the traumatic events.

General Treatment Strategies

As with other treatment for anxiety disorders, cognitive–behavioral methods have been used and found to be effective in treating PTSD in children and adolescents as compared to supportive psychotherapy. CBT approaches typically have included cognitive therapy, exposure, and anxiety reduction techniques. In general, greater effect sizes have been seen with adolescents compared to children.

Panic Disorder

General Treatment Goals

Because the primary factor in panic disorder is the child's fear of the physical sensations that accompany a panic attack or of the attack itself, treatment is focused on reducing the frequency of attacks or associated anxiety sensitivity by addressing somatic symptoms and faulty cognitions. Goals may include helping the child to manage the physical sensations or fears when they occur or to cope with situations that may serve as triggers for attacks.

General Treatment Strategies

Most psychotherapeutic treatments for panic disorder in children and adolescents are based on cognitive and cognitive–behavioral methods (Chambless & Ollendick, 2000). The specific primary modes of intervention have been panic control treatments that include three components: (a) relaxation training and learning how to breathe to reduce neurobiological sensitivities, (b) interoceptive exposure for heightened somatic symptoms, and (c) cognitive restructuring to alter faulty misinterpretations that are related to somatic symptoms (Barlow, 1988). Some evidence of effectiveness of panic control treatments is available (e.g., Barlow & Seidner, 1983; Ollendick, 1995), but more research is needed. Nevertheless, CBT and anxiety reduction strategies appear to have evidence to support their use in treatment of panic disorder in children and adolescents.

Case Example

The case of Andrea was presented in Chap. 8 that described the presenting problems and the clinical assessment of her anxiety symptoms using a multimethod approach. Using Friedberg and McClure's (2002) approach, a description of an intervention approach using CBT methods will be described for Andrea, drawing upon the referral information and the assessment data derived. The reader is referred to Chap. 8 to review the specific assessment results and discussion. Friedberg and McClure's approach considers six variables in conceptualizing a CBT intervention, followed by a three-step formulation of the treatment plan. This approach will be presented with regard to developing a CBT treatment plan for Andrea.

Presenting Problems

Cognitive symptoms—worry, concentration problems, memory difficulties, inattention,

Behavioral symptoms—"fidgety," distractions, off-task, anxious in some social situations, socially withdrawn, reserved

Physiological symptoms—muscle tension, flushing of the skin and shaking during public performances, some sleep problems

Test Data

The formal and informal assessment data derived from the clinical interview and the parent, teacher, and child reports reveal high levels of internalizing symptoms of anxiety and somatization. Of particular interest are the discrepancies among the informants with regard to symptomatology. For example, the teacher reports a very high level of anxiety ($T=96$), which is uncommon in a school setting and indicates that the symptoms are highly evident. The mother's corresponding report of anxiety was also at a high level ($T=76$), which is clinically significant. Andrea's self-reports on the *MASC*, *PIY*, and *BYI* are at lower levels and do not necessarily correspond with the interview information and her own subjective report of symptoms. Discrepancies among data are not uncommon in children and adolescents and may reflect difficulties in their ability to report subjective symptoms.

Andrea's self-reports on the *MASC* are most consistent with her interview and history, and the Anxiety scale of the *BYI* indicates generalized anxiety. The *MASC* results are consistent with the *BYI* Anxiety scale with elevations on Physical Symptoms (Tense/Restless$=68$, Somatic/Autonomic$=71$, Total$=70$), Harm Avoidance (Perfectionism$=62$, Anxious Coping$=72$, Total$=70$), Social Anxiety (Humiliation/Rejection$=59$, Performance Fears$=67$, Total$=64$), Separation Panic$=65$, Total$=68$, and Anxiety Disorder Index$=68$. Thus, the preponderance of the assessment data indicates that Andrea has a Generalized Anxiety Disorder with onset beginning at a young age.

Cultural Context Variables

Andrea comes from a stable middle-class family with two siblings who have similar anxious patterns. The parents appear to have a stable marriage that provides some reduction of risk of the development of contributing external stressors. There are no major socioeconomic stressors, financial problems, or cultural factors that appear contributory to Andrea's anxiety. However, both parents have some histories of mild to moderate mental health issues, which could have some effect on parenting behaviors, ability to provide emotional support, and recognition of Andrea's symptoms and needs. The fact that the mother admits she is a "worrier" and tends to be overprotective may create conditions where she reinforces avoidance behavior, does not allow Andrea to take some risks and develop social competence skills, and may encourage dependent behavior. Consequently, her mother tends to be directive, rather than encouraging Andrea to develop problem-solving skills. Her father is described as being "laid back" and is less involved in Andrea's difficulties, which may send conflicting messages to Andrea about abilities, competence, and self-esteem. Andrea may not perceive her father as a sense of social and emotional support and sees her mother as being overcontrolling and a "helicopter" parent. The fact that her siblings have similar behaviors and patterns suggests that there may be a genetic or biological basis for some symptoms and that the children imitate and adopt the behaviors of each other. If complex family dynamics are present, progress in treatment could be hindered, requiring consideration of family therapy or parent training.

History and Developmental Milestones

Andrea met all typical developmental milestones at expected ages, and there is no evidence of developmental, language, cognitive, or motor difficulties. Her cognitive ability is in the low average range, and achievement is consistent with her ability. Overall academic performance is at about the sixth grade, which is consistent with her classroom performance and reports by teachers. The pattern of concern is that Andrea has shown a tendency toward anxious and withdrawn behavior since childhood, which suggests that she may have a strong predisposition to anxious symptomatology and disorder. With a positive family history for some mild to moderate mental health problems, Andrea is at greater risk for developing emotional and behavioral difficulties. Factors associated with parenting, family dynamics, and sibling relationships may play a role in her symptoms as discussed above.

Cognitive Variables

The initial interviews with Andrea revealed several cognitive distortions that contribute to her anxiety and interfere with her ability to cope with the symptoms and regulate her emotions. She has developed some negative schemata that trigger automatic thoughts when confronted with anxiety-producing situations. Given the apparent age of onset, the negative schemata developed over many years and are likely highly ingrained as persistent patterns. Andrea also demonstrates several cognitive distortions including mind reading ("I actually think I'm a little weird and other kids think the same thing about me."), catastrophizing ("I also get nervous when I have to talk in school, like when giving an oral report because I am afraid that I will make a fool of myself."), personalization ("When things happen, I always figure either it's my fault or that I have disappointed my mom and dad or one of my teachers."), and labeling ("worrier," "dumb"). She also has other characteristics of anxiety, such as fear of negative evaluation, low self-esteem, and believes that she cannot do anything to change her situation (learned helplessness).

Behavioral Antecedents and Consequences

Andrea becomes anxious when asked to perform in public or when she tries to enter a social group. Behavioral symptoms include being "fidgety," withdrawal, and becoming very quiet. Physiological symptoms include muscle tension, flushing of the skin, and increased heart rate. She expects that she will fail and that others will make fun of her. Concerns about social rejection cause her to be reluctant to initiate contact with others. She is eager to please others, so she is compliant and obedient around adults, which is reinforcing to her because it reduces anxiety. Compliance and allowing her mother to be overprotective with little resistance reduce her anxiety while also reinforcing the parental behavior. Parental overprotection inhibits Andrea's initiative to attempt new experiences, further reinforcing her feelings of incompetence. Consequently, having fewer social competence skills reinforces maternal overprotection behaviors. Because she has cognitive schemata that most things are her fault, she tries to avoid things where she is likely to fail and cause problems. When events happen, she is quick to accept blame, apologizes, and becomes withdrawn.

Provisional Formulation

Andrea shows multiple signs of chronic generalized anxiety that has pervasive effects across family, social, and academic spheres. Although she has a few friends and is accepted by her peers, she tends to have some social anxiety that inhibits her ability to develop a wide circle of friends. She has a fear of negative evaluation in social situations and with regard to some school tasks, which impairs her ability to perform. By assuming that most negative outcomes are her fault, she has developed an expectation that they will continue to occur in the future and that she will not be able to cope with them. Although she has average cognitive ability, her anxiety interferes with her development of problem-solving and coping skills, which contributes to continued feelings of lack of competence and belief that her situation will not improve. The presence of cognitive, behavioral, and physiological symptoms that she may not always recognize as being interrelated may affect her ability to cope with anxiety. She also demonstrates an attributional bias for threat, by tending to view social and performance situations as likely to lead to negative outcomes.

Pressures to perform at school in both social and academic areas increase feelings of trait anxiety that may be exacerbated by situations that raise anxiety, such as performing and the need to be perfect in some tasks. Because she struggles in school tasks, she may perceive herself as being incompetent, leading to lowering of academic self-esteem and increased apprehension about social acceptance as a student. Although Andrea's teacher did not indicate that Andrea is viewed as incompetent, the high ratings on the behavior rating scales indicate that she is perceived as impaired in self-regulation, leadership, and adaptive skills, with a high degree of internalizing symptoms.

Andrea's patterns indicate that intervention should focus on helping her to recognize and understand her cognitive, behavioral, and physiological symptoms, their interrelatedness, and how they interfere with her functioning and impair her ability to develop social relationships and to perform at school. Therapeutic goals would include helping her to manage symptoms at a nonimpairing level, improving social skills, reduction of the fear of negative evaluation, reduction of her threat attribution, improved feelings of competence, reduction of tendencies to blame herself for all problems, and always expecting negative outcomes. Interventions in the school setting for social skill problems and performance anxiety are indicated.

Anticipated Treatment Plan

1. Andrea should receive relaxation training to help her cope with anxious symptoms when under stress, such as in performance situations where fear of negative evaluation is likely to be highest.
2. Cognitive therapy using a manualized treatment approach that consists of educational components to learn coping strategies, followed by in vivo practice of newly learned skills. Emphasis should be placed on helping Andrea to recognize and reduce her negative cognitive, behavioral, and physiological symptoms, their interrelatedness, and effects on her social and academic functioning.
3. Involvement of the parents as facilitators of the manualized treatment program, by providing opportunities and situations to allow Andrea to practice newly learned skills. Direct parental involvement in the treatment is not indicated, but participation in a psychoeducation group regarding managing of behavior may be helpful.
4. Teach Andrea social skills in how to enter groups, participate effectively, and reduce discomfort.
5. Teach Andrea coping strategies to reduce anxiety associated with public performance, such as rehearsal, relaxation exercises, and organization.
6. Pleasant event scheduling, increasing involvement in social and community groups, and the development of hobbies and interests.
7. Work with Andrea's parents on positive behavior management skills, with emphasis on reduction of overprotective behaviors and reinforcement of dependent behavior. This therapy should be done separately and not as part of Andrea's program.
8. Work with Andrea's teachers on how to respond to her anxious behaviors, reinforcement for effort, providing advance organizers, and use of self-monitoring techniques.

Expected Obstacles

Initially, Andrea may be hesitant to participate in therapy because she views problems as her fault and that things will not change. However, she wants to be less anxious and to be more successful socially, so she likely will become engaged in the process and do the homework assignments.

A potential obstacle may be parental behavior, specifically maternal overprotection and "hovering," where Andrea's compliant and passive style may be reinforcing to her mother. It is possible that her mother may like the dependent behavior and feel needed by Andrea; therefore, she may be reluctant to change her behavior. She does seem to recognize, however, that Andrea has problems that are also seen in her siblings, so she may be willing to relinquish the overcontrol and overprotectiveness. The lack of involvement and apparent relative passivity of the father should be addressed, with attempts to involve him in the therapeutic process. His role as a male model to a preadolescent girl may be pivotal in her overall success and adjustment as a teenager and adults.

Finally, resistance to intervention at school should be explored. If the teachers do not see Andrea as having problems but as noncompliant and resistant, it may be difficult to engage them in a change process. Also, the nature of the school-based intervention should be considered and adapted to the level of feasibility and cooperation of the teachers. The teachers must be active participants in the development of the interventions and agree to the feasibility and implementation of the final treatment plan.

Andrea presents as having chronic, generalized anxiety that has onset in early childhood and is maintained and exacerbated by environmental variables, including parental behavior. The case is intended to demonstrate that conceptualization, assessment, and treatment of anxiety are complex and that the clinician must consider multiple variables simultaneously. Interventions should be multilevel and involve all settings where anxiety impairs functioning. In Andrea's case, parents should be involved as change agents, but, at this time, formal family therapy is not indicated, because there does not appear to be significant parental or family psychopathology, unless new information emerges.

Conclusion

Child and adolescent anxiety disorders are complex, requiring the clinician to consider the various contexts, assessment approaches, and interventions from a comprehensive, multidimensional perspective. Because anxiety disorders tend to be pervasive and show symptoms across multiple settings, interventions often will require working with parents, teachers, community agencies, medical providers, and others. The current research literature indicates that cognitive–behavioral and behavioral methods have much promise for treating anxiety disorders and should be considered to be a primary intervention approach. If medications are indicated, they should be combined with therapeutic methods to provide the best chance of symptom alleviation and improvement in psychological functioning.

Chapter 11
Interventions for Depression and Mood Disorders

Although anxiety, depression, and mood disorders share some common origins, characteristics, and symptoms, there are differences in how treatment is conceptualized, developed, and implemented. A distinguishing developmental difference is that, while anxiety is a normal experience in all persons, depression does not have this characteristic. Although it is common for children, adolescents, and adults to have periods of "feeling down," feeling "blue," "sad," or "having the blahs," they are not chronic or severe and do not impair functioning to a significant degree. Often, they are situation specific and last only a few hours or days. Although anxiety has some specific developmental "markers" (e.g., stranger anxiety and separation anxiety in infancy), there are not similar developmental manifestations of depression and mood in children and youth. Of course, adolescence is a time when teens are frequently described as "moody" and irritable and may have more periods of unhappiness, but their functioning typically is not so impaired that intervention is needed. Apart from the teen years, there are not specific ages or circumstances in which mood problems are manifested in almost all children.

The vast majority of adolescents experience good social, personal, and psychological development, despite the "moodiness" that occurs in many, if not most, teenagers at some time. Therefore, interventions are warranted when individual circumstances indicate that the child is having mood and depression problems that impair functioning. Depression can be *chronic* where the onset is more insidious and lasts for an extended period of time, often without an identifiable precipitating event, or *acute* when an identifiable triggering event is known, such as loss of a loved one or experiencing trauma.

Similar to treatment for anxiety disorders, the primary evidence-based interventions shown to have probable efficacy are behavioral, cognitive–behavioral, and pharmacotherapy approaches. The reader is referred to Chap. 10 for an overview of the principles and techniques of cognitive–behavioral therapy (CBT), as well as to various books that discuss it in more detail (e.g., Friedberg & McClure, 2002; Reinecke, Datillio, & Freeman, 2006). In a manner similar to CBT treatment for

T.J. Huberty, *Anxiety and Depression in Children and Adolescents:*
Assessment, Intervention, and Prevention, DOI 10.1007/978-1-4614-3110-7_11,
© Springer Science+Business Media, LLC 2012

anxiety disorders, the focus in depression is on faulty beliefs, attributions, and negative self-talk that perpetuate a depressive perspective by the child. Some of these characteristics create difficulties for the clinician to establish a therapeutic relationship and rapport with the child, such as low self-esteem and feelings of hopelessness that improvement is possible.

The Initial Interview with the Depressed Child or Adolescent

Although the initial presentation of the depressed child may have some similarities to the anxious child, there are differences that the clinician will observe. Because most children who are refereed for psychological services are inexperienced with treatment, they often do not know what to expect. As discussed in Chap. 10, the clinician should determine what the child has been told about why he or she is being seen and what expectations are present. Like the anxious child, the depressed child is likely to feel discomfort, apprehension, and take personal responsibility for the problems. The depressed child may feel threatened but is less prone to have an attribution for threat seen in anxious youth. Rather, a negative attributional bias is more likely, where the child sees personal circumstances as being negative, unrewarding, and hopeless. These children also may be less likely to talk readily at the outset, creating challenges for the clinician in establishing rapport and dialogue. The depressed child may be less aware or able to describe internal affective states than does the anxious child. This potential limitation may make it more difficult to conduct the initial interview if the child is young or otherwise has less well-developed expressive language skills. Some clinicians ask children to draw pictures of objects or people, such as houses, trees, people, family, and friends. These projective techniques often are used as diagnostic measures of social–emotional functioning, despite a significant lack of evidence of psychometric reliability and validity for most of them. Thus, they should not be used as diagnostic indicators for the depressed child, but they may be helpful as a means to conduct a more thorough clinical interview by discussing items the child may draw and discuss.

The clinician should be alert for manifestations of signs of Beck's (1987) three-factor description of the depressed child or adult as having a negative view of self, the world, and the future. Consistent with attributional theory, the depressed child also will show much self-blame and responsibility (internal locus of control), see almost everything as being negative (global), and as being fixed and relatively immutable (stable). Clinical assessment of the child's beliefs and attributions forms the basis for CBT and other interventions.

As with treatment for anxiety, it is important that the clinician determines what the depressed child has been told about why he or she is being seen. Depending on what the child has been told or is capable of understanding or expressing, he may not be able to respond to the question "What have you been told about why you are here?" If the child does not respond to this question, a follow-up question could be "Your parents tell me you have been sad or unhappy lately and are concerned about you.

I would just like to talk with you about why they brought you here." Some depressed children may show signs of irritability or "crankiness" rather than classic symptoms of depression, and it may be easier for the child to talk about these feelings, especially in young children who tend to have more difficulty expressing mood states. Similarly, a statement such as "Your parents tell me you have been kind of unhappy or upset lately about some things and I would like to talk with you about that. Do you feel that is true?" If the child says "yes" or some affirmative answer, then say "Would it be o.k. if we talk about it a little bit?" Then proceed to conduct a semistructured interview appropriate to the child's developmental level. If the answer is "no," then more time is indicated to talk about topics that are less directly relevant until sufficient rapport and dialogue have been established.

Cognitive–Behavior Therapy for Depression and Mood Disorders

Cognitive–behavior therapy has been found to be an effective treatment for depression and mood disorders in children and adolescents. Because some of the primary symptom patterns for depression and mood problems are similar in children and adults, the basic principles and techniques can be utilized for both groups. For young children and preadolescents, the specific treatment methods will require adaptation and modification for their developmental levels.

The central focus of CBT approaches to treating depression is the presumption that the child or youth has negatively biased cognitions that reflect negative beliefs about the self, the world, and the future, i.e., Beck's (1987) model of the three factors that characterize depression. The presence and severity of these negative cognitions contribute to the initiation and maintenance of depressive mood that are manifested as cognitive, behavioral, and physiological symptoms. The CBT approach incorporates strategies to help the child recognize and evaluate the negative biases and faulty beliefs for their veracity and their effects on functioning. As treatment progresses, the client also learns other cognitions and beliefs that replace or diminish the negative ones. CBT also incorporates behavioral techniques to engage the child in activities that produce pleasant outcomes, which addresses the view that depressed persons receive little positive reinforcement from the environment. By combining cognitive and behavioral approaches, the therapist helps the child to change belief systems and also participate in activities that produce pleasurable outcomes, thereby changing experiences from negative environmental input to positive experiences.

Depending on the age of the child and other factors, the parents may be directly involved in the behavioral component by giving the child opportunities to participate in fun activities, such as seeing a movie, going to an amusement park, or playing games. Typically, the cognitive component of CBT involves direct work with child, and the parents have indirect involvement but are kept informed of the treatment program. Obviously, because depression may involve greater risk of suicidal ideation, parents would have to be informed if the therapist determined that their child is at imminent risk of self-harm, consistent with the laws of the particular state. (*Note:* When working with any anxious or depressed child, the therapist must have full knowledge of state laws regarding the limits of confidentiality and reporting requirements regarding minors when issues of harm to self or others arise.) CBT also seeks to improve emotion regulation problems and deficits in social regulation skills that often accompany moderate to severe depression.

Most treatments that address child and adolescent depression focus on one or more of the following primary areas: (a) mood monitoring, (b) cognitive restructuring, (c) behavioral activation, pleasant activity scheduling, and goal setting, (d) relaxation and stress management, (e) social skills and conflict resolution training, and (f) training in general problem-solving skills (Kaslow & Thompson, 1998; Kazdin & Weisz, 1998). It is common to address more than one of these areas in treatment, particularly if depression is accompanied by high levels of anxiety, anger, or other mood regulation problems.

Monitoring Moods

Because moods tend to vary in intensity, duration, and frequency over a variety of situations, monitoring them is an important part of the treatment process for at least three reasons: (a) to help the child to recognize moods and their variations, (b) to improve the ability to link cognitive, behavioral, and physical symptoms to mood states, and (c) it assists in the ongoing assessment of treatment effectiveness by providing feedback and information to both the child and the therapist. Most manualized treatment programs have checklists that ask the child to evaluate moods between treatment sessions. Monitoring of moods involves having the child rate the range of moods over a period of time, such as a day, on most days of the week. Additional information might include what the child was doing, the location, and the time of day.

Appendix E provides an example of a mood monitoring form that may be useful when nonmanualized CBT methods are being used. This form provides a format for the client to record the occurrences of specific mood identified in collaboration with the therapists with criteria for defining the moods. The client should record the day of the week, the time, and what he or she was doing at the time. This information will help to determine if certain moods tend to recur on a regular basis and the client is asked to rate the intensity of the mood on a ten-point scale. The client is then asked to record what he or she did to alleviate the intensity of the mood. Finally, the client is asked to rate how well the effort worked to alleviate the symptoms. This format may help the client to identify moods, rate them, and then evaluate how well the effort worked to regulate the mood. This type of ongoing feedback may be helpful to the client to identify emotions/moods, severity, what was done (if anything), and a personal rating of how well it worked. In ongoing therapy sessions, the form could be reviewed at each session to assess what the client is experiencing and the effectiveness of personal efforts.

Another method to monitor moods is to ask the child to keep a daily "mood diary," in which daily activities, moods experienced during the day, antecedents and consequences of mood states, coping methods used, and an informal evaluation of their effectiveness. In addition to providing information to the therapist, self-collected data can be useful as therapeutic feedback about mood experiences.

Cognitive Restructuring

The origin of the term "cognitive restructuring" is credited to Ellis (1962) and to Beck (1976) where Socratic questioning and rational disputation are used to alter and replace maladaptive or distorted thinking. Kendall and Hollon (1979) and Meichenbaum (1977) refined the term and began applying it to the treatment of anxiety and depression in children and youth. The overall goal of cognitive restructuring therapy in depression is to alter the irrational beliefs and cognitive biases that contribute to and maintain depressive symptomatology. Table 11.1 describes some of the major cognitive symptoms of depression and general goals for cognitive restructuring.

Table 11.1 Depressive cognitive distortions and general treatment goals

Cognitive distortion	General treatment goal
"All-or-none" thinking—thinking in extremes rather than considering a middle ground in situations; often uses words such as "always" or "never", e.g., "I always do the wrong thing" or "I can never do things right"	Improve cognitive flexibility and ability to generate and evaluate situations at multiple levels, rather than only at extremes; recognize that "all-or-none" thinking leads to inaccurate beliefs and increases stress
Catastrophic thinking—expects that almost all events will have worst possible outcome, e.g., "If I don't do well on this test, I will never get to college and will be a failure"	Improve thinking skills to understand that not all negative events are predictive or causal in the outcomes of future events and not all will be catastrophic
Mental filter—focusing primarily on selected aspects of a situation rather than evaluating all positive and negative aspects, e.g., noticing only specific negative characteristics	Improve ability to evaluate all aspects of a situation and not focus on one (usually negative) that may support a negative bias or self-perception
Discounting the positive—minimizing or ignoring positive aspects of a situation and focusing on the negative aspects	Improve ability to look at both positive and negative aspects of a situation and increase emphasis on positive aspects
Overgeneralization—takes an isolated event and assumes that most or all future similar events will have similar negative outcomes, e.g., "I did not do well in that situation, so I will not do well in others like it"	Improve ability to evaluate each situation differently and that not all situations are alike or will necessarily have the same outcomes
Personalization—assumes responsibility for things that are beyond personal control, e.g., child believes that misbehavior led to parents' divorce	Improve ability to accurately evaluate and determine that some things are beyond personal control and that the person did not cause the events, although it may seem that way due to proximity or circumstances

(continued)

Table 11.1 (continued)

Cognitive distortion	General treatment goal
Jumping to conclusions—drawing inferences or conclusions without evidence; may include "mind reading' where people believe they understand the motives and intentions of others, although there is no evidence; may include "fortune telling", which is the tendency to have rather rigid expectations for outcomes that are not easily dissuaded. Example: "I didn't do well on that test, so everyone thinks I am dumb"	Improve ability to engage in problem-solving and look at alternative explanations for outcomes, rather than making a quick judgment; improve ability to appreciate multiple perspectives and that "mind reading" and "fortune telling" can lead to inaccurate conclusions
Emotional reasoning—person experiences a feeling and assumes it is true about him/her as a person,, e.g., "I feel dumb, so I must be dumb"	Improve ability to understand how thoughts and feelings are related and that each can affect the other and lead to inaccurate self-perceptions
"Should" perspective—person has a repertoire of "should statements" that imply that he or she *must* have certain characteristics or behaviors that always apply and are not changeable, e.g., "I must always be perfect and anything less is not acceptable"	Improve ability to accept less than perfection and that "should statements" contribute to unrealistic expectations that will be impossible to achieve and can lead to further stress and frustration
Labeling/mislabeling—person applies labels to himself or mislabels self as an explanation for outcomes; labels/mislabels tend to be difficult to change and the person may be resistance to changing them; e.g., "I am a loser, so I will not get anywhere in life"	Improve ability to focus on the specific situation; analyze it individually and not explain it as a function of a label that is considered accurate and unchangeable

Rational disputation is a therapeutic process using Socratic questioning techniques aimed at understanding the client's belief system and helping him or her to recognize, understand, and change irrational beliefs. Using questioning and non-evaluative statements, the therapist helps to "dispute" the irrational beliefs and replace them with rational ones that the child can accept and incorporate into cognitive schemata. The following dialogue demonstrates how this process might work for Andrew, a depressed adolescent, who has faulty beliefs about his general academic ability:

Therapist: Andrew, you said something about not doing well in school.

Andrew: Yes, I am not doing well and I have to be the stupidest kid in school. I can't do anything well.

Therapist: Can you give me some examples of why you believe you are the stupidest kid in school?

Andrew: Well, I get mostly C's and D's, kids make fun of me because I can't read very well, and I don't have any friends. So, when you put all that together, that makes me a big loser. I get really depressed about it sometimes and I begin to think "What's the use?" I will never do well or have any friends.

Therapist: So, you think all of these problems happen because you are stupid?

Andrew:	Absolutely. I'm not good at school, can't make friends, and have always had trouble with grades. I would like to have a girlfriend, but I don't even know how to talk to girls. So, when I put all that together, it seems pretty obvious to me that I'm a loser, am stupid, and I don't see how anything will change. It's really kind of a slam dunk, don't you think?
Therapist:	I'm really more interested in what you think, because that can have a lot to do with what you do and how you see yourself. Let's talk about school a bit. You said that you don't do well in school, correct?
Andrew:	Yeah, that's right. It has really gotten worse since about eighth grade.
Therapist:	Earlier, you said you said you always did poorly in school, but you just said that it's gotten worse. So, there was a time before that when you did better in school?
Andrew:	Well, yeah, in elementary school, I actually did pretty well, getting mostly B's, some A's, and an occasional C. So, I guess it wasn't always bad. It just seems like once I got into middle school, it started getting harder and I just couldn't do it and it became pretty obvious that I was kinda dumb. I also had a lot more friends than I do now.
Therapist:	So, you haven't always felt stupid and in fact did pretty well and had more friends a few years ago. Could it be that it's not so much a matter of you being stupid but that things have changed for you and have gotten harder?
Andrew:	Well, things have certainly changed, but, you're right. I did well for awhile but I don't know why it's much harder now.
Therapist:	So, do you think it's possible that things have just changed and you need to work on them, rather than just being due to you feeling stupid? Maybe what used to work well doesn't work so well now?
Andrew:	Well, that's true, when you put it that way. I hadn't thought about it by looking at what I had done before. I was just looking at what is going on now and it seems pretty bad. It's when I start thinking about what is going on now that I start getting all depressed again.
Therapist:	So, do you think it's possible that a lot of what is going on with school is that things have changed and you need new ways of doing things, rather just because you think you are stupid?
Andrew:	Well, you've got me to thinking that maybe it is more about needing to make some changes, because I've done better before. But, I'm still not convinced that I'm not dumb.
Therapist:	Well, rather than focusing on being dumb, how about if we focus on developing some ways to work on these problems and see if things improve? If things improve, do you think it might help you see yourself as more capable than you think?
Andrew:	Maybe. At least, I'd like to give it a try.
Therapist:	Let's work on a plan together to see what we can do. Now, I would also like to talk about your concerns about friends and maybe having a girlfriend. You said that you don't have many friends.
Andrew:	That's true. Most kids don't like me and make fun of me or just ignore me most of the time.

Therapist:	What makes you think that kids don't like you?
Andrew:	Well, they get real quiet when I come around and they won't talk to me.
Therapist:	So, the fact that they don't talk to you tells you that they don't like you?
Andrew:	Well, sure! Wouldn't you think the same thing?
Therapist:	I'm not sure what I would think in that situation, but I can see how you might come to that conclusion. What do you think it is about you that they don't like?
Andrew:	They just think I'm a dork and a loser and don't want to be around me. It's mostly at school.
Therapist:	Has anyone ever said things to you like you're a dork and a loser?
Andrew:	Yeah, a couple of kids have said things like that.
Therapist:	You said a couple of kids. How many kids are in your school that you see a lot?
Andrew:	Oh, probably, two or three hundred.
Therapist:	So, are you concluding that most kids think you are a dork or a loser on the basis of the comments of a couple of kids out of two or three hundred?
Andrew:	Well, yeah, I guess. I have really only heard it a little.
Therapist:	So, am I correct in saying that you have concluded that most kids think you are a dork or a loser on the basis of the comments of a couple of kids?
Andrew:	Right.
Therapist:	So, based on what you just said, you don't really know if most kids think you are a dork and a loser. Is that right?
Andrew:	Well, that's right. I really don't know for sure.
Therapist:	O.k. Let's assume that most kids don't think that you are a dork and a loser. What might be some alternative explanations for why you feel you are having problems with other kids?
Andrew:	I don't really know. It just seems that when I am around no one seems to like me.
Therapist:	How do you know that?
Andrew:	Well, when I approach a group, no one will talk to me.
Therapist:	So, when you approach a group, no one talks to you and you think that they don't like you. When you do that, do you initiate conversation first?
Andrew:	No, I wait for them to say something first, but they don't, which shows they do not like me.
Therapist:	Do you think it's possible that they think you do not like them or feel uncomfortable talking and they don't know what to do or say? That might be one possible explanation.
Andrew:	I hadn't really thought about it that way. I guess it's possible that they do not know what to do or say when I am to around.
Therapist:	So that is one possibility. What other possible explanations could there be?

Andrew: Well, maybe they think I am not interested in what they are doing and are talking about. That might explain why they don't talk to me. Maybe I need to work on some stuff.

Therapist: So, there are at least two possibilities for why things do not go well with others and you think that maybe there is something you are doing or not doing that might help explain the problem. Do I have that right?

Andrew: That's right.

Therapist: So, it would seem we could work on looking at alternative reasons for some of these problems and things you could do to help improve them. How does that sound to you?

Andrew: It's worth a try. What do we do?

Therapist: How about if we identify some of the major things that bother you, talk about what you think and do, and see if we can come up with some things to try?

Andrew: O.K.

Analysis of the Dialogue

In this example, Andrew is showing some cognitive distortions, and the therapist is using Socratic questioning to elicit irrational beliefs to help Andrew become aware of and begin to change them. He exhibits a negative view of himself (i.e., is "stupid" or "dumb"), the world (i.e., he is not having much success in anything), and the future (i.e., "I will never do well or have any friends"). There are some suggestions that he feels the situation is hopeless and will not change and that he gets depressed when he thinks about it. He also shows that his beliefs reflect a highly internal locus of control and are stable and global.

Andrew states that he is "the stupidest kid at school," which reflects his negative view of himself and conclusion that no one could be as "stupid" as he is. He shows cognitive distortions of labeling and overgeneralization. The therapist engages in disputation by asking Andrew about his prior experiences and finds that he has had success in the past and points out a discrepancy between what Andrew believes and what is fact. After Andrew realizes that his belief may not be accurate, the therapist proposes that they work on developing some strategies to address the problem, to which Andrew agrees.

Next, Andrew states that he is a "dork" and a "loser," and the therapist begins asking questions about his beliefs and why he thinks others think of him this way. Through questioning, the therapist discovers that Andrew has overgeneralized that others think of him as a "dork" and a "loser" on the basis of one or two peers out of a few hundred. Andrew is using the cognitive distortions of labeling, emotional reasoning, and mind reading. Again, the therapist uses questioning to point out the discrepancy between the distorted belief and actual evidence.

Finally, the therapist explores the issue of social interactions and Andrew's perception that others do not like him. In this approach, the therapist attempts to help

Andrew consider the possibility that there may be alternative explanations for situations and that the reasons for events are not always as they seem. The therapist helps guide Andrew's thinking to come to the conclusion that perhaps his behavior is a factor in social relationships and that there may be things he can do to improve the situation. At no time does the therapist make a value judgment or imply that Andrew is wrong in his beliefs. The focus remains on eliciting automatic thoughts, distortions, and faulty beliefs that can be discussed and addressed in the therapeutic process. The therapist suggests they work together on the problems they have discussed and obtains Andrew's consent to collaborate. The Socratic questioning process has shown some evidence of helping to modify Andrew's cognitive distortions and irrational beliefs.

Linking Cognition, Behavior, and Physical Symptoms to Mood States

One of the central objectives in CBT is helping the client to recognize and understand the associations among cognitions, behaviors, and physical responses. Recognizing these links, however, is only a start, and specific interventions are developed in a collaborative manner between child and therapist using CBT techniques. These links are established through participation in therapy sessions where emphasis is placed on using Socratic questioning and discussion to help the child understand that the three areas are interrelated. For example, emphasis might be placed on helping the depressed adolescent to understand that withdrawing from social situations (behavior) is related to the belief that others do not like him (cognitive) that may lead to stress and tension (physiological). Other components of CBT programs typically include homework rehearsal, practice, homework assignments, and behavior change strategies that facilitate the linking of cognition, behavior, and physical symptoms. Manualized treatment programs typically include an education component accompanied by homework, followed by implementation and practice of learned strategies in various settings.

Behavioral Activation, Pleasant Activity Scheduling, and Goal Setting

Behavioral Activation

A common characteristic of depressed people is that they lose interest in things they formerly enjoyed and show less physical activity, initiative, and involvement in groups, hobbies, and projects. This loss of interest and activity can lead to further social isolation and unhappiness, increasing depressive symptomatology.

Behavioral Activation Therapy (BAT) is a technique to treat depression that has shown promise of effectiveness when CBT does not work. Jacobson, Martell, and Dimidjian (2001) and Martell, Addis, and Jacobson (2001) developed BAT as a treatment to work with depressed adults who were not successful with CBT or were otherwise not deemed appropriate candidates for CBT. BAT proposes that when CBT does not alter the depressed person's thinking, a focus on directly altering their behavior in a positive way can be effective. BAT focuses on conducting a functional analysis of the depressed person's behaviors. After the functional analysis is completed, the client is taught to recognize avoidance patterns that maintain the depressive symptoms and to increase participation in activities that may lead to more positive reinforcement and improved mood. BAT has been shown to be effective in treating depressed adults, but there is little evidence about whether it works with children and adolescents. Nevertheless, some of the principles and techniques of BAT may be considered when working with youth because the majority of symptoms of depression in children and adults are similar.

Pleasant Activity Scheduling

Because depressed children and youth often do not enjoy activities and hobbies, pleasant activity scheduling (PAS) can be a valuable tool to address the anhedonia, social withdrawal, and fatigue associated with depression (Friedberg & McClure, 2002). One strategy to increase a child's participation in fun activities is to conduct an interview to determine what kinds of tasks the child might enjoy. Initially, it may be difficult to generate a list of possible activities, because the depressed child often does not think about positive events or deriving enjoyment from the environment. If the child has some difficulty with this task, it may be useful to ask what she or he used to enjoy and to rank the level of enjoyment on a five-point scale. If several tasks can be ranked this way, then the therapist can discuss ways to reengage the child in one of the higher-ranked tasks. Another strategy is to generate a list of possible pleasant activities common to peers and ask the child to rank each one on a five-point scale. From the highest ranked items, one or two can be selected as short-term goals in which to involve the child. Depending on what activities are chosen, the parents may need to be involved in implementing the choices if matters such as financing or travel are involved. PAS should be a part of most treatment programs for depression, whether it is an integral part of a systematic program or as a component of an individualized approach.

Goal Setting

This strategy is intended to help the depressed child or adolescent to set therapeutic, personal, social, academic, or occupational goals. Depressed children tend to have difficulty setting goals because they have difficulty focusing on what they want to achieve, are not future-oriented, or set unrealistic goals that are nearly impossible to achieve. Because they cannot set attainable goals, feelings of failure continue that exacerbate the depression.

Street et al. (2004) discuss the concept of conditional goal setting (CGS) as related to depression in children. CGS theory suggests that depressed people feel that they can be happy only if specific goals are obtained. These "conditional goal setters" are more vulnerable to depression because they engage in an unhealthy pursuit of this goal, believing that happiness can only be achieved with its attainment. This belief is an example of all-or-none thinking because achievement that is less than what is expected is unacceptable. Alterations of this cognitive schema include acceptance of less than perfection and that happiness can be achieved with less than complete attainment of goals.

Despite the difficulties that depressed children may have with goal setting, it is an important aspect of treatment. Younger children likely will have more difficulty with this task due to a greater tendency to focus on the present, so goal setting will more often focus on short-term, objective goals, which may be focused on fun activities and pleasant activity scheduling. For adolescents, goals can include objective aspects but can also focus on topics such as education planning, social activities, and other tasks that have longer-term trajectories.

Some characteristics of therapeutic goals include:

- Clearly defined
- Specific
- Attainable
- Short-term
- Measurable

Some examples of therapeutic goals are

- "I want to be less depressed."
- "I want to fight less with my parents."
- "I would like to enjoy things more."
- "I would like to worry less about what others think of me."
- "I would like to be less of a perfectionist."
- "I want to be with other people."

When setting therapeutic goals, it is important that they be operationalized and measured in ways that are meaningful to the client. For example, if a youth states that "I want to be less depressed," a goal could be developed that the child would have fewer episodes (frequency) of feeling depressed, episodes that are less severe (intensity), do not last as long (duration), or are a combination of these indices. After these criteria are determined, appropriate methods of measuring them would be developed, such as daily checklists or logs that are reviewed during therapy sessions. These techniques could be used as self-monitoring devices after therapy has ended.

Relaxation and Stress Management

It is well known that adolescence is a developmental period when increased stress is a common experience for youth. Depressed children and adolescents typically experience stress and anxiety in addition to typical events of adolescence. Efforts to treat and prevent worsening of depression often incorporate relaxation and stress management training (SMT). Relaxation training involves learning forms of systematic desensitization and deep muscle relaxation, which is often used in treating anxiety (see Chap. 10).

SMT is often used in business, industry, and other settings to help employees maintain performance and to reduce effects of stressful working conditions. SMT has been found to be an effective component for treating stress associated with adolescent depression and preventing a relapse of symptoms (e.g., Clarke & Lewinsohn, 1995). SMT programs typically address the child or adolescent's coping skills and include activities and instruction about how to improve the ability to respond to and control stress. These programs focus on the person's sense of self-efficacy, perceived stress, identification of stressors, coping skills, and recovery abilities. Pincus and Friedman (2004) suggest that SMT programs should include active coping instruction, relaxation, recovery, and distraction components, and Clarke (2006) emphasizes a stressor-dependent approach, where the focus is on controllability of stressors. SMT programs and procedures are often an important and effective component of intervention programs for children and youth, especially for adolescent girls who are at higher risk for depression.

Social Skills and Conflict Resolution Training

Social Skills Training

Children and youth with depression often have significant difficulties demonstrating adequate social skills, which may contribute to increased isolation, loneliness, and inability to derive enjoyment from the environment. It is possible that deficient social skills contribute to interpersonal problems, leading to social isolation or rejection. Poor social skills exacerbate depressive symptoms that interfere with the ability to interact socially.

Therefore, social skills training may be a valuable adjunct to treatment of depressed children.

Social skills training programs abound in the professional literature and in commercial and programmatic offerings. In general, social skills training programs have six components that are similar to the problem-solving model described below.

1. *Identify social skills deficits*—In this step, the clinician systematically evaluates and determines what social skills deficits exist. A thorough assessment is accomplished through several means:

   - Semistructured interviews—These interviews should be conducted with teachers, parents, and others who know the child well and can describe social skill strengths and deficits and how they are manifested in various settings. The child should also be interviewed to assess his personal perspective on social skills. It is common for discrepancies to exist among informants, which may be due to personal biases, variation in familiarity with the child, and the tasks, demands, and contingencies of various settings.
   - Standardized rating scales and checklists—These measures provide objective data by informants on the type and severity of social skills deficits. One of the most well-established standardized rating scales is the *Social Skills Improvement System* (*SSIS*; Gresham & Elliott, 2008), a revision of the *Social Skills Rating System* (Gresham & Elliott, 1990). The *SSIS* contains scales to measure the social skills of Communication, Cooperation, Assertion, Responsibility, Empathy, Engagement, and Self-control. The *SSIS* also contains scales to assess child psychopathology and academic performance. Other formal and informal social skills checklists are available to conduct a systematic assessment of social skill deficits.
   - Observation—Systematic observation of the child in various settings using coding systems is an effective but often time-consuming method of direct assessment of social skills. However, direct observation may be the most appropriate method to identify social skill deficits that occur in specific settings.

2. *Determine if the deficits are performance or skill deficits*—Performance deficits are those where the child knows how to perform a skill but does not perform it reliably or accurately. Depressed children or youth may not have the motivation to perform acquired skills perhaps because they perceive it to be pointless and will not lead to positive outcomes. Therefore, the treatment approach focuses on helping the child to perform the skill appropriately in a manner that leads to accomplishment. Skill deficits are shown when the child does not know how to perform a social task. In these situations, the child may have to be taught how to perform and practice the skills.

3. *Generate a list of possible intervention strategies*—The clinician works with the child and others to develop a range of strategies that may be considered for the specific skill deficit and setting. The strategies could include individual work with the child or group social skills training. From the list of strategies, an assessment of likelihood of success and acceptability to all persons involved is made.

4. *Select the intervention strategies*—From the generated strategies, one or more with a high probability of success are selected, and plans are made to implement them. To the extent appropriate, the depressed child should be involved in this step to determine the degree of motivation and ability to participate in the intervention.

5. *Implement the strategies*—The strategies are implemented according to the established plan with appropriate monitoring and ongoing evaluation.

6. *Monitor, evaluate, and modify the program as necessary*—Almost all behavior intervention plans will require some modification as they progress and should be based upon ongoing monitoring, data collection, and evaluation across settings. Changes are made according to the data generated from the ongoing assessment.

Conflict Resolution Training

Depressed children and youth often have interpersonal difficulties that may include anger and impairments in the ability to resolve interpersonal conflicts. They may benefit from training in conflict resolution aimed at anger reduction and the ability to work cooperatively and to resolve everyday conflicts. Conflict resolution training is based on the principles and procedures of mediation, which involves bringing two or more parties into a problem-solving mode so that each party receives a satisfactory outcome and avoids future conflict. When mediation is necessary, the parties have reached an impasse and cannot resolve the deadlock without help. Failure to resolve a conflict may lead to additional confrontation, avoidance, violence, or other nonproductive outcomes.

The key skills necessary to resolve conflict are perspective taking and the ability to listen actively to the positions and perspectives of others, skills that often are impaired in children and adolescents with depression. Deficiencies in emotion regulation, mood variations, cognitive distortions (e.g., "all-or-none" thinking), and difficulty anticipating and appreciating future outcomes are among additional characteristics of depressed children that inhibit the ability to resolve conflicts. Conflict resolution training with depressed children and adolescents must address the cognitive factors associated with impaired conflict resolution skills and that younger children are be less able to engage in perspective taking and problem solving. One of the characteristics of depressed children is the tendency toward all-or-none thinking that may lead to being able to perceive and evaluate only one or two options. Due to its mediation-oriented perspective that requires looking at multiple perspectives and options, conflict resolution training initially may be difficult with depressed children and youth but nevertheless is an important skill to target and develop. The process of helping depressed children to see multiple perspectives through conflict resolution training may be slow at first but is an important tool for the clinician to draw upon.

Developing General Problem-Solving Skills

Many depressed children and youth have difficulty engaging in effective problem solving, often due to a combination of cognitive deficiencies, lack of experience, and social difficulties. Training in general problem-solving skills by working with the child on specific tasks may help to increase social and personal success. Although many approaches exist, a five-step model will help to improve problem-solving skills. These steps are:

1. *Problem identification*—In the first step, the therapist works with the child to identify the problem to be solved in objective terms. For example, a depressed child might say that he does not know how to make friends. Although this presenting problem may be an accurate self-report, it is not sufficient to develop an action plan to improve the ability to make friends and improve social relationships. Rather, the therapist would work with the child to identify a specific problem, such as not knowing how to initiate a conversation.

2. *Generation of possible strategies*—In this phase, the therapist helps the child to generate ideas about how to initiate conversations. This phase is often called "brainstorming" because all ideas are considered with no initial judgment made as to their feasibility or likelihood of success. For the depressed youth, this phase may have added benefits in helping to improve cognitive flexibility, reduce the tendency toward "all-or-none" thinking, and improve the ability to generate alterative solutions to problems.

3. *Selection of a strategy or action plan*—From the alternatives generated, the therapist and child select a strategy or action plan that has four characteristics: (a) is acceptable to the child and others who might be involved, (b) is able to be implemented effectively, (c) has a high likelihood of success, and (d) can be readily evaluated to determine if it is successful. It is especially important that the selected strategy has a high likelihood of success because many depressed children have a low sense of self-worth and often feel like failures. Selecting a strategy that does not succeed may worsen the child's feelings of low self-worth and self-efficacy. Thus, small increments of improvement should be a primary goal as therapy progresses.

4. *Implementation of the strategy or action plan*—After a strategy is selected, the therapist and child collaborate to develop a specific plan of how to implement it, including (a) what resources or help is needed, (b) the specific tasks the child is to do, and (c) the schedule or timetable for implementation. The therapist then helps the child to write down the plan and outline the specific tasks and behaviors to be performed.

5. *Evaluation of the success of the strategy or action plan*—Finally, the therapist and child should determine how progress will be measured. This is a particularly important part of the problem-solving process because depressed children may have unrealistic or biased expectations of what constitutes success. Thus, the evaluation method should be easy to do and have realistic success criteria that are acceptable to the child. As the child becomes successful and has objective data to show success, the therapist can continue to help develop solutions to other problems using this five-step approach. Progress is evaluated using self-reports, checklists, homework assignments, rating scales, and similar measures. The depressed child may or may not try or evaluate some strategies as planned, perhaps due to lack of motivation, opportunity, or other factors. These occurrences are not treated as failures or relapses, but as tasks and topics to be addressed in subsequent sessions. It is common for depressed children and adolescents to be inconsistent with implementation and evaluation.

Developing Conflict Resolution Skills

The ability to resolve interpersonal conflicts is an essential skill for effective social and psychological functioning for all people, even if they are not depressed. For children who are depressed, they may need direct instruction in conflict resolution skills, and many of these skills are embedded in intervention programs such as *Taking ACTION* (Stark & Kendall, 1996) and *Adolescent Coping with Depression Course* (CWD-A; Clarke, Lewinsohn, Rohde, Hops, & Seeley, 1999; Lewinsohn, Clarke, Hops, & Andrews, 1990).

Although detailed description of conflict resolution programs will not be described here, the Conflict Resolution Network (www.crnhq.org) lists 12 conflict resolution skills that lead to more effective outcomes:

1. *The win/win approach*—how to solve problems as partners rather than opponents
2. *Creative response*—transforming problems into creative opportunities
3. *Empathy*—developing communication tools to build rapport. Using listening to clarify understanding
4. *Appropriate assertiveness*—applying strategies to attack the problem, not the person
5. *Cooperative power*—eliminating "power over" to "power with" others
6. *Managing emotions*—expressing fear, anger, hurt, and frustration wisely to effect change
7. *Willingness to resolve*—naming personal issues that cloud the picture
8. *Mapping the conflict*—defining the issues to chart common needs and concerns
9. *Development of options*—designing creative options together
10. *Introduction to negotiation*—planning and applying effective strategies to reach agreement
11. *Introduction to mediation*—helping conflicting parties to move toward solutions
12. *Broadening of perspectives*—running meetings in conflict resolving mode

Cognitive–Behavior Therapy Programs for Depressed Children and Youth

Several evidence-based CBT programs for child and adolescent depression have been developed and been supported in research trials. One of the first manualized treatment programs shown to be effective is the *Adolescent Coping with Depression* course (CWD-A; Clarke, Lewinsohn, Rohde, Hops, & Seeley, 1999; Lewinsohn, Clarke, Hops, & Andrews, 1990). The program is designed to be used as a group treatment for youth who are currently depressed and provides 16 sessions of two hours each. The program manual and adolescent workbook are available from http://www.kpchr.org/public/acwd/acwd.html and may be used in research and clinical practice without charge. The program is based on principles of cognitive–behavior therapy and includes components about learning to relax, improving communication skills, learning how to solve problems, looking to the future, improving social skills, pleasant events scheduling, conflict resolution, and preventing relapse of symptoms. It is conducted in two sessions per week for eight weeks. The 16 sessions are:

1. Depression and Social Learning
2. Self-Observation and Change
3. Reducing Tension
4. Learning How to Change
5. Changing Your Thinking
6. The Power of Positive Thinking
7. Disputing Irrational Thinking
8. Relaxation
9. Communication, Part 1
10. Communication, Part 2
11. Negotiation and Problem Solving, Part 1
12. Negotiation and Problem Solving, Part 2
13. Negotiation and Problem Solving, Part 3
14. Negotiation and Problem Solving, Part 4
15. Life Goals
16. Prevention, Planning, and Ending

There is an evidence-based companion program that is used with parents of youth taking the *CWD-A* course comprised of nine two-hour sessions designed to help parents work with their depressed adolescent by providing information and strategies. The *CWD-A* and parent sessions are conducted separately, with the exception of two joint sessions with the adolescent and the parents. The instructor's manual and parent workbook may be obtained at http://www.kpchr.org/public/acwd/acwd. html. Like the *CWD-A,* the program may be used for research or clinical work without charge. The nine sessions are:

1. Introduction and Communication, Part 1
2. Adolescent Lessons and Communication, Part 2
3. Adolescent Lessons and Communication, Part 3
4. Adolescent Lessons and Problem Solving, Part 1
5. Adolescent Lessons and Problem Solving, Part 2
6. Adolescent Lessons and Problem Solving, Part 3

Lewinsohn, Clarke, Hops, and Andrews (1990) randomly 59 depressed adolescents to either the *CWD-A* program alone consisting of 14 two-hour group sessions, *CWD-A* plus parent group of 7 weekly sessions, or a wait-list control group. At the conclusion of treatment, 43% of the adolescent only group and 48% of the adolescent-plus-parent group no longer met diagnostic criteria for depression, compared to only 5% of the control group. Both groups showed lower scores on self-report depression measures as compared to the control group. Treatment effects were maintained at 1, 6, 12, and 24 months. Interestingly, the adolescent-plus-parent group did not have significantly better outcomes than the adolescent only group, suggesting that active parent involvement in therapy for depressed adolescents may not necessarily produce better results. Adolescents with more significant cognitive distortions, higher depressive symptomatology, and comorbid anxiety disorders tend to have poorer outcomes (Clarke, Hops, Lewinsohn, Andrew, & Williams, 1992).

In the subsequent study by Clarke, Lewinsohn, Rohde, Hops, and Seeley (1999), using the same design as Clarke et al. (1990), 65, 69, and 48% of adolescents only, adolescents plus parents, and controls, respectively, did not meet criteria for depression or dysthymia at the conclusion of treatment. The design included one or two booster sessions for those participants who remitted to diagnostic criteria prior to the end of treatment. These sessions did not reduce the rate of depression recurrence in these children, but they did increase the rate of recovery for those who had not yet recovered by the end of the acute treatment phase. These studies indicate that the CWD-A not only produced immediate therapeutic benefits but that the positive effects were maintained over time.

Taking ACTION is a manualized CBT intervention program for younger depressed children developed by Stark and Kendall (1996). It is primarily designed for girls aged 9–13 who have unipolar depression, dysthymia, or depressed mood. The authors assert that the treatment model and procedures are appropriate for all ages with appropriate developmental adaptations. It is used in a group format of about 4–8 children or can be used individually. There are 18 child sessions of about an hour each and 11 family sessions. The first eight child sessions are conducted twice a week for four weeks to provide more rapid symptom relief and then one hour per week for the subsequent ten weeks. The first eight sessions are primarily educational, and the remaining sessions are focused on altering distorted cognitions, practicing of learned strategies, pleasant activity scheduling, and problem-solving skills. The significant family involvement is designed to address complex interactions and communications that may contribute to the development and maintenance of depressive cognitions and symptoms. The program includes separate workbooks for children and parents, as well as separate therapist training manuals. Consistent with other manualized intervention programs, "*Taking ACTION*" includes homework assignments, check-in procedures at each session, and the opportunity to practice newly learned skills. The program has four primary components: (a) affective education, (b) coping skills training, (c) problem-solving training, and (d) cognitive interventions. The third component, problem-solving training, forms the core of the "*ACTION*" component:

*A*lways Do Something to Feel Better.
*C*atch the Positive and Let the Negative Go.
*T*hink of It as a Problem to be Solved.
*I*nspect the Situation.
*O*pen Yourself to the Positive.
*N*ever Get Stuck in the Negative Muck.

The child sessions with objectives are summarized as follows:

1. Introduction and Establishing Rules

   - Introduction of Therapist and Participants
   - Address Participants' Thoughts and Feelings about Participation and Shape Expectations
   - Set Rules for the Group
   - Assess Current Severity of Depressive Symptoms

2. Building Group Cohesion and Identifying Emotions

   - Discuss Therapist's Expectations
   - Build Group Cohesion and Establish Labels for Emotions
   - Prepare Participants for Homework Assignment

3. Introduction to ACTION

   - Discuss Participants' Concerns and Set an Agenda
   - Continue to Build Group Cohesion. Help Children Learn How to Recognize Emotions and Understand Relationship Among Thinking, Feeling, and Behaving
   - Introduction to Taking ACTION
   - Begin to Link Mood and Engagement in Pleasant Events
   - Introduce New Feelings Diary

4. Pleasant Events Scheduling

   - Extend Participants' Understanding of Mood–Thoughts–Behavior Relationship
   - Extend Participants' Understanding of ACTION
   - Extend Pleasant Events Schedule

5. Introduction to Problem Solving

   - Extend Mood–Behavior–Thought Relationship
   - Introduce the Group to Problem Solving

6. Problem Solving and Coping

   - Increase Engagement in Pleasant Events
   - Extend Participants' Understanding of Problem Solving; Review of Each of the Six Steps

7. Overcoming Avoidance of Problem Solving

   - Extend Participants' Understanding of How to Use Problem Solving
   - Begin Building a Positive Sense of Self
   - Introduce the Mood Scale to the Pleasant Events Schedules

8. Application of Problem Solving to Mood Disturbance

   - Application of Problem Solving to Mood Disturbance
   - Case of the Missing Solution
   - Assess Participants' Sense of Self

9. Application of Problem Solving to Daily Hassles

   - Apply Problem Solving to Daily Hassles
   - Continue to Build a Positive Sense of Self

10. Formal Introduction to Cognitive Restructuring

   - Spontaneous Use of Problem Solving
   - Rationale for Cognitive Restructuring
   - Help the Children to Learn how to Tune into Their Thoughts
   - Continue to Build a Positive Sense of Self

11. Catching Negative Thoughts

   - Practice Catching Thoughts
   - Introduction to Cognitive RestructuriNg
   - Continue to Build a Positive Sense of Self

12. What is the Evidence

   - Improve Participants' Understanding of how to use Cognitive Restructuring
   - Improve the Children's Ability to Catch Their Own Thoughts
   - Continue to Build a Positive Sense of Self

13. Alternative Interpretation

   - Introduce Alternative Interpretation
   - Continue to Build a Positive Sense of Self
   - Establish Standards in a Concrete Manner
   - Introduction to Self-Evaluation

14. There are Many Ways to Interpret Things

   - Extend the Point that There are Many Ways to Interpret Things
   - Identify an Area for Self-Improvement
   - Establish Goals
   - Break the Goals into Subgoals
   - Help the Participants to Start Working Toward Self-Improvement

15. What If

   - Introduce What If? = What is Going to Happen?
   - Practice Using What If?
   - Continue to Work Toward Self-Improvement
   - Use Problem Solving and Cognitive Restructuring To Facilitate Change

16. Working Toward Self-Improvement: Gaining a Sense of Self-Efficacy

   - Continue to Work Toward Self-Improvement
   - Use Problem Solving and Cognitive Restructuring to Facilitate Change
   - Begin Preparing for Termination

The program is well grounded in CBT theory, principles, and procedures and has empirical support for its effectiveness (e.g., Birmaher et al., 1996). The program is highly "user-friendly" and is easily adapted to the needs and circumstances of the child. Although the program is designed for girls, it can be used with boys and can be implemented in school or clinical settings.

Interpersonal Psychotherapy

Interpersonal psychotherapy (IPT) is an alternative to traditional CBT for the treatment of depression that was originally developed for use with adults (Weissman, Markowitz, & Klerman, 2000). IPT is based on the assumption that depression occurs in an interpersonal context and that it affects social relationships, which, in turn, affect mood. Thus, IPT focuses on depressive symptoms that occur in interpersonal interactions and relationships. There is ample clinical and research evidence that depressed adults, adolescents, and children have difficulties with interpersonal interactions, including the fact that they often lose the emotional and social support of others, worsening the depressive symptoms. The IPT perspective of depression emphasizes three components: (a) symptom formation, (b) social functioning, and (c) personality characteristics, with the primary therapeutic focus being on the first two areas. By decreasing depressive symptomatology and improving social relationships, the client's mood, social support, and interpersonal functioning improve. IPT takes a problem-solving approach in which the client and therapist identify specific problems to be solved and they collaborate to develop communication and problem-solving skills. As these skills are learned, they are practiced during therapy sessions, and the client applies them to improving significant relationships in the community.

IPT with Adolescents

IPT has been adapted for use with adolescents where the focus on relationships increases significantly compared to childhood, such as romantic and sexual relationships, peer influences, family interactions, and other situations that emphasize significant interpersonal interactions. IPT for adolescents (IPT-A) has many similarities to CBT, with an emphasis on therapist–client collaboration, structure and planning, active involvement, and learning through teaching and instruction. Like CBT, IPT-A is time limited and has a set number of sessions with additional sessions as needed. Young and Mufson (2008) summarize the components of IPT-A as typically being 12 weekly sessions, and 16 sessions can be used if indicated. Three phases are described in IPT-A:

Initial Phase (Sessions 1–4)

- Confirm the diagnosis of depression.
- Education about depression and assigning a "limited sick role."
- Introduce IPT-A principles and the structure of treatment.
- Conduct an inventory to identify interpersonal problem areas.
- Develop a treatment contract.

Middle Phase (Sessions 5–9)

- Further clarification of identified problems
- Identification of strategies to target problems
- Implementation of selected interventions

This phase focuses linking affect to interpersonal events, analysis of communication skills, role playing activities, homework assignments, dealing with grief issues, dealing with interpersonal disputes, and addressing interpersonal deficits.

Termination Phase (Sessions 10–12)

In this final phase, the therapist and adolescent focus on several topics:

- Review of progress
- Changes in interpersonal functioning linked to improved mood and decreased symptomatology
- Identification of effective strategies and the importance of continuing to use them after treatment ends
- Discussion of areas that continue to need improvement and work
- Discuss warning signs of depression
- Appropriate termination procedures
- Meet with the parents, if possible, to discuss progress, effective strategies, relapse signs, and the fact that some depressive symptoms may remain

IPT-A is designed to work with individual clients, and there is sufficient research to indicate that it is an efficacious treatment for adolescent depression. Studies by Mufson et al. (1994), Mufson, Weissman, Moreau, and Garfinkel (1999), and Mufson, Dorta, Wickamaratne et al. (2004) have supported the efficacy of IPT-A. Rosselló and Bernal (1999) compared the effectiveness of CBT and IPT-A with Puerto Rican adolescents and found that CBT and IPT-A produced a greater reduction in symptoms, an increase in self-esteem, and better social functioning than occurred in the control group. IPT-A showed a greater effect in meeting recovery criteria than did CBT (82% vs. 52%). Limited research exists on using IPT-A in a group format, although Mufson, Gallagher, Dorta, and Young (2004) found no difference between individual and group use of IPT-A, suggesting that a group format may be an efficient and effective delivery method.

Positive Psychotherapy for Adolescent Depression

Traditional forms of psychotherapy have focused primarily on negative symptoms, such as distorted cognitions, low affect, depression, poor social skills, high levels of anxiety that impair functioning, and mood problems that reflect psychopathology. Treatment focuses on the alleviation of these symptoms to help people to become more functional, with an acceptance that not all symptoms may be alleviated equally or that they will dissipate completely. There is also an implicit assumption that by alleviating symptoms, people will become happier, have greater self-esteem, and that many of their problems will be eliminated or lessened significantly with participation in therapy. Not surprisingly, Ryff and Keyes (1995) reported that measures of psychopathology show modest, negative correlations with measures of happiness and personal well-being. From a positive psychology perspective, good mental health is not only the absence of psychopathology but also happiness, well-being, and life satisfaction (Ryff & Singer, 2002).

From the positive psychology perspective, treatment should focus not only on symptom alleviation but also on promoting happiness, life satisfaction, and positive well-being. An emphasis on positive psychology also has implications for prevention of psychopathology or at least at a lower level of severity. Research on the effectiveness of positive psychotherapy (PPT) is not as well developed as for CBT and other well-established therapies. There is evidence that positive emotions serve as a protective factor against depression (Gillham & Reivich, 1999) in adults, but substantial similar data regarding children are fewer.

It is beyond the scope of this discussion to describe PPT in detail, and the reader is referred to Ryff and Singer (2002), Seligman (2002), and other resources on the applications of positive psychology to the treatment of depression and other forms of psychopathology. However, Rashid and Anjum (2008) provide a summary of a fourteen-session sequence of PPT that demonstrates the nature and structure of the approach:

1. *Orientation*—Lack of positive resources maintains depression
2. *Engagement*—Identifying signature strengths
3. *Engagement/pleasure*—Cultivation of signature strengths and positive emotions
4. *Pleasure*—Good versus bad memories
5. *Pleasure/engagement*—Forgiveness
6. *Pleasure/engagement*—Gratitude
7. *Pleasure/engagement*—Midtherapy check

8. *Meaning/engagement*—Satisfying instead of maximizing
9. *Pleasure*—Optimism and hope
10. *Engagement/meaning*—Love and attachment
11. *Meaning*—Family tree of strengths
12. *Pleasure*—Savoring
13. *Meaning*—Gift of time
14. *Integration*—The full life

Treatment of Pediatric Bipolar Disorder

The majority of research studies on the treatment of depression and mood disorders in children and adolescents have focused primarily on unipolar depression, dysthymia, or subclinical mood problems. There is less research on the efficacy of psychosocial treatments for pediatric bipolar disorder; thus, it is less clear which treatments are effective with children and adolescents. Due to the high degree of comorbidity in bipolar disorders, the likelihood that at least one parent has an active mood disorder and that families with children who have bipolar disorder tend to be more dysfunctional, the exact course of treatment and effects of specific treatments can be challenging to define. Over the last few years, a primary treatment focus has been the use of pharmacotherapy for treating adult and child bipolar disorder. Medications used to treat adult bipolar disorder are commonly used with children and youth, but their effectiveness has been understudied in randomized, controlled trials, and they are often used "off label" in that adult dosages are adjusted to work with children without specific research knowledge of effects in children (Johnston, 2009, personal communication). Given the difficulties and controversies surrounding pediatric bipolar disorder, much needs to be known about the efficacy of drug treatment for pediatric bipolar disorder.

Although there are few studies of the efficacy of psychotherapy and psychosocial treatments of bipolar disorder, there is evidence that treatments used for unipolar disorder may be effective. Miklowitz and Scott (2009) conducted a review of 19 studies of randomized clinical trial studies that included adults and children who received various treatments, including psychoeducational approaches focusing on providing information and training to parents about working with children having bipolar disorder. Miklowitz and Scott concluded that psychosocial treatments of bipolar disorder from the prior meta-analyses found that disorder-specific therapies (CBT, IPT, family, and group) enhanced the effectiveness of mood stabilizers (OR = 0.57; 95% CI: 0.39–0.82) over 1–2-year periods. They concluded that psychosocial therapies have significant value as adjunctive to medication treatment and resulted in reductions in recurrence, hospitalizations, and functional impairments. Included in the review was a study by Mendenhall, Fristad, and Early (2009) that provided a combination of didactic information, stress management, communication skills, and strategies to address mood escalation in 175 children with bipolar disorder (70%) and unipolar disorder (30%). The treatment format was a multifamily group model in which the children participated with their parents. Over the course of a year, the children in the treatment group showed greater improvement in mood symptoms than did children in the wait-list control group. No data were reported on recovery or recurrence, and an additional outcome was parents' increased ability to advocate for their children's health and mental health needs.

An interesting aspect of the Miklowitz and Scott (2009) review was that the authors identified factors that mediated and enhanced the effectiveness of the psychosocial treatments. These factors appeared to be influential in determining the degree of success of the various treatment modalities. These mediating factors were:

- Acquiring emotion regulation skills
- Acquiring behavioral and less pessimistic attitudes toward the self in relation to the illness
- Improving family relationships and communication
- Improving social skills
- Decreasing self-stigmatization and increasing acceptance of the disorder
- Increasing social and treatment supports
- Enhancing medication adherence
- Stabilizing sleep/wake cycles and other daily routines
- Improving ability to identify and intervene early with relapses (p. 111)

Miklowitz and Scott suggest that attending to these mediators may help with decisions about which treatments to implement, their effectiveness, and cost-effectiveness. Thus, therapies may be more effective if they include consideration of these mediating factors in the overall treatment protocol. Although the review suggests that CBT and psychoeducational approaches can be effective for the treatment of pediatric bipolar disorder, the authors state that more research is needed on the effects of psychosocial treatment on disorder onset in young children.

Interventions for Suicidal Children and Youth

Psychopathology of various forms increases the risk for suicidal ideation and attempts, with depression, substance abuse, and conduct disorder being primary precursors of higher risk in adolescents. Girls are more likely to have depressive disorders and males to have conduct disorder, each of which raises the risk for suicidal ideation and attempts by sex, respectively (Shaffer et al., 1996). Children and youth who have depression and mood disorders are at greater risk of thinking about and attempting suicide, although the psychopathology and factors leading to this risk originate many years earlier.

Research on treatments for suicidal youth is limited, due to obvious problems with conducting randomized clinical trials that would assign suicidal youths to a wait-list or control group. Thus, most research has been with adults. Some research has suggested that dialectical behavior therapy (DBT) using cognitive and behavioral strategies can be effective in treating suicidal behavior. DBT targets the problem of poor emotion regulation that is found in depressed persons who are more prone to attempt suicide. Henriques, Beck, and Brown (2003) considered suicidal behavior to be the problem rather than only a symptom and developed a brief cognitive intervention for suicide attempters aged 18 and older. The program consists of ten sessions that begin with identification of thoughts and beliefs that occurred prior to the suicide attempt. Then, cognitive and behavioral strategies are applied to help individuals develop more effective ways of thinking about and evaluating their situation and responding to distress. Typical cognitive–behavioral methods may also be useful in reducing suicidal ideation and attempts by targeting distorted beliefs and feelings of hopelessness.

Rathus and Miller (2002) used a variation of DBT to treat adolescent suicide attempters who had at least three features of bipolar disorder. This program includes 12 sessions of twice per week meetings with the adolescent and parents for family skills training. Participants had better adherence to treatment and had fewer hospitalizations than those receiving the standard treatment. The youth also showed less suicidal ideation, symptom severity, and overall distress, although the reductions were not significantly different from the control group.

Thus, the research indicates that initial therapeutic approaches should focus primarily on the suicidal behavior and less on the underlying psychopathology. Once the risk for suicide has lessened and is not considered imminent, attention can be directed toward the broader range of psychopathological symptoms. Variations of cognitive therapies have promise to treat suicidal ideation and attempts and should be considered as one approach to treatment.

Treating the Anxious–Depressed Syndrome

It is well established in clinical practice and research that comorbidity between anxiety and depression is common in children and adolescents, occurring in up to 75% of cases (e.g., Kovacs, 1990), which has been described by some authors as an anxious–depressed, narrow band syndrome (Achenbach & Rescorla, 2001). Consequently, it is often challenging to distinguish between the two disorders and raises questions whether to attempt to treat them separately or as a mixed syndrome.

If a child has high levels of anxiety and depression, there are several possible implications for treatment:

1. High levels of anxiety tend to complicate treatment of depression.
2. High levels of anxiety and depression tend to be associated with poorer therapeutic and developmental outcomes than occur with either disorder by itself.
3. High levels of anxiety predispose the child to fears, phobias, and panic attacks that may require immediate intervention before depression can be addressed effectively.

4. High levels of depression may impair the child's ability or motivation to participate in treatment, making it more difficult to treat either condition.
5. The presence of both disorders increases the risk for the development of other disorders, such as panic disorder, substance abuse, and aggression.
6. Treatment processes may be similar for both conditions but may need to be tailored and adapted for the symptoms of the condition that requires the most attention.
7. As treatment progresses and the symptoms of one disorder subside, attention to the other one may become more feasible if it does not remit simultaneously.

When treating the anxious–depressed syndrome, there may be an inclination to treat the anxiety first, assuming that it most likely preceded depression. Conversely, treatment of the depressive disorder may seem more appropriate if the child is having difficulty making friends, enjoying being with others, or otherwise showing behavioral dysfunction. Although it is beyond the scope of this chapter to address treatment of the anxious–depressed syndrome in detail, the following are suggested as an initial plan to address the symptoms:

1. Conduct an assessment of suicidal risk. If there is imminent and purposeful suicidal ideation, this should be treated first to reduce the possibility of an attempt.
2. Through assessment, attempt to determine which symptoms are the most impairing and contributing to the other disorder. For example, if the clinician determines that the child has a depressed mood due to high levels of anxiety associated with feeling a loss of control, treatment of the anxiety symptoms may simultaneously reduce the depressive symptoms exacerbated by the anxiety.
3. Maintain ongoing assessment of the intensity, frequency, and duration of symptoms for each condition and develop a monitoring system for them.
4. Develop a treatment protocol to address the most problematic symptoms/behaviors or cognitive distortions and emphasize them in the initial phases of treatment.
5. As treatment progresses, continue to evaluate symptom severity and the increase or decrease in other symptoms and treat as appropriate.

Pharmacotherapy for Child and Adolescent Depression

Although considerable controversy exists as to whether there is sufficient research on the effectiveness and appropriateness of the use of medications with children and adolescents, pharmacotherapy is a rather common practice for the treatment of youth depression. The chart in Appendix F lists some medications commonly used to treat child and adolescent depression.

The US Food and Drug Administration (FDA) has advised physicians that antidepressants may increase the likelihood of suicidal ideation or attempts and has requested that warnings to this effect be included on the labels of these medications. These warnings are to include information that depressive symptomatology may increase in children and adolescent, especially in light of the lack of research on both the short-term and long-term efficacy of these medications.

Selective serotonin reuptake inhibitors (SSRIs) have been evaluated extensively with research paradigms that are in randomized, double-blind studies using placebo control groups. Emslie et al. (1997) studied the effects of 20 mg of fluoxetine and found that 50% of depressed and 33% of the placebo group showed significant improvement. Later, Esmlie et al. (2002) found that fluoxetine showed "much" or "very much" improvement of self-reported depression ratings in 52% of depressed youth, compared to 37% of the placebo control group. Following release of this study, the FDA approved the use of fluoxetine to treat children and adolescents who have major depression.

Other studies have been conducted using antidepressants to treat child and adolescent depression. Keller et al. (2001) compared the effects of paroxetine and imipramine to a placebo group and found effects of 66, 48, and 48%, respectively. Wagner et al. (2003) found sertraline to be significantly more effective than a placebo. Ryan (2003) reviewed several studies using tricyclic antidepressants and concluded that they were not more effective than a placebo. All of these studies were at least eight weeks in duration and had sample sizes ranging from 174 to 500.

Evidence of Efficacy of Combined Pharmacotherapy and Psychotherapy

There is literature suggesting that a combination of medication and psychotherapy is more effective for treating depression than is either one alone, but this research has been conducted primarily on adults. Randomized clinical trial studies on the separate and combined effects of therapy and medication for treating depression in children and adolescents are limited, but some studies have been conducted. One of the best studies was the Treatment for Adolescents with Depression Study (TADS; Treatment for Adolescents with Depression Team, 2004) that compared the singular and combined effects of cognitive–behavioral therapy and fluoxetine on 439 adolescents (mean age = 14.6) with major depressive disorder over a 12-week treatment period. Adolescents considered at high risk for suicide were not included, although 29% did show suicidal ideation at baseline. Fluoxetine and placebo were administered in a double-blind condition, while CBT alone and CBT with fluoxetine were provided in a nonblind condition. Primary outcome measures were self-reports of depression, and a global clinical index was used as a responder analysis rated as "much improved" or "very much improved."

The results indicated response rates as follows:

- Fluoxetine alone = 60.6% (N = 109)
- Fluoxetine with CBT = 71.0% (N = 107)
- CBT alone = 43.2% (N = 111)
- Placebo = 34.8% (N = 112)

Fluoxetine with CBT was significantly different from placebo ($p = 0.001$), while treatment with fluoxetine alone and CBT alone was not different from placebo ($p = 0.10$ and $p = 0.40$, respectively). Fluoxetine with CBT was superior to fluoxetine alone ($p = 0.02$) and CBT alone ($p = 0.001$). Analyses were conducted on the week 12 data, which yielded slightly different results: (a) fluoxetine with CBT and fluoxetine alone were superior to placebo ($p = 0.001$ and $p = 0.002$, respectively) while CBT was not superior to placebo ($p = 0.97$), (b) fluoxetine with CBT was superior to CBT alone ($p = 0.001$) but not to fluoxetine alone ($p = 0.13$), and (c) fluoxetine alone was significantly more effective than CBT alone ($p = 0.001$). The finding that CBT was not significantly different from placebo was unexpected, given that the authors cited other studies indicating that CBT has shown approximately a 60% efficacy rate in treating adolescent depression. The authors suggested that the lower effectiveness of CBT may have been due to differences in the CBT program, although it was effective in reducing suicidality in both the CBT alone group and the CBT with fluoxetine group. The group receiving CBT alone was comprised of adolescents showing more severe and chronic depression and higher rates of comorbidity, with half having one or more comorbid disorders. Thus, the adolescents in that group may not have responded as well to the treatment compared to previous studies.

The study authors also reported adverse harm-related events associated with each treatment condition that included suicide attempts. Thirty-three (7.5%) of the 439 participants had an adverse harm-related event, and 24 (5.5%) had a suicide-related adverse event.

	CBT with fluoxetine	Fluoxetine alone	CBT alone	Placebo
No. of events	15 (8.4%)	22 (11.9%)	10 (4.5%)	10 (5.4%)

These data suggest that treatment with fluoxetine was associated with an increased risk of harm-related or suicide-related events up to twice as often compared to CBT alone or placebo, which were equal. The fact that CBT with fluoxetine showed a lower frequency of adverse events suggests that CBT may have had a protective or mitigating role in reducing the risk of adverse events.

There were also psychiatric adverse events in some patients that included symptoms such as mania, irritability/depressed mood, agitation/restlessness, anxiety/panic, sleep problems, fatigue/sedation, or other problems (i.e., tremors, abnormal behavior, and feelings of abnormality). The number of events and patients involved by treatment condition is reported below.

	CBT with fluoxetine	Fluoxetine alone	CBT alone	Placebo
No. of events	16 (15%)	23 (21%)	1 (1%)	11 (9.8%)
No. of patients	12 (11.2%)	20 (18.3%)	1 (0.9%)	8 (7.1%)

These data suggest that there was a greater risk of adverse psychiatric events with the use of fluoxetine, but less so with CBT and fluoxetine together or CBT alone. It is possible that CBT helped to lessen the chances of adverse effects with fluoxetine, given that CBT alone was associated with only one adverse event. Although fluoxetine alone was associated with adverse psychiatric events at twice the occurrence of placebo may raise questions about its use, fluoxetine alone and with CBT nevertheless produced better outcomes than placebo.

Further, the authors found that fluoxetine was associated with reduced suicidal ideation at a level comparable to placebo, indicating that the medication did not increase suicidal ideation. Suicidal ideation decreased significantly in all treatment groups, with the fluoxetine and CBT combination showing the most reduction. Seven participants attempted suicide, although no attempts were successful. The authors concluded that fluoxetine with CBT produced the best outcomes. The number of suicide attempts was too small to link to effects or noneffects of any treatment condition. Although CBT with fluoxetine was superior to either treatment alone, only 37% of the subjects in that group achieved remission, leaving about two-thirds with significant symptomatology. A potential limitation of the study was the use of self-reports of depression and suicidal ideation, which may not have assessed all areas that might have been affected by the treatments, such as distorted cognitions and feelings of self-efficacy.

Other evidence exists to suggest that pharmacotherapy and psychotherapy together are more effective than either alone in treating adolescent depression, while other studies have found no difference or even that psychotherapy alone is more effective. Brent (2006) and Weisz, McCarty, and Valeri (2006) suggest that the CBT program used in the TADS study was not optimally developed and delivered, which may help explain its less than typical effectiveness outcomes. In a recent review of the literature, Sommers-Flanagan and Campbell (2009) concluded that psychotherapy should be the "...frontline treatment for youth with depression and that little scientific evidence suggests that combined psychotherapy and medication treatment is more effective than psychotherapy alone" (p. 111). Thus, considerable controversy and conflicting evidence remain about the relative roles of psychotherapy and medication in treating youth depression, and decisions on whether to use one or both will depend on multiple factors, including comorbidity, family issues, adherence to treatment, and severity of symptomatology. At the least, however, psychotherapy using CBT approaches to treat child and adolescent depression has significant support with little risk of adverse effects.

In a meta-analysis of relapse in unipolar depression with adults, Vittengl, Clark, Dunn, and Jarrett (2007) found that without continuation of cognitive therapy for acute depressive episode, relapse occurred in about 54% of cases within two years. Further, they found that cognitive therapy reduced relapse significantly compared with acute-phase pharmacotherapy (22% reduction) or without medication (22% reduction). They concluded that patients, clinicians, and those who develop treatment guidelines should consider that cognitive therapy may have preventive effects not seen with medication treatment. In cases of mild to moderate depression, an initial course of treatment may be a cognitive therapy approach, while more severe cases may warrant consideration of medication and psychotherapy.

Considerations for Developing Interventions for Child and Adolescent Depression

Despite inconsistencies in the research literature about what are the best approaches to treating child and adolescent depression, there are some procedures and considerations that clinicians can use to help the youth, their families, and others to make decisions about what to do and how to formulate a treatment plan that may involve questions about medications:

- Conduct a thorough developmental history.
- Complete appropriate psychological assessment.
- Try to determine the protective factors that may help facilitate treatment.
- Try to determine risk factors that may hinder treatment and if they can be lessened.
- Assess for suicidal risk. If risk is high, an initial course of treatment may be to address the suicidal ideation and behavior before treating underlying or comorbid psychopathology.
- Assess for comorbid psychopathology, which is likely to be present and determine which symptoms must be addressed first.
- Consider whether referral for medication management is appropriate.
- If medication is used, the clinician should maintain close collaboration with the prescriber to monitor overall progress and whether changes in medications or dosages are having desired or untoward effects.
- Develop a method for ongoing monitoring and evaluation of the treatment program while in progress and at termination of therapy.
- The clinician should consider whether any or all of the following are indicated to be included in the treatment plan:

  - Social skills training
  - Problem-solving training
  - Pleasant activity scheduling
  - Behavioral activation
  - Goal setting training
  - Conflict resolution training
  - Relaxation training and stress management

Considerations for Parent Involvement in Treatment of Child and Adolescent Depression

As is the case with anxiety, there is little doubt that parents should be involved in treatment of child and adolescent depression. However, most treatment programs work with the child directly, unless a family therapy approach is used. Most individual and group treatment programs emphasize CBT approaches, such as

Taking ACTION (Stark & Kendall, 1996) or the *Coping with Depression-Adolescent* manualized treatment program (Clarke et al., 1999; Lewinsohn et al., 1990). Many programs include parents as collaborators or as separate participants, such as the *Coping with Depression-Adolescent* program for parents of depressed adolescents (Clarke et al., Lewinsohn et al.).

A potential difference in consideration is that families of children with depression tend to be more dysfunctional with greater parental psychopathology than are families of anxious children. Therefore, the specific ways in which parents may be involved may require more planning and consideration. Similar questions to those posed in Chap. 10 for anxious children and youth may be useful in considering parental involvement for depressed children:

- Whether the parents have significant depressive disorders that might impact treatment
- Whether the parents are committed to positive outcomes for the child
- Whether the parents can serve as effective collaborators in treatment
- Whether there is significant family psychopathology, such as marital distress
- Whether there is significant parental psychopathology that is best addressed in adult treatment

Case Example

In Chap. 9, the case of Adam, a 12-year-old boy with depression associated with family and school problems was presented. Data about the family history and from a psychological assessment are presented that describe Adam having a mood disorder that is related to dysfunction at home and social and academic problems at school. The complex family dynamics contribute to the development and maintenance of his depressive symptoms, and a plan for treating the marital discord and family dysfunction is beyond the scope of this chapter. However, these factors are important in conceptualizing an intervention approach for Adam from a CBT perspective using the framework presented by Friedberg and McClure (2002) that considers six variables and a three-phase treatment formulation plan.

Presenting Problem

Cognitive Symptoms—anger, frustration, concentration problems, "all-or-none" thinking, negative attributional bias, negative view of the world, self, and the future

Behavioral Symptoms—withdrawal, aggression, impulsiveness, distractibility, avoidance, underperformance in school-related tasks

Physiological Symptoms—sleeping problems, muscle tension, psychomotor agitation, low energy

Test Data

The data presented in Chap. 9 indicate that Adam is experiencing depressive mood ($T=78$) that is pervasive across home and school and is associated with aggressiveness, home and family difficulties, and school-related problems. He experiences anhedonia ($T=71$), problems with locus of control ($T=78$), attention problems ($T=67$), conflicts with peers ($T=77$), impulsivity ($T=72$), and noncompliance ($T=71$). There are discrepancies among the informants, with generally more severity reported by the mother across internalizing and externalizing dimensions. He has a negative attitude toward school that likely is related to his academic problems, lack of social engagement, and deficits in social skills. His adaptive skills are impaired across home and school settings, and he reports poor relationships with others. The comorbid externalizing symptoms, including ADHD, exacerbate his problems at home and school and contribute to difficulties in social relationships. Thus, the results of the assessment indicate that Adam has a mood disorder and also has externalizing problems that include oppositional behavior, impulsivity, noncompliance, and inattention. Interventions will need to focus simultaneously on all of these areas. For the purpose of this chapter, the focus will be on CBT approaches to addressing his depressive mood and negative attributional style.

Cultural Context Variables

Adam comes from a lower middle class family where there are some financial stresses, but the family is not impoverished. The primary contextual variable is that the family is experiencing some stressors associated with marital difficulties, sibling disagreements, maternal depression and paternal relationships, and lack of family support for Adam's emotional needs. These factors could interfere with the effects of a CBT intervention because family support to carry out the various activities may be absent or inconsistent. Furthermore, Adam may not be able to practice learned strategies at home or may not receive recognition and reinforcement for his efforts to participate in and benefit from the therapy.

History and Developmental Milestones

Adam met all developmental milestones as expected and showed no delays in cognitive, language, motor, or other areas. His current family situation appears to be a contributor to his difficulties at home and at school. Although a formal cognitive and achievement assessment was not completed, his academic history suggests that he is of at least average ability and can do at least grade level work. Due to his apparent lack of motivation, effort, and performance, he is achieving in the bottom fourth of the class, below his expected level. His current social difficulties and coexisting depressive mood suggest that he is at significant risk for the development of psychological disorders, specifically major depression. He is at the age when depression tends to have its onset (Mash & Barkley, 2003), which puts him at greater risk of social, personal, and academic problems in subsequent years.

Cognitive Variables

Interviews with Adam revealed some cognitive distortions that often occur in children with depressed mood. Although he was reluctant to talk and to be forthcoming, he did make some statements that provide inferences into his cognitive schemas. When asked about his difficulties with aggression and peer relationships, Adam seemed to lack awareness of his role in confrontations and difficulties with others. He stated that "Other kids don't like me because they think I'm stupid" (mind reading) and that "I am the reason for the problems between mom and dad" (personalization). When asked about his relationships with his parents, he stated that "I should be a better kid and not cause so many problems for them" (should statements) and that "No matter what I do, it's always wrong. I can't do anything right" (dichotomous thinking). When discussing problems at school, Adam reported that it is not worth trying to work hard because he always seems to fail at everything (overgeneralization) and that everyone is smarter than he is (comparing). He does not believe that the situation will improve (hopelessness) and feels unable to do anything to improve it (helplessness). These cognitive distortions are consistent with Beck's (1967) conceptualization of depression as the child having negative views of self, the world in general, and the future. These distortions may become the focus of intervention techniques to replace automatic negative thoughts with positive cognitions.

Behavioral Antecedents and Consequences

Adam's negative mood and irritability are triggered and exacerbated at home when conflicts among family members arise, and he feels unable to control the associated stress. His primary method of coping with the family problems is to become angry or to withdraw and avoid confrontations and negative interactions as much as possible. The consequences of his angry reactions lead to negative responses from his parents, including yelling at him, loss of privileges, and continued arguments. Moreover, Adam does not receive positive feedback or is given positive alternatives for his behavior, which exacerbates his symptoms over time. The withdrawal behaviors reduce the confrontations, but Adam does not develop effective ways to communicate his emotions and thoughts to family members.

At school, Adam's anger and depression contribute to confrontations with others at school, as well as withdrawal and lack of involvement when asked to comply with assignments, tasks, and to participate, which tend to precipitate negative reactions. Confrontations with peers seem to be triggered when he perceives that he is being teased, ridiculed, or excluded. His common reactions of withdrawal or aggressive behavior lead to discipline by the school and exclusion by peers. Consequently, he does not learn effective social skills or obtain positive feedback from others that will help him to develop emotion regulation skills.

Provisional Formulation

Adam shows many symptoms of dysthymia and depressed mood, including withdrawal, anhedonia, negative mood, hopelessness, social skills deficits, and interpersonal relationship problems that are pervasive across home and school. He has few friends and is not successful at school in either social or academic spheres, due to lack of motivation, effort, or interest. Although he has at least average academic ability, his lack of effort and performance at school leads to underachievement and low grades. He experiences low self-esteem and lack of self-efficacy in nearly all aspects of his life, with home problems being major contributors to the development, exacerbation, and maintenance of the symptoms. Home and school are not effective avenues to help him develop emotion regulation skills, and he often reacts with anger and withdrawal when confronted with problems. He has a negative attributional style that is seen often in children with depressed mood, which inhibits the development of insight and problem-solving skills. He is experiencing several cognitive, behavioral, and physiological symptoms that are characteristic of children with depressed mood and occur across multiple settings.

Adam feels pressure to perform at school and to comply with academic and social expectations of teachers and peers. Although he may appear to be unmotivated at school, his lowered performance is partially the result of his depressive symptoms that include low energy, fatigue, loss of interest in tasks, sadness, irritability, difficulties concentrating and sustaining attention, and low task persistence. These symptoms also may be related to his diagnosis of ADHD, although it may be difficult to determine which of the symptoms are related to ADHD or to depressive mood.

An intervention program for Adam should focus on his depressive symptoms at home and at school and include components to help him function better in both settings. Using a CBT program such as *Taking ACTION* (Stark & Kendall, 1996) that includes specific tasks and structure would help Adam to recognize his cognitive, behavioral, and physiological symptoms and begin to understand how they are related. It would be important to help him learn to understand not only how his anger is related to his situation but also how expressing anger inappropriately leads to more problems for him at home and at school. Therefore, the treatment plan for him should include a component to address self-management of his anger and aggressive behavior. He also needs to become more aware of how his behavior contributes to his social problems and begin to develop strategies to improve his social skills. The therapist should also determine if Adam has skill deficits or performance deficits with regard to his social interactions.

Anticipated Treatment Plan

1. Although Adam does not show clinically significant levels of anxiety on the psychological assessment measures, training in relaxation methods may be useful to help him calm himself when he begins to experience anger and frustration.
2. Adam should receive a CBT-manualized treatment program intended to reduce depressive symptomatology, such as *Taking ACTION* (Stark & Kendall, 1996) or the *Adolescent Coping with Depression Course* (Clarke et al., 1999; Lewinsohn et al., 1990). A CBT program should emphasize helping Adam to understand the interrelatedness of his negative attributions and schemata, depressive mood, behavioral patterns, anger, and aggression.
3. The parents should be involved in a program to help address Adam's depressive symptoms, but not as active participants in treatment sessions with Adam, given the apparent family dysfunction and marital difficulties. These issues should be addressed separately, and parent involvement should be adjunctive, such as using the *Group for Parents of Depressed Youth* (Clarke et al., 1999; Lewinsohn et al., 1990), a companion program to the *Adolescent Coping with Depression Course* (Clarke et al., 1999; Lewinsohn et al., 1990). The parents should be involved in assisting Adam to practice new skills learned in treatment, such as transporting him to social events.
4. Involve Adam in pleasant activity scheduling that he can do with peers and family members. Encourage him to become involved in group activities and hobbies in which he shows some interest.
5. Involve Adam in social skills training activities, such as groups and psychoeducational activities.
6. Develop and implement anger management strategies that Adam can use when he become angry and feels the urge to act out.
7. Work with Adam's teachers to help them understand his depressed mood, anger problems, and how to respond to them in the classroom. They may benefit from some direct training in depression and anger problems.
8. Develop and implement classroom management strategies at school as an alternative to subjecting Adam to punitive discipline.
9. Develop social relationships at school that include "buddy systems," peer tutoring, and social skills training in the school setting.

Expected Obstacles

Initially, Adam may be resistant to participating in therapy, due to lack of motivation, insight, hostility, and unwillingness to admit to problems. His negative attributional style may inhibit the ability or desire to explore options for his behavior, especially if he views problems as being caused by others. His view of his family situation may indicate feelings of helplessness and hopelessness that significant change can occur. Initially, his parents may not be able to be effective participants in the treatment and may need to be treated simultaneously while serving primarily as support for activities that Adam will need to engage in to reduce his depressive symptomatology. Adam's coexisting anger issues may also inhibit initial progress using a CBT approach.

In the school setting, it may be difficult to develop a partnership with Adam's teachers to develop classroom-based interventions to help with issues of interpersonal relationships with other students and task completion. They may not be familiar with the nature of depressive disorders and their relationship with academic performance and peer relationships. Therefore, some in-service training and consultation may be necessary initially to give them information about Adam's difficulties. It will also be necessary to evaluate the degree of acceptability that school personnel have about school-based interventions and the extent to which they will participate.

Adam presents as a child with chronic depressive symptoms and developing mood disorder that have pervasive effects across home and school settings and interfere with personal, social, and academic functioning. Treatment should involve direct work with Adam using CBT techniques, as well as working with the parents separately and interventions at school. As Adam's depressed mood improves, it may be possible to involve the parents more directly in treatment if their own treatment shows progress and there is evidence that they can be helpful in his progress.

Conclusion

Like anxiety disorders, depression and mood disorders are complex and require a multifaceted approach across a variety of settings and contexts. Because children with depression are more likely to have one or both parents with psychopathology than is the case with anxiety disorders, the implications for treatment are more challenging. Children with moderate to severe depression are likely to have comorbid anxiety disorders, as well, which may complicate treatment. Moreover, because depression is associated with increased risk for suicidal ideation, special care must be taken to address this possibility. Untreated depression is associated with negative outcomes, including social dysfunction, academic problems, and significant anhedonia. Long-term implications into adolescence and adulthood are associated with vocational, interpersonal, and social dysfunction, as well as increased risk for substance use. Therefore, systematic interventions including various forms of psychotherapy, psychoeducation, and family treatment for depressed children and adolescents are indicated, which may include medications. With effective treatment, however, outcomes for these children can lead to positive developmental trajectories.

Chapter 12
School-Based Interventions

Conceptualizing School-Based Interventions

When considering interventions for mental health problems in schools, the application of traditional models with emphasis on symptoms and disorders may not feasible or desirable. Generally, formal DSM-IV diagnoses are not needed in schools, unless services are being delivered by professionals who are receiving health insurance reimbursement or are working for agencies that require diagnoses. These models focus on internal pathology as the primary source of problems and as the focus of treatment. Adelman and Taylor (2010) suggest that such an emphasis, while not discounting the presence of internal pathology in some children, creates a narrow perspective on problems and ways to approach them. They suggest that the majority of children's emotional and behavioral problems are due primarily to sociocultural and economic factors. Relatively few children have diagnosable mental disorders, and Adelman and Taylor suggest that complex classification systems that focus on "…personal pathology has skewed theory, research, practice, and public policy" (p. 11). Rather, mental health in schools should take a broader perspective and focus on the following:

- Provide programs to (a) promote social–emotional development, (b) prevent mental health and psychosocial problems, and (c) enhance resiliency and protective buffers
- Provide programs and services to intervene as early after the onset of behavior, learning, and emotional problems as is feasible
- Enhance the mental health of families and school staff
- Build the capacity of all school staff to address barriers to learning and promote healthy development
- Address systemic matters at schools that affect mental health, such as high stakes testing, including exit exams, and other practices that engender bullying, alienation, and student disengagement from classroom learning
- Develop a comprehensive, multifaceted, and cohesive continuum of school–community interventions to address barriers to learning and promote healthy development (p. 12)

T.J. Huberty, *Anxiety and Depression in Children and Adolescents:*
Assessment, Intervention, and Prevention, DOI 10.1007/978-1-4614-3110-7_12,
© Springer Science+Business Media, LLC 2012

Because emotional and behavioral problems in schools most often are related to both academic and nonacademic factors, a traditional mental health approach that emphasizes therapy to change the child's behavior and cognitions often is not sufficient. Schools create conditions that may tend to trigger, cause, or exacerbate emotional and behavioral difficulties, but they also provide opportunities to treat and prevent the onset or worsening of problems. The importance of school-based interventions becomes more salient because many of the problems seen by community mental health providers are due to referrals by teachers and other school personnel. In the school setting, approaches toward intervention typically involve behavior intervention teams that engage in problem-solving, collaborative efforts. For example, many schools have "teacher assistance teams" or a similar program where children who present with emotional and behavioral problems are discussed by a group of teachers and others who generate suggestions for addressing the behaviors. Often, these approaches are effective, but in those cases where the problems are severe or chronic, school psychologists and other mental health personnel may be needed. The intervention plans developed often are focused on behaviors that occur within the classroom as well as in other school settings.

Schools provide opportunities to develop and implement interventions for a variety of emotional and behavioral problems, including anxiety and depression. Although schools may not have the facilities and personnel to provide traditional psychotherapy services, they can be instrumental in helping to address a range of mental health problems. In general, schools are not therapeutic settings, because they must address developing literacy and other skills while simultaneously recognizing that educational outcomes are influenced by mental health factors of children and youth. Nevertheless, schools are ideal settings to address mental health problems of children and youth for several reasons: (a) there are more opportunities to identify problems early in their development, (b) it is easier to address the inextricable relationship between academic and emotional/behavioral problems in the school than is possible in community-based services, (c) it is easier to implement interventions at the onset of problems rather than waiting until they become severe, (d) prevention programs can be established, (e) the vast majority of all children attend public or private schools, increasing the likelihood of working with a larger proportion of the school-age population, and (f) parents may be more willing to participate in school-based mental health services rather than going to a community mental health provider. Schools have a major role in providing mental health care to children and youth. In the US Surgeon General's Report on Mental Health (US Department of Health and Human Services, 1999), it was reported that approximately 70% of all mental health services provided to children occur in the public schools. Hoagwood and Johnson (2003) indicate that schools provide up to 75% of mental health services to children and youth in schools.

It is possible to use traditional psychotherapeutic methods in the school setting, and they may be appropriate at times to help children deal with specific personal issues and symptoms. Schools, however, provide opportunities to approach mental health problems from individual, systemic, family, ecological, and family perspectives. Thus, school-based interventions tend to be less focused on traditional conceptualizations of mental health problems as resting within the individual, but to view them in terms of how they affect social, personal, and academic functioning. This chapter will focus on school-based interventions from a problem-solving, multiple level intervention approach, which may include psychotherapy and counseling, behavioral interventions, and consultation to teachers, parents, and others.

Identification of Mental Health Problems in the School Setting

Schools are often referred to as being a "setting," suggesting that they are different from the home setting. In fact, schools can be considered to comprise multiple *settings*, i.e. one classroom is a setting with unique circumstances, stimuli, and contingences that may be very different from another classroom setting, requiring different approaches. Many school-based interventions require that modifications be made in these various settings to account for variations across them. Consequently, identification of problems must take into account the various settings that schools provide.

The first step in identification of mental health problems is to devise a method that has the potential to accurately identify those children who have or are at risk of developing difficulties over time. For children who have primarily externalizing problems, identification is easier because the behaviors are readily observable. Internalizing problems, however, tend to be covert, and they are not readily identified unless severe. Mild to moderate cases tend to go unnoticed or be seen as "laziness," apathy, or lack of ability by the student. Thus, a systematic approach is necessary to increase the probability of accurate identification of all children with mental health problems that impact social, personal, and academic functioning. The system must also be capable of identifying comorbid conditions so that misdiagnosis or nondiagnosis does not occur.

A common method to identify mental health problems in schools is to implement multiple-gating procedures (MGP), which begin with screening large groups or populations, followed by identification of children who are at risk of developing difficulties. Perhaps the most well-established and empirically supported MGP is the Systematic Screening for Behavior Disorders (SSBD) by Walker and Severson (1992). The SSBD has a three-stage procedure that begins with a teacher rating all students on a scale that includes items for both internalizing and externalizing symptoms. Thus, a teacher rates an entire class of students with a scale that can be completed in a few minutes for each child. After the data are collected and scored, the three students with the highest scores on the internalizing and externalizing scales are assessed further with two teacher rating scales. Walker and Severson concluded that identifying the top three students for further assessment is likely to identify those students with the most significant problems in both internalizing and externalizing dimensions. Cutoff score criteria are set in the second stage to identify those children who should be referred for Stage III in-depth psychological evaluations. The SSBD also includes structured observations in school and non-school settings.

A variation of this approach is to use well-established and psychometrically adequate behavior rating scales such as the *Child Behavior Checklist–Teacher Report Form* (CBCL–TRF; Achenbach & Rescorla, 2001) or the *Behavior Assessment System for Children, Second Edition* (BASC-2; Reynolds & Kamphaus, 2004). A teacher would be asked to complete a form for each student in the class, similar to Stage I of the SSBD. Using a standard score of 60 as a cutoff criterion would be used as an indicator of the presence of psychopathology. Children at or above this score would be referred for more in-depth screening or psychological evaluation that would include additional rating scales, observations, and self-report measures.

Another method of universal screening is the *Devereux Student Strengths Assessment* (DESSA; LeBuffe, Shapiro, & Naglieri, 2009), a 72-item measure of social–emotional competencies related to resilience in children from kindergarten through eighth grade. It is completed by teacher, parents, or other caregivers who rate a child on the items. It is well standardized on a representative US sample and yields a total score and eight subscales: Self-Awareness, Social Awareness, Self-Management, Goal-Directed Behavior, Relationship Skills, Personal Responsibility, Decision-Making, and Optimistic Thinking. Reliability and validity are acceptable. The scale is purported to give an overall indication of social–emotional competence and to be useful in helping to inform instruction and intervention. As a relatively new measure, more research is needed, but the DESSA has promise as a universal screening measure that may provide a starting point for identifying children who are at risk of social–emotional problems.

Because internalizing disorders are more difficult to identify and there is a greater risk of underidentification, another variation is to increase the number of children considered for further screening and evaluation. Some research suggests that up to 20% or more of adolescents have subsyndromal levels of internalizing symptoms that cause impairment, although they may not meet DSM-IV diagnostic criteria for a mental disorder (e.g. Costello et al., 1996). Failure to identify these children could result in several Type II errors, leaving them to continue to "suffer in silence" and be at risk for further development of psychopathology. At the elementary level, the frequency of symptoms tends to be lower than in adolescence, and prevalence of anxiety or depression is approximately equal between boys and girls. At adolescence, however, there is an expected ratio of about 2:1 girls to boys. A gating procedure in a high school class of 30 students with a prevalence rate of 20% would yield approximately four girls and two boys who have subclinical or clinical symptoms that should be evaluated further. Another advantage of lowering the cutoff for subsequent gating steps is the possibility of early identification, monitoring, and prevention of psychopathology. In cases where high risk is identified, more thorough psychological assessment using a multimethod approach would be indicated, with possible referral to school-based or community mental health providers.

Gating procedures are the most efficient and accurate methods of identifying children and youth in the school setting who may have or be at risk for psychopathology. Effective use of multiple-gating procedures requires a commitment by school systems, including school boards, administrators, teachers, support personnel, parents, and others. There must be awareness, understanding, and commitment to screening children at all grade levels and to be prepared to provide necessary services. It is also necessary to be certain if school policy or state laws require parental consent for teachers to rate children on psychological dimensions in a multiple-gating screening procedure.

School-Based Interventions from a Three-Tier Perspective

Interventions for emotional and behavioral problems in schools, including anxiety and depression, have been approached from a three-tier model that conceptualizes treatment from universal to individual, intensive approaches. At the first tier, all children are the recipients of intervention services, which are preventive in nature. Reading programs for all children is an example of a Tier I academic intervention that all students receive in elementary grades. The preventive aspect of a universal reading program is that it forms the basis for much of the tasks of education and helps to decrease the risk of academic failure and its consequences, such as dropping out of school. An example of a Tier I intervention for behavior is a school-wide positive behavior support system that is provided to all students to help facilitate social and personal functioning. Tier I interventions are considered to be sufficient for approximately 80% of students in general education (e.g. Walker & Shinn, 2010).

Tier II interventions focus on students who have been identified as being at risk for or having mild to moderate academic and behavioral problems and have been referred for services. Some children who have been identified through a multiple-gating procedure are likely to be given services, such as counseling, social skills training, and behavior management programs. This tier is considered to comprise about 15% of students (e.g. Walker & Shinn, 2010).

Tier III interventions are provided to students who have significant emotional or behavioral problems that require more intensive services, such as individual or group therapy or special education. Interventions at a Tier III level are more intense and require more resources than does Tier II. The preventive nature of Tier III interventions is to remediate problems so that they do not become severe or contribute to the onset of other symptoms or disorders. The percent of children needing Tier III services is often considered to be about 5%, and some have considered it to represent special education services, i.e. if Tier II interventions are not successful in the general education program, the next level of intensity of services would be special education (Tier III). Walker and Shinn (2010), however, suggest that Tier III interventions are not necessarily special education programs, but only reflect the need for more intensive services. Figure 12.1 provides a graphic representation of the three-tier model and is a common type of format for demonstrating the relationship of the three tiers and the respective percentages within each level (cf. Walker & Shinn, 2010). Ostensibly, effective intervention at earlier levels reduces the likelihood that intervention will be needed at the other tiers or, at least, the intensity of resources will be less.

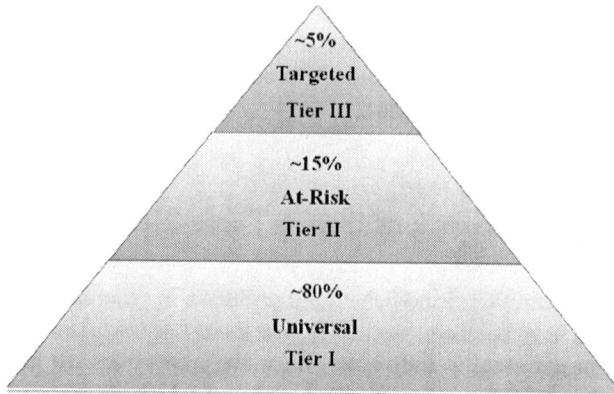

Fig. 12.1 Three-tier model of school-based interventions

Three-Tier Interventions Within a Problem-Solving Approach

Although the three-tier model is useful as a way to conceptualize and design intervention programs, it is not sufficient alone to develop specific interventions. In traditional psychotherapy, either the child or the parents/family is the "client." In a school setting, the "client" is, in effect, both the child and the teachers and other personnel who likely will be involved in the design, implementation, and evaluation of behavioral intervention programs. Thus, many school personnel must take some "ownership" and responsibility for the integrity and outcomes of interventions. A problem-solving approach that is collaborative and focused on outcomes allows all who are involved to arrive at mutually agreed upon intervention plans. Problem-solving models are especially useful for Tier III interventions that often require more intensive services and collaboration, but are also useful for Tier II problems. Several problem-solving models have been described in the literature to address anxiety and depression in the schools (e.g. Huberty, 2008, 2009). For the purposes of this chapter, a five-phase model will be presented that is similar to the model presented in Chap. 11 regarding working with depressed children and youth.

Problem Identification

In this phase, a consultant or intervention specialist, such as a school psychologist, meets with the teacher and others to define the problem(s) that are to be addressed. It is common for initial discussions about behaviors to have four characteristics: (a) many problems are presented, (b) the behaviors are initially described in general or nonspecific terms, (c) the frequency, intensity, or duration are not well defined, and (d) if there are several behaviors, those that are of the most concern are not identified clearly. Through collaborative discussion, use of rating scales, observations, interviews, and behavioral history, the behaviors that are to be focused upon are identified. An important aspect of this phase is that all collaborators are in agreement about: (a) the specific behavior(s) to be addressed, with no more than two or three at one time, (b) the frequency, intensity, or duration of the behaviors, and (c) the behaviors are prioritized in terms of their importance and impact.

Generation of Alternative Interventions

After the problems are identified in Phase 1, the collaborators engage in generation of possible alternative interventions, often referred to as "brainstorming." In this stage, all possible approaches are presented without evaluation so that all participants have an opportunity to provide input. Although some alternatives may not seem feasible, it is important that they not be dismissed without discussion or evaluation. This process assures that all input is considered, and there is increased commitment to the process.

Selection of Interventions

In this phase, the team members evaluate the generated interventions and achieve a consensus on the techniques that will be implemented. Key considerations are (a) the feasibility and practicality of the approaches, (b) the likelihood of success, (c) whether the interventions can be reliably and validly measured, (d) whether the interventions can be implemented, and (e) whether the chosen interventions are acceptable to all persons involved. If any of these criteria are not met, the interventions are not likely to be effective and will not be implemented as planned or given sufficient opportunity to be effective. If there is a lack of consensus on the interventions, it may be necessary to return to the Problem Identification phase and reconsider the possible interventions or reduce the scope of the initial interventions and work with a more limited range of behaviors. It is essential that agreement among the collaborators be achieved before considering intervention approaches. If agreement is not achieved, implementation is more likely to be inconsistent, ineffective, and, perhaps, unintentionally "sabotaged." The intervention plan should be constructed as a positive approach, rather than as being predominantly negative. Negative consequences (e.g. the child not earning an opportunity to participate in a preferred activity) may be provided as part of the program, but the overall plan should be stated and delivered in a positive manner.

Implementation of Interventions

After agreement about the interventions has been achieved, the participants determine how they will be implemented. Each person's role is defined with clear descriptions of what will be done in each setting to address the behaviors, with an emphasis on as much consistency as possible within and across settings. A written plan should be developed, agreed upon, and copies shared with all participants. The plan should contain a description of the behaviors to be addressed, who is responsible for implementation, the desired positive replacement behaviors, specific techniques that will be used to promote positive behaviors, and, to the extent necessary, procedures for addressing disruptive behaviors. Then, the interventions are implemented according to the plan.

Evaluation of Interventions

In a problem-solving approach that focuses on specific behaviors, it is necessary to develop methods for evaluating the interventions both formatively and summatively. In general, evaluation of intervention success should be done using the same or similar methods that were applied at baseline and the Problem Identification phase. If the problems have been redefined, it may be necessary to supplement existing data with new data. A component of the intervention plan should include procedures for ongoing monitoring and evaluation (formative evaluation) so that changes can be made, if necessary. It is often more the rule than the exception that intervention programs need to be modified after they have been implemented. If changes are necessary, the participants may need to meet to reconsider the situation, which may include review of the Problem Identification phase, generation of new alternatives, selection of other interventions, implementation changes, and revised methods of evaluation. When the plan is completed, a final evaluation is conducted (summative evaluation).

This problem-solving approach has several characteristics to recommend its use in schools: (a) it promotes a focus on operationalizing of problems in behavioral terms, (b) it facilitates communication among the participants so that all are in agreement, (c) it is consistent with the current emphasis on evidence-based interventions, (d) it leads to evidence-based interventions, (e) its procedures and outcomes are easily communicated to teachers, parents, and others, and (f) the interventions generated are replicable to establish their effectiveness. The approach can be used in all tiers and is especially useful with intensive, individualized interventions in Tier III.

Direct, Indirect, and Systems Approaches to Interventions

Interventions delivered in schools can be of three types: (a) direct services to children, (b) indirect services in the form of consultation to teachers and others who assume the primary responsibility for delivery of services, and (c) system-wide approaches that include both intervention and prevention elements. Direct and indirect services are especially useful at Tiers II and III, while systems approaches have both direct and indirect aspects that serve to remediate existing problems and prevent occurrence or worsening of problems. These approaches are consistent with a developmental psychopathology perspective of altering trajectories and creating new pathways for the development of positive behaviors.

Direct Services

Many of the therapeutic approaches described in Chaps. 10 and 11 are designed to treat specific problems and symptoms and can be implemented in schools. The child is the client or recipient of the services and the focus is on alleviation of symptoms. Therapeutic goals are based on perceived strengths and deficits and the techniques that are applied build upon strengths and enhance resilience while simultaneously mitigating and correcting dysfunctional behaviors, beliefs, cognitions, and skills. CBT techniques can be used with individual children, even if formal, manualized interventions are not feasible. Cognitive–behavioral and behavioral techniques can be applied readily in schools and can be adapted to the specific symptoms presented by the child and the setting circumstances, such as multiple problem behaviors across classrooms. Direct services to children may include teachers and parents as implementers as resources to provide contingencies for positive behavior, provide monitoring of progress, and to support the interventions. Teachers often are involved in helping to establish direct intervention programs.

Social Skills Training

There is no doubt that effective social skills are essential for the development of interpersonal relationships, competence, social and academic success, and ultimate success in adulthood. Effective social skills serve as protective factors, while ineffective skills are risk factors for a wide range of academic, social, and personal problems that are inextricably intertwined. There are many causes of social skills problems, including:

- Cognitive and learning problems
- Language problems
- Genetic and neurological problems
- Mild to severe psychopathology
- Parental psychopathology and associated problems
- Exposure to abuse
- Dysfunctional home environments
- Chronic exposure to highly stressful and unpredictable situations

Over the last two decades, there has been increased interest in teaching social skills to children who have identified skill and performance deficits. If training is successful, children with deficits should be more resilient, less vulnerable to psychopathology, and better able to develop a positive developmental trajectory. Effective instruction in social skills should also help alleviate or mitigate competing problem behaviors. Although there are many programs to teach social skills and research studies to investigate their effects, a remaining question has been whether the effects are long lasting and will generalize beyond the training situation.

In a review of meta-analyses of studies of social skills interventions, Gresham (2010) considered studies of children who were considered to have emotional or behavioral problems. The studies adequately defined social skills for purposes of research, and they focused on one of three skill development areas: (a) social interaction, (b) prosocial behavior, and (c) social–cognitive skills. Six of seven meta-analyses found an overall effect size of $r=0.29$, which indicated that approximately 65% of the children in social skills training group improved compared to 35% in the control groups. These data indicate that social skills training produced significant improvement. A review of a meta-analysis of 35 studies, however, found an effect size of $r=0.10$, although Gresham indicates that the analysis had some methodological limitations. Gresham concludes from these studies that social skills training is effective, although it is likely a Tier II intervention. He lists several interventions at each of the three tiers that include (a) the "Good Behavior Game," positive behavior support, and class-wide interventions (Tier I); (b) behavioral contracts, self-management, and differential reinforcement methods (Tier II); and function-based assessment and replacement behavior training (Tier III). Formal psychotherapeutic interventions would be used primarily at Tier III, although elements of them could be used at Tier II. There is relatively little information about whether the learned social skills are generalized and maintained over time. Even less is known about children in special education and whether they benefit from social skills training and whether any benefits persist for a significant time beyond the intervention.

Gresham (2010) addresses the lack of research support for generalization of social skills training and suggests there are three major reasons for these outcomes: (a) failure to adequately prepare for generalization and maintenance, (b) failure to match instructional methods with specific deficits, and (c) failure to target socially valid behaviors. Gresham also suggests that newly learned skills may not be sufficiently strong enough to compete with older and more well-established competing behaviors. This imbalance between new skills competing with older and established behaviors may help explain why new skills do not tend to generalize to other situations and may also deteriorate over time.

Indirect/Consultation Services

School-based consultation is the provision of indirect services to teachers and other school personnel to solve academic and behavioral problems in the school setting. Because consultation is an indirect service (i.e. the services are not provided directly to students), a variety of models have been presented to address mental health and emotional/behavioral problems. There is a large literature base on consultation models and delivery methods, which is too extensive to review here. There are two characteristics that should be considered in successful consultation: (a) the consultation model used and (b) the relationship between the consultant and the consultee.

Consultation Model

A variety of consultation models in mental health and education have been developed and implemented in a range of settings. A behavioral consultation approach using the problem-solving model described above is one of the most useful models in schools, due to its focus on behaviors, its collaborative nature, clearly identified steps, flexibility, inclusion of an evaluation component, and focus on positive outcomes. It is also an efficient approach, because much can be accomplished in relatively brief periods of time and each stage can be revisited as needed. In school settings where teachers' time is often limited, the behavioral consultation approach is an effective avenue for problem solving.

Consultant–Consultee Relationship

Successful consultation in the schools requires that a collaborative and mutually respectful relationship between the consultant and the consultee be established and maintained. This relationship is especially important in working with emotional and behavioral problems, due to their complex nature and that interventions often require ongoing collaboration between the consultant and the consultee. The collaborative approach is in contrast to the "expert" model, where an "expert" dominates and highly directs the interchange between the consultant and the consultee. Critics of the collaborative approach, however, suggest that it lacks definition and specificity (Erchul, 1992, 1999; Schulte & Osborne, 2003). Some research has suggested that greater directiveness results in better outcomes in consultation, which would appear to contradict a collaborative approach (e.g. Gutkin, 1996; Houk & Lewandowski, 1996; Rhoades & Kratochwill, 1992). Studies that have addressed the degree of consultant directiveness have found that it is at least as effective as, if not more than a nondirective, nonexpert approach (Houk & Lewandowski; Rhoades & Kratochwill; Witt, Erchul, McKee, Pardue, & Wickstrom, 1991). Erchul (1992) concluded that collaboration is not necessarily absent if the consultation process tends to be dominated by the consultant. Gutkin (1999) asserted that collaboration and the use of an expert model are not opposites, but that collaboration can occur when a consultant tends to dominate the process. Rather, the opposite of collaboration is coercion, which is likely to be ineffective or nonproductive.

Thus, consultation can be collaborative, and the process can range from being directive to nondirective. Gutkin (1999) and Erchul (1999) concluded that consultation can be effective with high degrees of direction or nondirection, depending on the individual situation. Successful consultation is a combination of both approaches, which may vary during the consultation process. For example, in the beginning, the consultant may be relatively nondirective as she tries to conceptualize the Problem

Identification phase but may become more directive in helping to generate options for intervention, helping to evaluate the likelihood of effectiveness for an intervention, developing the specific procedures for implementation, and designing evaluation methods. In this process, however, the consultant must obtain the cooperation, agreement, and "buy-in" from the teacher if the consultation process is to lead to effective outcomes. Thus, there is no single approach that is appropriate for all situations, but a collaborative approach with varying degrees of directiveness is more likely to be successful. Much of the success in collaborative consultation depends on the skill of the consultant to operate on the directive–nondirective continuum as the situation dictates.

Systems Approaches to Intervention

Systems approaches to behavioral interventions focus on working with the largest number of children and generally include early identification, intervention, and prevention. Consequently, system-wide approaches are conducted primarily at the Tier I level, although they can be adapted for Tier II and Tier III problems. The most widely known, implemented, systematic, and evidence-based approach toward addressing behavior problems in schools is positive behavior support.

Positive Behavior Support Programs

Positive behavior interventions and support (PBIS) programs are intended to serve all children in a school setting and incorporate strategies to address instructional and behavioral problems and to prevent their occurrence or recurrence. PBIS has three basic principles that guide its implementation and operation: (a) emphasis on evidence-based practices, (b) facilitating change in discipline practices, and (c) increasing schools' ability to sustain effective practices over the long term (Coyne, Simonsen, & Fagella-Luby, 2008; Sugai & Horner, 2006). When used across an entire school system, PBIS is often referred to as school-wide positive behavior support (SWPBS) and is a decision-making process that focuses on four elements: (a) data for decision-making, (b) measurable outcomes that are supported by data, (c) practices with evidence that outcomes are achievable, and (d) systems that efficiently and effectively support these practices (OSEP, 2010). The percentages of children served at each level with SWPBS are similar to Fig. 12.1. For SWPBS to be effective, it requires that teachers, principals, and others show a commitment to the program and seek positive outcomes for students, rather than relying primarily on negative approaches. The principles and practices of SWPBS are too extensive to present here, and the reader is referred to Frey, Lingo, and Nelson (2010), who provide an excellent overview, as well as to the Technical Assistance Center for Positive Behavioral Interventions and Supports sponsored by the US Office of Special Education Programs (http://www.pbis.org/school/what_is_swpbs.aspx).

Interventions for Anxiety and Depression in the School Setting

All of the approaches discussed above and in previous chapters can be implemented in some manner in the school system, despite the responsibilities of schools to teach academic content. However, it is clear that the two areas are inseparable and that problems in one area are likely to cause or exacerbate problems in the other area. Thus, treating anxiety and depression in the school setting should be part of a comprehensive approach that includes consideration of internal pathology, sociocultural factors, economic factors, academic variables, social relationships, and other factors that operate singly and in combination to create conditions that require interventions in the school setting.

Direct Services for Anxiety and Depression

Many, if not most, of the interventions described for anxiety and depression in Chaps. 10 and 11 can be implemented in the school setting. Programs such as *Coping Cat* (Kendall & Hedtke, 2006) for anxiety and *Taking ACTION* (Stark & Kendall, 1996) for depression can be used in their entirety in schools in either individual or group formats. These types of programs would be used at Tier II and Tier III levels to treat symptoms and to prevent worsening of academic and emotional/behavioral problems. Other procedures that can be implemented include:

- Pleasant activity scheduling
- Reinforcement approaches
- Social skills training
- Self-monitoring
- Relaxation training
- CBT techniques

Because the major therapeutic approach espoused in this book is cognitive–behavioral therapy, the techniques can be adapted and applied to school settings. However, when applied in schools, the clinician is likely to encounter distorted thinking that is related to both academic and emotional/behavioral/social difficulties. Table 12.1 provides a summary of some cognitive distortions that may be seen in anxiety and depression that are related to school problems and some example self-statements based on eleven common thinking distortions presented by Menutti, Christner, and Freeman (2006).

The examples presented in this table should not be construed as exhaustive or specifically characteristic of anxiety or depression. It is common for anxious children to have negative thoughts often associated with depression (e.g. negative labeling) and for depressed children to have anxious thoughts (e.g. worry, perfectionism). This overlap is especially common in children with symptoms of both conditions. These thoughts often occur in many children and youth at some time and should not

Table 12.1 Examples of cognitive distortions regarding academic and social situations

Distortion	Description	Academic example	Social example
Dichotomous ("all or none") thinking	Child thinks of situations in absolutes rather than on a continuum	"Nothing less than an 'A' is acceptable"	"No one likes anything about me"
Overgeneralization	Child infers from one circumstance that other negative outcomes will occur	"If I fail this exam, I will not graduate from high school"	"I did not do well in that group activity and I will not do well in others"
Mind reading	Child believes he knows what others think about him, despite lack of evidence	"Mrs. Smith did not say that I did good work, so she must think I didn't do very well"	"Johnny was laughing when I got there, so he was laughing about me"
Emotional reasoning	Child assumes that what he believes is true, despite lack of evidence	I did not do well on that test, so I am not a good student"	"Because I was not selected to be part of the team, I am not a good player"
Disqualifying the positive	Although an experience would be considered positive by most people, the child discounts it based on a negative cognitive template	"Although I got an 'A' on the test, it was a fluke"	"Even though I was picked for the baseball team, I won't get to play much because I am not that good"
Catastrophizing	Child predicts catastrophic outcomes about the future, which may affect willingness to try	"There is no reason to study for this test, because I will fail it anyway"	"There is no reason to try to get into the group because I will fail and everyone will reject me"
Personalization	Child assumes that he is the reason for a negative outcome, despite lack of evidence	"Our group did not do well on that assignment, and it is all my fault"	"My friend is depressed because I did not sit with him at lunch"
Should statements	Child has a cognitive template that he must or should do certain things	"I should always be at the top of the class and must stay there to be successful"	"I should always be what other people expect me to be"
Comparing	Child frequently compares himself to others	"My brother was smarter than I was in school and I will never be that good"	"I can never be as good as my friend Aaron when it comes to talking with girls"
Selective abstraction	Child focuses on one perceived negative aspect of a situation and ignores the rest	"Even though I got a good grade on my speech, I could have done some things a lot better, so it really wasn't that good"	"Even though people in the group talked with me, they really don't like me that much"
Labeling	Child applies a negative global label to self rather than focusing on specific behaviors or situations	"I did not do well on that test, so I am a poor student"	"I am a total loser because I say the wrong thing so often"

be a cause for concern unless they become patterns that interfere with academic or social functioning. As children reach adolescence, they are more likely to engage in social comparisons, worry about school and social relationships, and have negative attitudes and thoughts at times, all of which are developmentally typical. Unless they are frequent and impairing, however, they may not require intervention other than what would be done for most children. Nevertheless, a definite and repeated pattern may indicate that anxiety or depression is emerging or is not yet identified.

Table 12.1 also is intended to indicate that there often is commonality between academic and social/emotional/behavioral concerns. Children who have cognitive distortions related to academic problems are also likely to have distortions related to social and personal issues, demonstrating the frequent overlap among them. They may have cognitive templates that are pervasive across academic, social, and personal areas. Therefore, when school personnel see evidence of cognitive distortions in one area, there is a likelihood of distortions in another area. Although there may be some basis for the belief, the cognitions are distorted to the point of being irrational and unrealistic.

There is evidence to suggest that interactions in schools may contribute to the development of negative attributional style (NAS) associated with childhood depression. Haines, Metalksy, Cardamone, and Joiner (1999) discussed interpersonal pathways about how attributional styles contribute to the development of depression in children. They suggest that three interpersonal domains are likely to have significant influences on the development of NAS: (a) parent–child relationships and family experiences, (b) peer relationships, and (c) teacher–child relationships. Haines et al. suggest that children who have chronic, intense, and negative experiences in these domains are at increased risk of developing NAS that is associated with depression. They cite research by Peterson and Seligman (1984), suggesting that the type of feedback children get from teachers may contribute to the development of NAS by affecting the process of the acquisition of contingent self-worth. This concept posits that children's self-worth is contingent on the feedback they receive from significant others in their environment, including peers and teachers (Burhans & Dweck, 1995). Children typically seek positive feedback from others, and, if received, their self-worth is enhanced. Conversely, if they receive negative feedback from others, their self-worth is negatively affected, leading to feelings of helplessness. Because NAS and learned helplessness are associated with depression, children who constantly receive negative feedback that lowers self-worth are at greater risk of developing a mood disorder. Although NAS and helplessness are associated with depression, it is reasonable to propose that they are generalizable to other disorders in which the feedback children receive can be factors in behavior (e.g. conduct disorder). Given that peers at school and teachers are major sources of feedback, the school setting creates an environment that may either enhance self-worth or increase the risk of the development of NAS and depression. Thus, children who may have a predisposition to anxiety or depression have a higher likelihood of developing NAS and low contingent self-worth if they receive negative feedback at school. Consequently, school-based intervention and prevention programs should include consideration of sources of negative feedback from teachers and peers in design and implementation.

Indirect/Consultative Services for Anxiety and Depression

Teachers and other school personnel may feel less comfortable in addressing anxiety and depression in the classroom, because the behaviors may be perceived as mental health problems for which they may not feel prepared. Because the symptoms tend to be covert and are not disruptive, teachers may feel more comfortable with externalizing behaviors which are readily observable. Thus, a first step in consulting with teachers is to provide them with information about anxiety and depression and emphasize that the focus will be on behaviors and how to change them. It should be communicated that they are not expected to be therapists or counselors, but that they can play a significant role in helping to alleviate the stresses and behaviors associated with anxiety and depression. It may be necessary to provide some in-service training, printed information, or Internet resources regarding the symptoms, interventions, and impact of anxiety and depression on academic and social performance. During the consultation process, it will be important that teachers understand the nature of anxiety and depression and that they can be an integral part of intervention in the school setting.

The five-step behavioral consultation process described above can be applied to cases of anxiety and depression, either individually or in small groups. Because the symptoms tend to be pervasive across settings, it likely will be necessary to involve multiple teachers, aides or paraprofessionals, and specialists to identify the behaviors and operationalize them, generate alternatives, select an intervention, implement it, and collect evaluative data. Because several people may be involved, there may be a need to make slight modifications to the intervention program to accommodate setting differences, but the changes should not be major ones. Consistency of interventions is essential for anxious and depressed children who tend to be sensitive to the actions and attitudes of others and have attributional biases of threat or negativity.

Problem Identification

How the problems associated with anxiety and depression are identified will depend upon how they are conceptualized. If they are seen as behaviors to be addressed in the classroom, a functional approach to identification is appropriate. If a focus is to include the child's subjective experience and distorted cognitions, then methods to access these thoughts and feelings will be included, for example, counseling and social skills training. An example of a behavioral interview dialogue for an anxious child between a consultant (Ct) and a teacher consultee (Ce) is provided to demonstrate the Problem Identification phase:

Ct: Mrs. Jones, you have expressed some concerns about Jennifer in your classroom. Could you tell me more about her?

Ce: Well, she just seems nervous and uncomfortable in the class.

Ct: Can you give me some examples of what you mean by "nervous" and "uncomfortable?"

Ce: Well, she sits in the classroom and fidgets a lot, avoids eye contact, has few friends, does not volunteer, and seems like she wants to withdraw.

Ct: How does she perform academically?

Ce: Well, she is capable of doing the work, but she often turns in assignments late or not at all. When I ask her about that, she says it is not good enough to turn in, so she doesn't.

Ct: How about relationships with others?

Ce: Well, she is not rejected by others, but seems afraid to try to make friends. Other students have tried to include her and make her feel a part of the class, but there hasn't been much change. Whenever someone asks her to join their group, she starts getting nervous. I don't know why, however. I think they have sort of given up, but no one says that they don't like her.

Ct: How do you know she is nervous? What behaviors do you see?

Ce: Well, she starts looking away, does not say much, and gets red in her neck and face. She just looks uncomfortable and I really feel sorry for her, but I don't know what to do.

Ct: So it seems as if she has some academic and social problems. Is that right?

Ce: Yes, but I think the academic problems are mostly about not doing the work. Everything I know about her is that she can do the work at least as well as others, but does not do it consistently.

Ct: Which behaviors do you see as being the most problematic?

Ce: Well, I see two major things that I think if they could be improved, some of the other things would fade away over time. Those two things are getting her to turn in work that is fine, even if it is not perfect, and the other is for her to participate in a group comfortably.

Ct: Well, it seems as if Jennifer is kind of anxious, and it is showing up in both her academic performance and social areas.

Ce: I don't know very much about how to work with students who have psychological problems.

Ct: Well, even though she may be anxious, we can still focus on the behaviors that are causing problems in your classroom. We don't need to think of her as having psychological problems to address them, but just to think about replacing some of the behaviors she is showing with others that help her progress. If we can get improvement in those behaviors, then she may be able to participate more, improve her social relationships, and be less anxious.

Ce: I guess that makes sense. Where do we start?

Ct: Well, you said that two behaviors that concern you are her turning in work and interacting more with others. How about if we start there and see if we can generate some ideas on how to go about improving on these behaviors?

Ce: Sounds good to me.

Analysis of the Dialogue

This example intends to demonstrate how the consultant tries to determine the nature of the problem, operationalize it, address the teacher's concerns about dealing with "psychological problems," and develop a collaborative relationship. Obviously, more time would be needed to explore and define the problem than is presented here, but the goal should be to arrive at a consensus about the behaviors that are to be the focus of intervention. In the beginning, the consultant is somewhat of an "expert" and is being rather directive, but is working toward developing a collaborative relationship with the teacher who has indicated willingness to participate. The consultant may also need to provide the teacher with some information to help her better understand the symptoms and correlates of anxiety and depression problems, even if they do not meet criteria for a diagnosis of a mental disorder. As long as the behaviors are causing impairment, a formal diagnosis is not necessary to begin developing an intervention. In fact, it is helpful if the teacher sees Jennifer as needing help to solve some school-based problems, rather than having "psychological problems" or a mental disorder. Finally, it is important to communicate to the teacher than she can be instrumental in helping Jennifer to deal with her symptoms in the classroom.

Generating Interventions

It is important for the teacher to have significant input into generating ideas for interventions for anxious or depressed children, with guidance from the consultant. Given the covert nature of some symptoms, however, it may be difficult to identify interventions, requiring more guidance from the consultant. In Jennifer's case, the behaviors chosen for intervention are common to many types of problems, and it may be easier to generate options. Because a central characteristic of anxiety and depression is difficulty with regulating emotion, the consultant may suggest strategies to help the student with self-regulation skills. For example, if a problem behavior was that the child gets upset easily when confronted with an anxiety-producing task, generated interventions may focus on the manifestation of the behavior, but also in how to help create conditions to prevent their occurrence. A functional behavioral assessment may be an effective way of eliciting information for interventions. Interventions focused on self-regulation skills are consistent with the notion presented in Chap. 4 that caretakers such as parents and teachers can be instrumental is helping children learn to regulate emotions.

Selection of Interventions

After the interventions have been determined, the teacher and consultant should jointly decide which one(s) will be implemented. As described above, the criteria for selection of interventions should be (a) the feasibility and practicality of the approaches, (b) the likelihood of success, (c) whether the interventions can be reliably and validly measured, (d) whether the interventions can be implemented, and (e) whether the chosen interventions are acceptable to all persons involved. Although all interventions should be positively based, those used with anxious and depressed children especially should avoid having punitive or negative evaluation components. These children are especially sensitive to criticism, negative feedback, and are likely to expect to fail. If they perceive these conditions to be present, they may not respond well to the intervention. If an intervention has a negative component, such as response cost in a token reinforcement program, there should be ample opportunity to recover the tokens and progress toward improved behavior. The interventions should include discussion of what to say to the children and how to respond when they make statements that appear to be cognitive distortions. For example, if a child says "I am really stupid because I flunked the test" (labeling), a response could be that "I can see why you might feel that way, but you have done well on many other tests and projects, so maybe it was just this one that was more difficult." A list of statements that the child has used in the past could be generated, and the consultant and the teacher can discuss possible responses that tend to refute the belief without causing confrontation or sending a negative evaluation message.

Implementing the Interventions

Implementation of the interventions should follow a specific plan that is written and distributed to all who are involved with the child, including teachers, aides, specialists, and others. The plan should include the methods, timelines, materials, needed resources, and other elements necessary to increase the likelihood of success. For anxious and depressed students, it is important that the program be followed closely so that consistency and predictability is evident, which will help to reduce perceived stress. If the program itself causes anxiety or negative responses, its potential effectiveness may be undermined.

Evaluation of the Program

The program should contain a description of how the program is to be evaluated. Some objective information will be readily available, such as increases in completion of assignments. Teachers can record information such as number of times the child initiates a social interaction, increases in number of times a student voluntarily participates in class, time on task, frequency of negative vs. positive statements, or how often cues are needed to be given by the teacher. To the extent appropriate, the child should also self-record data, such as time on task, self-ratings of anxiety over several weeks, or subjective evaluations of social comfort or interactions.

Systems Approaches to Addressing Anxiety and Depression

Screening for anxiety and depression will identify those students who may be at risk for problems, which likely will then become the focus of Tier II and Tier III interventions. However, psychoeducational programs can be used with large groups of students, such as individual classrooms or entire grade levels. Published programs or learning modules designed to address symptoms or correlates of anxiety and depression can be used with large numbers of students. In schools, it is important to address not only the symptoms but also related academic concerns, such as completing assignments or developing and sustaining interpersonal relationships. It is recommended that the interventions chosen be empirically supported, using either published programs or specific techniques, such as CBT or behavioral interventions. Examples of learning modules or programs include stress reduction, relaxation training, social skills development, and study skills. These types of programs or modules can be presented in brief sessions in classrooms, each lasting a few minutes. In these situations, they would be considered to be Tier I interventions but could also be used at Tier II and Tier III levels.

One of the most well-developed programs that can be used as a curriculum is *Strong Kids: A Social and Emotional Learning* Curriculum (Merrell, Carrizales, Feuerborn, Gueldner, & Tran, 2007) for students from preschool through 12th grade. It is composed of five volumes: *Strong Start: Pre–K, Strong Start: Grades K–2, Strong Kids: Grades 3–5, Strong Kids: Grades 6–8,* and *Strong Teens: Grades 9–12.* The curriculum is designed to be delivered in schools by teachers without the assistance of mental health professionals. The overall goal of the program is to facilitate children learning about social and emotional functioning that helps to promote resilience and adaptation. A primary focus of the curriculum is to help children how to identify emotions in themselves and others. It has a strong cognitive–behavioral basis with an emphasis on understanding the associations among thoughts, feelings, and actions and to identify irrational thoughts that can be replaced with more rational thoughts. The two *Strong Start* volumes are composed of 10 lessons each, and the *Strong Kids/Strong Teens* have 12 lessons each. Contained in the lessons are topics such as learning how to relax, reduce stress, and develop effective problem-solving skills. Instructional methods include role playing, group discussions, and practice and reinforcement of learned skills during the school day (Merrell & Gueldner, 2010). The program is well developed, is based on solid theory and research, and is presented in formats that are appealing to teachers, mental health professionals, and students. The program can be used as a prevention curriculum, as well as an intervention with children who have been identified as being at risk for anxiety and depression, although the latter may require the participation of mental health professionals.

A recent study using the *Strong Kids* (SK; Merrell, Carrizales, Feuerborn, Gueldner, & Tran 2007) curriculum was conducted by Harlacher and Merrell (2010) using a sample of 106 3rd and 4th grade students in a public school system. The purpose of the study was fourfold: (a) whether the SK program would lead to an increase of SEL knowledge, (b) to determine if the program would lead an increase in the use of SEL skills, (c) whether gains in knowledge and skills be maintained over a few months, and (d) whether children who received the SK curriculum would show better social functioning after a few months compared to children who did not receive the program. The study was completed over a school semester using twelve once per week sessions and a booster session that were administered by the students' teachers. Follow-up data were collected approximately two months later. Results indicated that students who received the curriculum improved on all measures from pretest to posttest and when compared to those who did not receive the program. The authors concluded that the program was effective with regard to all of the research purposes and that it offered support for the effectiveness of SEL programs at the universal level of student support.

Conclusion

Schools present an opportunity to provide early identification, intervention, and prevention of anxiety, depression, and other mental health problems. Schools also present perhaps the best avenue for serving children, due to the fact that the vast majority of them attend school; thus, there is greater opportunity to reach a large percent of the school-aged population. Although community agencies and external mental health professionals provide valuable services, approximately 70–75% of mental health services are delivered in the schools (Hoagwood & Johnson, 2003; US Department of Health and Human Services, 1999). Schools face significant challenges in meeting the mental health needs of children and youth for many reasons, including having the responsibility for developing academic skills, the fact that many of the challenges they face are based in factors external to the school (e.g. socioeconomic pressures, cultural diversity issues), sufficient funding to provide programs and trained mental health professionals, and perceptions about whether schools should be actively involved in mental health care. Because many emotional/behavioral and academic problems are intertwined, however, it is essential that schools become primary sites for delivery of mental health services for all students, including those who are anxious and depressed.

The methods described in this chapter present some of the current best practices for providing services for emotional and behavioral problems in the schools. The three-tier intervention model provides opportunities to prevent problems before they begin or to identify emerging problems early in their development and prevent them from worsening or other problems from developing. A well-organized, comprehensive three-tier approach will prevent children from "falling through the cracks," which is common with anxious and depressed students who often do not attract attention. The problem-solving model is applicable to a wide range of problems and settings with individuals and groups. An emphasis on data-based problem solving where evidence is accumulated to demonstrate effectiveness provides important information for school personnel to improve services to children and enhance social–emotional and academic outcomes.

It should be noted that no one approach can solve all problems. Although the multitier model is logical and comprehensive, there likely will be some children who are not identified or who do not respond well to interventions within a tier. Some problems may have a genetic or biological basis, which could create greater challenges to address them in a school setting. Even children who have serious emotional and behavioral problems typically attend school and numerous approaches, and interventions may be needed to complement services the child is receiving elsewhere, such as psychotherapy or medication. Comprehensive service delivery for anxious and depressed students should encompass direct, indirect/consultation, and system-/school-wide approaches. Providing a wide range of services that have a significant impact will require the acceptance, cooperation, and collaboration of teachers, administrators, and community agencies and professionals working collectively on a common mission.

Chapter 13
Building Resilience Through Prevention

Resilience is a key concept in child mental health and is related to vulnerability discussed in Chap. 1. Although vulnerability can be difficult to change, children and adolescents can improve their ability to cope with problems. Determining how resilient a child is can be known only when encountering stressors and the degree of adaptation can be seen. Virtually, all mental health professionals have had or known of cases where a child is exposed to multiple or chronic stressors but is able to function quite well, thus being described as being "resilient." Conversely, many children have significant emotional and behavioral problems, but come from environments that are not significantly atypical and do not present severe stressors. There is no universally accepted definition of "resilience," but the definition proposed by Rutter (1990) provides a basis for its study and the implications for its development in children and youth. Rutter defines resilience as "maintaining adaptive functioning despite serious risk hazards" (p. 209). This definition implies that the resilient person is able to handle stress with minimal negative effects, although several people who are exposed to the same stressors may not be as able to adapt, i.e., they are less resilient. The factors that make some people more or less resilient than others are a combination of genetic, biological, and environmental variables.

If resilience is indeed a characteristic of adaptable people, key questions include (a) how does it develop, (b) can it be taught or developed in children and adolescents, and (c) if it can be taught or developed, how can it be facilitated in children to increase their ability to cope with stressors? If it can be taught and children improve their ability to deal with stress, they would be considered to have increased resilience. Programs designed to prevent the development or worsening of psychopathology represent attempts to develop resilience by teaching children how to solve problems, regulate emotions, and react appropriately to stressors. Prevention programs that focus on universal, selective, and indicated groups are involved in promoting resilience in children who are at risk of developing or have emotional and behavioral problems. Another perspective on prevention is to help children cope with stressful events and situation over which they have little control, such as

T.J. Huberty, *Anxiety and Depression in Children and Adolescents:*
Assessment, Intervention, and Prevention, DOI 10.1007/978-1-4614-3110-7_13,
© Springer Science+Business Media, LLC 2012

impoverished neighborhoods or dysfunctional families. This chapter focuses on the science and practice of developing prevention programs at the universal, selective, and indicated levels.

The Concept of Prevention and Developmental Psychopathology

Prevention of emotional and behavioral problems can be conceptualized from a developmental psychopathology perspective in four ways: (a) prevention of the onset of mental health problems or disorders when none existed originally, (b) prevention of the worsening of current problems or disorders in terms of symptom severity and intensity, (c) prevention of one disorder from evolving into another disorder, or (d) prevention of the development of comorbid disorders. If problems do exist, prevention programs also seek to (a) alter a negative developmental trajectory, (b) put the child onto a positive developmental trajectory, and (c) to mitigate possible long-term effects of a disorder. Prevention programs should focus on mitigating the effects of risk factors and enhancing the role of protective factors. Ultimately, prevention efforts should increase resilience and reduce the effects of vulnerabilities.

A Brief History of Mental Health Prevention Efforts

Although there has been much recent emphasis on prevention of mental health prob-lems, efforts have been made for several years. In 1998, the National Institutes of Mental Health (NIMH) produced a report that summarized two periods of emphasis in prevention efforts. The first period was identified as occurring in the 1930s as an outgrowth of the mental hygiene movement that began in the late nineteenth cen-tury. The focus changed from serving patients in asylums to including an emphasis on positive mental health of the general population and creating health-promoting environments. There was limited research on mental health prevention research, however. In the late 1960s, the second period began that included a stronger empha-sis on prevention research. Work on primary prevention continued for people not identified as having mental health disorders as well as with those considered at risk who would likely experience stress, such as from domestic violence, bereavement, or unemployment. In the 1970s, an increase was seen in research-based prevention efforts, and the NIMH concluded that there was sufficient research about prevention to conclude that a third period had begun (NIMH, 1998).

In 1994, the Institute of Medicine (IOM) released a report that identified three goals or desired outcomes of mental health prevention efforts: (a) reduction in the number of new cases of a disorder, (b) a delay in the onset of a disorder, and (c) reduction in the amount of time that early symptoms persist after onset and to stop or slow severity of symptoms to prevent meeting criteria for a mental disorder.

Thus, conceptualizations of prevention have existed for over a century, but the emphasis on research-based practices has received increased attention in the last two decades. In schools, the emphasis on prevention has increased significantly within the last decade.

Models of Prevention

The predominant model of prevention is a three-stage approach, similar to the three-tier model for interventions described in Chap. 12. Prevention is seen to have three levels: (a) primary, where the emphasis is on prevention efforts with an entire population, (b) secondary, with emphasis on working with at-risk populations, and (c) tertiary, where the emphasis is placed on working with subgroups of a population that have been identified as having mental health problems requiring intervention. Corresponding terms are often used to identify these levels: *universal* (primary), *selective* (secondary), and *indicated* (tertiary). The percentages of cases that presumably occur at each level are similar to the three-tier models discussed in Chap. 12. Some authors use different terms for the secondary and tertiary levels, such as *targeted* for the secondary/selective level. For the purposes of this chapter, the terms *universal, selective,* and *indicated* will be used.

Figures 12.1 and 13.1 represent a relationship that is more than similarity of design and percentages. If they are compared, it is quite easy to infer that prevention is a form of intervention and that intervention is preventive, i.e., if intervention is effective, it prevents or reduces the worsening of symptoms, delays or prevents the onset of comorbid conditions, alters negative developmental trajectories, prevents a disorder from evolving into another disorder, or prevents the development of comorbid disorders. Similarly, if prevention is effective, particularly in a high-risk group, then it interrupts and alters developmental pathways to create more positive, adaptive functioning. Thus, *prevention is intervention and intervention is prevention* if they result in altering negative developmental pathways or promoting positive development. If early identification and prevention are emphasized in young children, there is less likelihood that they will develop serious psychopathology and negative developmental trajectories.

It should be noted, however, that the percentages of 80, 15, and 5% that are frequently included in tier models are not absolute but should be considered as estimates, with many factors affecting the actual prevalence in each level. In some high-risk environments, such as impoverished neighborhoods and schools where more risk factors are present, a greater number of children may be represented at the second and third tiers/levels, and they may need more intensive services. In settings such as these, universal screening procedures should be more proactive and sensitive to identifying children at these levels. Generally, it is preferable to identify more children as being at risk through screening procedures, so that some are not "missed" ("false-negative" error). Failure to identify at-risk children who may have subsyndromal symptoms or are early into a negative developmental trajectory could

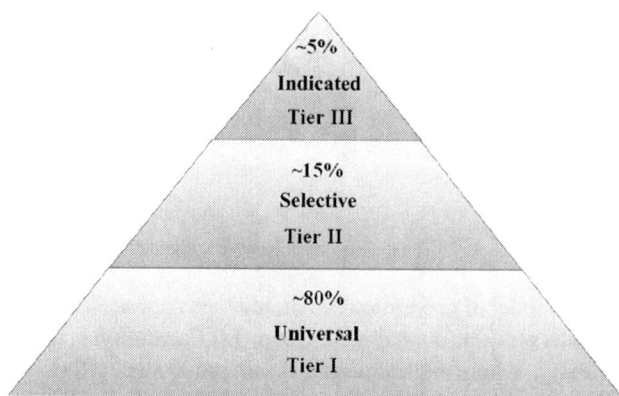

Fig. 13.1   Mental health prevention model

allow undetected problems to become worse and more difficult to treat. Although substantial alteration of the risk factors may not be possible, helping children to cope better with them is an important goal. To a great extent, prevention is relative to the circumstances of the child, and methods that are feasible in one setting may not be feasible in another setting.

Components of Effective Prevention Programs

Prevention programs can be challenging to establish, deliver, and maintain and require several elements to increase chances of success. Nation et al. (2003) conducted a review of reviews of prevention programs that focused on substance abuse, risky sexual behavior, school failure, and juvenile delinquency and violence to find common elements that help to define success. The authors found nine principles that are associated with effective prevention programs:

1. *Comprehensiveness*—programs should include strategies with multiple components that are applied in multiple settings and address a wide range of risk and protective factors related to the target problems
2. *Varied teaching methods*—a variety of teaching and intervention methods should be used, including active, skill-based components that involve the participants
3. *Sufficient dosage*—sufficient exposure to the program is necessary for an effect to be shown
4. *Theory driven*—the program and its components and strategies should have a scientific justification or logical rationale
5. *Positive relationships*—programs should emphasize the development of positive relationships among children and adults
6. *Appropriately timed*—programs should be delivered at the developmentally appropriate time in the children's lives to have the best opportunity for maximal effect

7. *Socioculturally relevant*—when designing prevention programs, they should be consistent with the cultural beliefs and practices of specific groups and local community norms
8. *Outcome evaluation*—systematic outcome evaluation is necessary to determine if a program, program components, or specific strategies were effective
9. *Well-trained staff*—programs must be implemented by staff who are competent, sensitive, and have received adequate training, support, and supervision

These nine principles serve as guidelines for the development, structure, operation, acceptability, feasibility, training, and interpersonal relationships necessary for a prevention program to be effective. They are applicable to community-based and school-based prevention programs that involve multiple components and should be grounded in the current research literature.

Many of the mental health prevention programs for children and adolescents have been conducted in schools, consistent with the perspective that more youth can be served at the universal, selective, and indicated levels. Several community-based programs have been developed that address mental health problems, substance abuse, eating disorders, and other problems, which are more difficult to implement in schools. Implementation is a particular challenge in prevention programs. Stith et al. (2006) conducted a review of the literature on issues surrounding implementation of community-based programs. These authors offered five recommendations for successful implementation of community-based programs: (a) a community must be ready to develop a prevention program, (b) coalitions must be developed within the community, (c) the programming must fit the community, (d) program fidelity must be maintained, and (e) adequate resources, training, and attention to evaluation are necessary.

Implementation is also a consideration in school-based prevention programs and the above recommendations are applicable. Payne and Eckert (2010) conducted a study to investigate the relative importance of provider, program, school, and community variables as predictors of the quality of the implementation of school-based prevention programs. They found that program structure characteristics were the best predictors of the quality of implementation, which was in contrast to the findings of other studies that provider characteristics were strong predictors. When provider characteristics and conscientiousness were considered alone, there was a significant relationship between them and program quality. The association was weakened to the point of nonsignificance for conscientiousness, however, when program structure was added to the analyses. Program structure included components such as standardized materials, supervision of the program, integration with typical school operations, a high level of quality of training, and implementation during normal school hours.

A literature review by Han and Weiss (2005) addressed the question of what factors best facilitate the sustainability of teacher implementation of school-based prevention programs. They concluded that four characteristics are essential to success: (a) acceptability to teachers, (b) the program must be effective and be able to change children's emotional and behavioral functioning, (c) the feasibility of ongoing implementation with at least minimal but sufficient resources, and (d) flexibility and adaptability. These findings are consistent with the nature of schools as complex entities that must simultaneously address administrative, academic, structural, and mental health issues. A school-based program that does not address these four characteristics is not likely to be accepted initially or maintained successfully after implementation.

Prevention of Childhood Anxiety Disorders

Prevention programs should focus on protective and risk factors in their rationale, goals, components, instructional methods, and outcome measures. Risk and protective factors for anxiety are discussed in Chap. 2, and those most relevant to prevention programs are presented here. There is a relative paucity of research about protective factors that are specific to anxiety, although there are general factors that are relevant to positive developmental outcomes, such as high cognitive ability, stable family relationships, presence of social support systems, and positive coping skills. Further, it is not known which of these and other general protective factors help to reduce the likelihood of developing an anxiety disorder. Although anxiety disorders tend to have genetic and family links, research shows that there is a greater likelihood that there is a transgenerational transmission of general tendencies for anxiety disorders rather than for specific ones (Eley, 2001). Thus, development of anxiety prevention programs that intend to build upon protective factors may be hindered by a relative lack of knowledge about what to emphasize to reduce onset of a pattern or disorder.

More is known about risk factors for anxiety disorders, although some of them are not modifiable (e.g., biological factors, sex). Costello, Egger, and Angold (2004) found that children with subsyndromal anxiety symptoms but who did not meet criteria for an anxiety disorder were twice as likely to have impaired functioning compared to those without symptoms. They also found that children who did not have an anxiety disorder during the eight-year study showed an average of about two symptoms compared to an average of 0.4 symptoms in those without an anxiety disorder. Children without a history of anxiety disorders but who developed at least one disorder during the study period had three times as many subsyndromal symptoms as those who did not have a disorder. These data suggest that identification of children with subsyndromal anxiety symptoms could be an important subgroup of children at risk for the development of an anxiety disorder.

Other risk factors include high degrees of autonomic reactivity, behavioral inhibition, parenting patterns, attachment problems, peer and community factors, alcohol and drug use (including smoking), and deviant peer associations and antisocial behavior. In these situations, it may be difficult to know if anxiety developed before, during, or after these factors emerged and whether they were causal. However, some of these risk factors could be targets of a prevention program for anxiety disorders. An often overlooked population for the prevention or mitigation of anxiety disorders is adolescents in the juvenile justice system, which tends to have a higher preponderance of minority youth. For example, separation anxiety disorder is high among Latino and African American youth who are in juvenile detention facilities (Teplin, Abram, McClelland, Dulcan, & Mericle, 2002). Although the initial focus would be to reduce symptoms, intervention would also have a preventive aspect by reducing the likelihood of worsening of symptoms or the development of comorbid conditions.

Prevention Programs

Universal Level

Implementation of universal prevention programs begins with a method to screen large populations such as the *Systematic Screening for Behavior Disorders* (SSBD; Walker & Severson, 1992) or the *Devereux Student Strengths Assessment* (DESSA; LeBuffe, Shapiro, & Naglieri, 2009) described in Chap. 12. The *FRIENDS* program (Barrett, Lowry-Webster, & Turner (2000a, b, c, d, e, f) described in Chap. 10 can be used with large populations and can be administered by teachers, psychologists, or other appropriately trained persons. It has been used with success as a prevention and intervention program, most often being implemented in schools. The program is recognized as one of the most effective prevention and intervention anxiety programs for children and adolescents. Several studies have shown it to have preventive and long-lasting effects (e.g., Barrett, Sonderegger, & Sonderegger, 2001; Barrett & Turner, 2001; Lowry-Webster, Barrett, & Dadds, 2001).

Selective Level

Programs specifically developed for the selective level are few and usually are delivered to children who have been exposed to trauma or other stressful situations. At this level, prevention involves intervening with children who have been identified through a screening or referral process because they have shown symptoms or otherwise been determined to be at risk. For anxiety disorders, the only program specifically designed for selective prevention is the *Macquarie University Preschool Intervention Program* (Rapee, 2002). Parents of behaviorally inhibited children, 3- and 4-year-old, were the participants and were assigned to either an intervention or monitoring/control condition. The intervention was primarily an education program with content about withdrawal, anxiety, parent anxiety management, instruction on modeling competence and independence in children, development of exposure hierarchies, and future child development. Follow-up ratings by parents at 12 months indicated significantly lower levels of inhibited behavior in the intervention group than in the monitoring/control group. Follow-up data beyond 12 months were not reported. This program appears to be effective and is a more appropriate method of intervention than is direct treatment or therapy with such young children. Its goal was to prevent long-term consequences of a temperamental variable of behavioral inhibition, suggesting that these patterns, though rather stable, can be influenced by well-designed interventions. Other anxiety programs that could be used at the selective level include the *Coping Cat* Program (Kendall & Hedtke, 2006) and various cognitive–behavioral programs that emphasize working directly with the child.

Indicated Level

Prevention of anxiety at this level is more similar to traditional psychotherapy with individual children or in small groups. Prevention is focused on reducing more severe symptomatology and reducing the likelihood of developing disorders, especially depression and related mood disorders. These children may have high subsyndromal levels of anxiety or have met criteria for an anxiety disorder. Children who are served at this level may show PTSD or panic symptoms, as well as signs of high anxiety sensitivity, generalized anxiety, or chronic stress.

Two randomized control trials for indicated prevention programs have been used with child samples. LaFreniere and Capuano (1997) conducted a study similar to the study of Rapee (2002) where parents of anxious and withdrawn children were the participants, and there was a control group. The program lasted six months and consisted of four phases: (a) assessment, (b) parent education about child development, (c) establishing specific objectives for the family, and (d) implementation of the intervention with eleven home visits. These visits included helping parents interact appropriately with their children, providing parent training, instruction in behavior modification techniques, and improving social support systems. Results indicated reduced parent stress and less anxious–withdrawn behavior by the children, although results about social competence between the two groups were confounded by initial high social competence of the children in the treatment group.

The *Queensland Early Intervention and Prevention of Anxiety Project* (Dadds, Spence, Holland, Barrett, & Laurens, 1997, 1999) included 128 anxious children who were assigned to a 10-week school-based intervention using the *Coping Cat* program or a control group. Follow-up at six, 12, and 24 months found significant differences in favor of the treatment at six and 24 months, but not at 12 months. Half of the children who had an anxiety diagnosis and did not receive the treatment maintained their diagnosis at 24 months. For children with anxiety symptoms but who did not have a formal diagnosis, there was little difference between the groups at 24 months, with 11% of the treatment group and 16% of the control group demonstrating an anxiety disorder. Thus, this study suggests that a program such as *Coping Cat* can be effective in reducing symptomatology.

Prevention Programs for Depression

Efforts to prevent depression are similar to those for anxiety, and there tends to be overlap among the universal, selective, and indicated levels. Research on the effectiveness of prevention programs for depression has shown mixed results. Many of the prevention programs have been delivered in school settings, and various outcomes have been found. Pössel, Horn, Green, and Hautzinger (2004) conducted a universal prevention program using cognitive restructuring, assertiveness training, and social skills instruction. They found that the level of risk was associated with different outcomes. Students with subsyndromal depressive symptoms showed a significant reduction in symptoms, while those participants with minimal symptoms showed little change. Students in the control group continued to show elevated symptom levels and, of those students whose depression scores were in the clinical range, only those in the control group showed a decline in symptomatology.

Prevention Programs

Universal Level

As with anxiety, universal prevention programs for depression may include children who have been identified as being at risk at the selective level. The *beyondblue* Schools Research Initiative is a relatively new program developed in Australia with a goal to use positive interventions that focus on more than skill acquisition by individual children. The program seeks to enhance protective factors as well as to develop individual resilience. It focuses on individual protective factors of (a) positive sense of self-worth, control, belonging, and purpose and (b) personal skills of problem solving, coping, and social skills. The program also addresses environmental protective factors that focus on safety and security, social support and positive relationships, and social connectedness and participation (Spence, Burns et al., 2005). The core/skill components are (a) emotional literacy and regulation, (b) stress reduction, (c) social skills training, (d) life problem solving, (e) cognitive skill building, (f) building social supports and connectedness, (g) participation in pleasant events, and (h) awareness of mental health issues and help seeking. The focus of each component changes, depending upon the grade of the student, and is used in grades eight through ten. This program is relatively new but is well constructed around principles of developmental psychopathology and developing positive, comprehensive, and integrated approaches toward prevention.

The research on efficacy of universal programs for prevention of depression has focused on immediate and long-term effects. Some studies have found significant reductions from baseline to postintervention using cognitive–behavioral techniques. Spence, Sheffield, and Donovan (2003, 2005) conducted a rigorous eight-week universal depression program that produced significant reductions in symptoms at the conclusion of the treatment, but they were not maintained at 1-year and 4-year follow-up. This study is an exception with regard to postintervention effects because most studies have not found similar effects and none has produced long-term reductions in depressive episodes (Seely, Rohde, & Jones, 2010). The reasons for the lack of effect are largely unknown, but may be related to several factors, such as whether mental health professionals or trained personnel (e.g., teachers) are more effective implementers, the length of time or intensity (i.e., dosage) of the intervention, rigor of the program, or if contextual factors such as school and family should be considered more fully (Spence & Shortt, 2007). Thus, at this time, there is little support for universal prevention programs for depression, although more research is needed.

Selective Level

The Penn Resiliency Program (PRP; Gillham, Jaycox, Reivich, Seligman, & Silver, 1990) is designed to focus on behavioral and cognitive–behavioral risk factors in adolescents that are associated with depression. The program has been used at the universal and selective levels; therefore, it is applicable to large groups of adolescents or those who have been determined to be at risk for depression. The program focuses on subsyndromal patterns with a goal of preventing in children aged 10–14, with the goal of preventing the development of depression that tends to onset in the adolescent years. The program can be implemented by teachers or school counselors, rather than relying on psychologists or external mental health professionals. An effective program would presumably prevent or reduce depressive symptomatology or reduce the likelihood of the development of diagnosable disorders. The PRP has two major components: (a) cognitive intervention and (b) social problem solving. The cognitive component is based in cognitive–behavioral theory with emphasis on how people interpret events and react to them cognitively, behaviorally, and emotionally and has five skill areas.

Cognitive Component

Skill 1: *ABC model*—*A* = Activating Event or Adversity, *B* = Belief or interpretation, and *C* = Consequence. Beliefs are seen as mediators between an activating event and the emotional or behavioral response.

Skill 2: *Recognizing cognitive (thinking) styles*—the model assumes that depressed adolescents have negative thinking patterns and explanatory styles that interfere with functioning.

Skill 3: *Cognitive restructuring*—learning to dispute negative thoughts by considering alternative explanations for events and improving the ability to evaluate information and evidence accurately.

Skill 4: *Decatastrophizing*—addresses catastrophic thinking characteristics of depressed adolescents, also termed "putting it in perspective," and youth learn how to consider the best, worst, and likely outcomes of events with emphasis on positive aspects.

Skill 5: *Hot seat*—combines several skills, including generation of alternatives, proper perspective taking, and searching for evidence.

Social Problem-Solving Component

Skill 6: *Assertiveness*—participants learn three behavioral approaches for dealing with interpersonal conflict: aggressiveness, passiveness, and assertiveness and the consequences of each approach and practice them in role-playing skits.

Skill 7: Relaxation—participants learn relaxation skills similar to those used to treat anxiety symptoms. The techniques include deep breathing, progressive muscle relaxation, and positive imagery.

Skill 8: Problem solving—participants learn a five-step approach toward problem solving: (a) stop and think to be sure their interpretation of a problem and others' perspectives is accurate, (b) identify their goals, (c) brainstorm possible solutions, (d) make a decision based upon likely outcomes and evaluating both positive and negative options, and (e) implement a solution.

The PRP has been used in several research studies with a variety of participants and generally has been found to reduce depressive symptoms that are maintained for several months, although variability across studies with regard to effectiveness has been shown. The first controlled study of the PRP included fifth and sixth graders who showed signs of depression or reports of family conflict. The results were quite promising, showing that explanatory style improved, with the improvement being maintained after three years (Gillham & Reivich, 1999). The participants reported decreased depressive symptoms at follow-up after two years, but not at three years. At the two-year follow-up, the results showed that PRP participants were half as likely as control group members to report severe depressive symptomatology, suggesting that the program prevented the development of severe symptoms (Gillham, Reivich, Jaycox, & Seligman, 1995).

Brunwasser, Gillham, and Kim (2009) conducted a meta-analysis of studies that used the Penn Resiliency Program (PRP) to prevent depression in children and youth. They found 17 controlled evaluations using the PRP program. The combined studies indicated fewer depressive symptoms at 8 and 12 months postintervention compared to those who did not receive treatment. Effect sizes ranged from 0.11 to 0.21. The authors concluded that there is sufficient evidence that PRP can prevent or reduce depressive symptoms up to one year after treatment. Research is needed with regard to the costs of PRP, whether a child's CBT skills mediate program success and whether the program is effective in the real world beyond the laboratory setting.

The PRP has also shown some effectiveness in reducing other problems. Some studies have found positive effects on anxiety symptoms (Gillham et al., 2006; Roberts, Kane, Bishop, Matthews, & Thompson, 2004). These findings are encouraging, given the overlap of symptoms of anxiety and depression. In an initial study of the effects of PRP on externalizing behaviors, reduction of behavioral problems was maintained for six months (Jaycox, Reivich, Gillham, & Seligman, 1994). Another study found significant preventive effects on externalizing symptoms after 30 months and that the effects were especially strong for those participants who showed prominent behavior problems at the beginning of the study (Cutuli, Chaplin, Gillham, Reivich, & Seligman, 2006). Overall, the PRP has shown much promise as a prevention program that has effects on many symptoms that improve resilience against the development of depression and mood disorders.

Indicated Level

The indicated level of prevention of depression most closely resembles typical therapeutic methods to reduce clinical levels of symptoms through working with individual children. Methods such as CBT and interpersonal psychotherapy discussed in Chap. 11 are used with children and adolescents who have been identified as having depressive symptoms or disorders. These methods will not be discussed again here, but their role in prevention is to reduce symptomatology and reduce the likelihood of the development of major depression or comorbid disorders.

Positive Youth Development Programs

The majority of mental health prevention programs have focused on deficit models, i.e., remediating or alleviating anxious or depressive symptomatology in children and adolescents that will lead to improved resilience and more positive developmental trajectories (Seligman et al., 2005). Most often, these programs have components that target risk factors, protective factors, and vulnerabilities of children known or suspected of having subsyndromal or syndromal patterns. Beginning with universal/primary prevention programs, the goal is to prevent the onset of mental health problems in individual children and adolescents. Although these approaches have merit and have been shown to be effective, an alternative approach is the development and implementation of positive youth development (PYD) programs.

In contrast to prevention programs that target deficits, PYD programs emphasize a positive approach toward developing competence in children and youth that will lead to adaptive outcomes. Although there is a focus on reducing problem behaviors and mental disorders, PYD programs have a central goal to enhance strengths and to develop skills to cope with situations. Roth, Brooks-Gunn, Murray, and Foster (1998) define PYD programs as "…developmentally appropriate programs designed to prepare children and adolescents for productive adulthood by providing opportunities and supports to help them gain the competencies and knowledge needed to meet the increasing challenges they will face as they mature" (p. 423). PYD programs are based in the positive psychology movement developed by Martin E.P. Seligman and his colleagues, where a primary goal is to take a positive approach toward the development of competence in a variety of domains, including social, personal, academic, and cognitive areas. There is an emphasis on strengthening protective factors that will offset or mitigate risk factors. Although environmental risk factors may not be modified, the child will become more resilient, adaptable, and able to cope with negative circumstances.

A primary focus of PYD programs is on developing a child's interests, strengths, abilities, and talents and to capitalize on a presumed innate capacity for resilience and the potential to develop resilience over time. Compared to the majority of prevention programs, PYD programs do not target specific areas or deficits, such as preventing anxiety or depression. Rather, the programs intend to develop a variety of skills that may be related to anxiety or depression, such as fostering self-efficacy, self-esteem, problem-solving skills, conflict resolution, and adaptability. By enhancing these skills, it is presumed that the risk of developing mental disorders is lessened.

Roth and Brooks-Gunn (2003) assert that PYD programs have three primary components: (a) goals, (b) atmosphere/environment, and (c) activities. These three components have subcomponents, which in the Goals area are referred to as the "five C's":

Goals

- Developing academic, social, and vocational *competence*
- Building *confidence*
- Strengthening *connections* to family, community, and peers
- Building *character*
- Strengthening *caring* and *compassion*

Atmosphere/Environment

- Supportive relationships between program participants and staff
- Empowerment through the development of autonomy and capability of participants
- Establishment of expectations of success
- Recognizing and rewarding positive behaviors
- Be of sufficient duration for effects to occur

Activities

- Opportunities to develop and improve skills
- Opportunities to engage in meaningful and challenging activities
- Broaden the horizons of the participants

Catalano, Berglund, Ryan, Lonczak, and Hawkins (2002) conducted a review of the literature on PYD programs and concluded that these types of programs seek to promote at least one of fifteen outcomes:

1. Promote bonding
2. Foster resilience

3. Promote social competence
4. Promote emotional competence
5. Promote cognitive competence
6. Promote behavioral competence
7. Promote moral competence
8. Foster self-determination
9. Foster spirituality
10. Foster self-efficacy
11. Foster clear and positive identity
12. Foster belief in the future
13. Provide recognition for positive behavior
14. Provide opportunities for prosocial involvement
15. Foster prosocial norms

If any of these components are a goal of a program, it is considered a PYD program. In this review, Catalano et al. selected 77 programs that met at least one of these 15 criteria, which were reduced to 25 programs that lasted at least nine months. The majority of these programs used random assignment and a consistent curriculum. In general, the programs achieved a high success rate on their stated goals, including improvements in competence, interpersonal skills, and school achievement and reductions in misbehavior, violence, truancy, and drug use. Although the programs reduced risk factors associated with depression, the authors could not identify whether depression was prevented or mitigated factors that might be associated with prevention. A number of well-known PYD programs exist, including Outward Bound, Big Brothers/Big Sisters, and the School Transitional Environment Project (STEP).

The research literature indicates that PYD programs can be effective from a positive perspective and are most applicable to Tier I and Tier II prevention, although some children with established disorders may be participants. Whether PYD programs can prevent depression and mood disorders per se is not known, but because many of them target behaviors that are symptoms or precursors to depressive disorders, they may have preventive value.

School-Based Prevention Programs

The majority of prevention programs have been developed and implemented in school systems because they provide the best opportunity to have an impact on the greatest number of children, especially at Tier I and Tier II levels. There is considerable similarity among school-based programs in both structure and the skills to be developed, such as social skills and problem-solving abilities. Universal programs are especially suitable for school systems because there are opportunities to work with children from diverse backgrounds and before problems become evident. Shochet and Ham (2004) assert that school-based universal programs have the advantages of (a) avoiding the effects of labeling that occur with selected programs where students are identified as being at risk, (b) participation rates are higher, and (c) numerous risk factors can be addressed simultaneously. Challenges to the development of prevention programs in schools include engaging administrators and teachers in the process, practical problems of incorporating the components in a systematic manner, and the costs associated with staff, materials, and operating expenses. Most programs have focused on prevention of depression, although elements of anxiety prevention are included, as well.

Merry, McDowell, Hetrick, Bir, and Muller (2004) performed a meta-analysis of school-based depression prevention program studies and found that, overall, the programs were effective in reducing scores on self-report measures of depression for selective groups, but not for universal interventions. The results were most positive following the intervention, but not over long-term follow-up, indicating some conflicting information about the efficacy of school-wide prevention programs. Spence, Sheffield, and Donovan (2005) conducted a randomized controlled trial of a universal prevention program for depression that was implemented by teachers of eighth grade students. High-symptom students showed a greater decrease in depressive symptoms and an increase in problem-solving skills than did children in the control group, where the patterns were reversed. After twelve months, however, the effects had dissipated. The authors suggested that the positive effects might reemerge and help students later as they encounter various stressors. However, the lack of significant differences remained over a four-year follow-up period. A similar study by Sheffield et al. (2006) found comparable results at follow-up, further suggesting that effects of a universal prevention program may not last in children who show little or no risk for depression. It may be that effects are more likely to be shown in children who already show symptoms and who benefit from more direct intervention at Tier II and Tier III levels. In these cases, prevention would focus on preventing the onset of a diagnosable disorder in children or an increase in symptoms.

More recently, Reddy, Newman, De Thomas, and Chun (2009) conducted a meta-analysis of school-based prevention and intervention programs for children who had emotional disturbance (ED). The definition of ED used by the schools was the one contained in the Individuals with Disabilities Education Act (IDEA; 20 U.S.C. § 1400 et seq.), the federal legislation that provides funding for special education services in the public schools. The studies reviewed included children with internalizing or externalizing problems or a combination of both patterns. The analysis did not permit evaluation of the specific interventions used. The results indicated that, in general, prevention and intervention programs were successful in alleviating early symptoms and reducing the severity of symptoms in children with more established problems. The authors found that less attention was given to internalizing problems; thus, the data were more limited. The programs were moderately effective in reducing internalizing symptoms in the school setting, but less information about effects in the home was available. The available data suggested that the prevention and intervention programs were minimally effective in reducing internalizing distress symptoms in the home. Reddy et al. concluded that, overall, prevention programs were less effective than intervention programs in reducing ED-related symptoms.

A noteworthy trend in these and other studies is that the programs addressed symptoms in the children, which reflects the deficit model of psychopathology. Because the majority of prevention programs focus on child symptomatology, relatively little is known about the nature of the school environment that may contribute to symptoms, whether and how these factors have a significant role in children symptoms, and whether changing some of these characteristics can have a positive, preventive effect. Also, emphasis needs to be placed on distinguishing the effects of intervention and prevention programs with regard to how schools create conditions that may serve as protective factors or, perhaps, exacerbate symptoms of anxiety and depression. Not only should effects on children and youth be assessed, but attention should also be given to looking at effects of these programs on teachers' feelings of self-efficacy, attitudes toward mental health issues of students, changes in attitude and behavior by teachers and others toward children with emotional and behavioral problems, and other variables associated with implementation of prevention programs.

Social–Emotional Learning Programs

In addition to the prevention approaches described above, social–emotional learning (SEL) concepts and programs have developed as a way to enhance the mental health of children and youth. In 1994, the Collaborative for Academic, Social, and Emotional Learning (CASEL; http://www.casel.org) was organized to initiate discussion, research, and practice on the development of programs to foster social and emotional learning that would help to facilitate the mental health of children and youth (Greenburg et al., 2003). The central premise of SEL is that skills that address emotional and social functioning can be taught to students, much like academic skills such as math or reading are taught. By learning these skills, it is presumed that children will become better able to cope with problems and stressors that they encounter, which is a major component of the concept of resilience. The intended outcome is to develop social competence through improved skills in emotional processing of information and adaptation to social situations that present challenges.

SEL is defined by CASEL as "…a process for helping children and even adults develop the fundamental skills for life effectiveness. SEL teaches the skills we all need to handle ourselves, our relationships, and our work, effectively and ethically" (n.d.). CASEL (n.d.) lists five core groups of social and emotional competencies:

Self-awareness—accurately assessing one's feelings, interests, values, and strengths; maintaining a well-grounded sense of self-confidence.

Self-management—regulating one's emotions to handle stress, control impulses, and persevere in overcoming obstacles; setting and monitoring progress toward personal and academic goals; expressing emotions appropriately.

Social awareness—being able to take the perspective of others and empathize with others; recognizing and appreciating individual and group similarities and differences; recognizing and using family, school, and community resources.

Relationship skills—establishing and maintaining healthy and rewarding relationships based on cooperation; resisting inappropriate social pressure; preventing, managing, and resolving interpersonal conflict; seeking help when needed.

Responsible decision-making—making decisions based on consideration of ethical standards, safety concerns, appropriate social norms, respect for others, and likely consequences of various actions; applying decision-making skills to academic and social situations; contributing to the well-being of one's school and community.

The competencies also consider developmental differences in children and youth and what skills should be expected at various ages. For example, for social awareness, elementary children should be able to recognize and label simple emotions such as sadness and anger. Middle school children should have the ability to analyze situations that trigger stress, while high school students should be able to understand how expressions of emotion affect other people (CASEL, n.d.). These varied expectations reflect typical developmental changes, ranging from rather concrete and basic skills to advanced cognitive skills of perspective taking of others, understanding the effect of one's behavior, and understanding that people have responsibility for how their actions impact others. SEL curricula consider the developmental level of the students and include components and instruction that are developmentally appropriate. Schools are logical places to implement SEL programs, because children are grouped in grades that are developmentally sequenced.

There is evidence that SEL is a predictor of resilience and that training is social–emotional skills can facilitate positive outcomes. SEL concepts and instruction are associated with positive school achievement (e.g., Capara, Babaranelli, Pastorelli, Bandura, & Zimbardo, 2000; Haynes, Ben-Avie, & Ensign, 2003) as well as on higher performance on standardized tests (Malecki & Elliott, 2002; Welsh, Parke, Widaman, & O'Neil, 2001). Although establishing causation between SEL and academic and behavioral functioning can be difficult, the research evidence suggests that SEL does have positive effects.

There is evidence that SEL also benefits educators through professional education in social and emotional education and classroom management, which helps to reduce frustration and anxiety (Elias, Parker, & Rosenblatt, 2006). Negative expectations can also be altered through participation in SEL activities by teachers learning how their expectations can affect achievement and behavior of students. Participation in SEL may help teachers to set realistic expectations of their students, which presumably helps improve student–teacher relationships. As these relationships improve, student academic performance and behavior also are enhanced. Children who come from difficult or impoverished backgrounds may elicit lower expectations for success from teachers and for themselves, resulting in lowered performance. By learning about setting higher, but reasonable expectations, teachers may produce greater levels of student performance than might have been expected initially (Elias et al.).

SEL Programs

Universal Level

Several prevention programs are available that have elements of SEL or are designed to be used as preventive interventions at the universal level working directly with children. Two well-developed programs are discussed here. The *Strong Kids* curriculum (Merrell, Carrizales, Feuerborn, Gueldner, & Tran, 2007) described in Chap. 12 is an example of a program that can be used at the universal level and has been shown to have positive effects on social and emotional learning of students. It could also be used for children identified as being at risk at the selective level, due to its strong focus on cognitive–behavioral concepts and strategies.

The *Promoting Alternative Thinking Strategies* (PATHS; Conduct Problems Prevention Research Group, 1999) is a curriculum with over 50 lessons designed to teach alternative thinking skills to enable children and adolescents to better address problems. It teaches participants how to identify emotions, develop skills in emotion regulation, learn social skills, and to be effective problem solvers. The PATHS program has been shown to be effective in promoting social competence and reducing behavior problems in children, including those who come from adverse environments (Kam, Greenburg, and Walls, 2003).

A recent study using a randomized clinical trial of a universal, school-based SEL program that included 1-year follow-up was conducted by Jones, Brown, Hoglund, and Aber (2010). It was developed for children in kindergarten through fifth grade and is focused on SEL and literacy development and has four primary components called the 4Rs: Reading, Writing, Respect, and Resolution. It is designed to link the teaching of social–emotional competencies with academic learning, under the assumption that the simultaneous and integrative approach leads to enhanced developmental outcomes. The program was implemented with third grade students who represented diverse racial/ethnic groups: Hispanic/Latino (45.6%), Black/African American (41.1%), non-Hispanic White (4.7%), and other (8.6%, e.g., Asian, Pacific Islander, Native American). Thirteen possible outcomes were assessed across three dimensions: (a) social–cognitive processes (e.g., hostile attributional biases), (b) behavioral symptomatology (e.g., conduct problems), and (c) literacy skills and academic achievement. Improvements were found on outcomes that included reduced self-reports of aggression and depression, as well as self-reports of aggressive fantasies, teacher reports of academic skills, reading achievement scaled scores, and school attendance. The results indicated that the program produced sustained improvement not only in social–emotional functioning but also in academic skills in children in general as well as those deemed to be at risk for social–emotional and academic problems.

Selective Level

At the selective level, programs described in Chaps. 10 and 11 that are used in therapeutic applications can be applied to address subsyndromal symptoms. These programs include *Coping Cat* (Kendall & Hedtke, 2006), *Taking ACTION* (Stark & Kendall, 1996), and the *Coping with Depression—Adolescents* course (Clarke, Lewinsohn, Rohde, Hops, & Seeley, 1999; Leonard, Goldberger, Raporport, Cheslow, & Swedo, 1990). The *Penn Resiliancy Program* (Gillham, Jaycox, Reivich, Seligman, & Silver, 1990) also has been used effectively at the selective level. Although some of these programs may be considered therapeutic interventions, they contain SEL elements through their emphasis on the development of social skills, problem-solving skills, emotion regulation, and coping strategies.

Indicated Level

At this level, prevention is focused on reducing established symptomatology and indicators of emerging disorders; thus, prevention is more therapeutic in nature. Some of the program described above can be used with some children and youth. An additional program that is more closely associated with this level is the *Coping with Stress* course by Clarke et al. (1995) and Clarke et al. (2001), although it has been used at the selective level (Clarke, Hawkins, Murphy, Sheeber, Lewinsohn, & Seely, 1995). It also has SEL elements with its emphasis on learning how to recognize emotions, distorted cognitions, problem behaviors, and the links among them, as well as learning coping and problem-solving skills, relaxation techniques, and alternative thinking processes.

Stice, Rohde, Gao, and Wade (2010) conducted a CBT-based prevention program for high-risk adolescents who had depressive symptoms but were not diagnosed with a disorder. Following completion of the program, the participants were followed at 1- and 2-year intervals. The randomized treatment conditions were a CBT group, group supportive CBT intervention, a CBT bibliotherapy condition, or an educational brochure condition (control group). In the study, authors noted that only 4 of 17 studies in a meta-analysis of CBT for adolescent depression produced sustained outcomes at one year with an average effect size of 0.08 (Stice, Shaw, Bohon, Marti, & Rohde, 2009). The authors were interested in determining which of the treatment conditions might prevent the worsening of symptoms over time. They found that the CBT group condition was more effective than the brochure condition at 1 year and the bibliotherapy at 1- and 2-year follow-up. The CBT condition was not superior to the expressive psychotherapy condition at 1- and 2-year follow-up. The CBT group and bibliotherapy conditions were associated with significantly lower risk for the onset of major or minor depression. This study provides support that evidence-based prevention programs can produce sustainable reductions in symptom severity or the likelihood of the development of depressive disorders in high-risk adolescents.

Preventing Child and Adolescent Suicide

In Chap. 1, an inverse relationship between resilience and vulnerability was presented, i.e., if vulnerability is low, resilience tends to be higher, while high vulnerability is associated with lower resilience. In perhaps no other circumstance is vulnerability high and resilience low than when a child or adolescent is seriously considering or has attempted suicide. At these times, the child feels overwhelmed with stress and does not see a way to overcome it, leading to feelings of helplessness and hopelessness that circumstances will ever change. Many cognitive distortions are likely operating, including "all-or-none" thinking as well as despair, sadness, and feelings of anhedonia. In these situations, the immediate goal is the prevention of suicidal behavior and a reduction in suicidal ideation. After the imminent risk of suicide is reduced, attention can be given to addressing the factors that contributed to the suicidal ideation and behavior.

Treatment and prevention of suicide are complex topics and cannot be covered in depth here. However, an understanding of suicidal behavior, epidemiology, and prevention strategies can be useful for the clinician in either school or clinical settings. Despite the obvious potential tragedy and seriousness of suicidal behavior, much can be done to prevent its occurrence and recurrence.

Epidemiology

Although clinically diagnosed depression is not present in all cases of suicide, it is a common correlate and is a factor in suicidal ideation and behavior. Epidemiological studies have found that suicide is rare in preschool children and is uncommon in young children under the age of 10, when the rate of suicide attempts starts to climb sharply, especially between ages 12 and 14. Many deaths by suicide occur in the 12–14 age range, and the rate increases markedly in the late teens, continues to increase into early adulthood in the 20s, and then again in later life (Gould, Shaffer, & Greenberg, 2003).

The US Centers for Disease Control (CDC) compiles statistics on adolescent health, including factors associated with death and injury. Suicide is the third leading cause of death in people age 10–24, with about 4,400 deaths each year, and accounts for about 12% of all deaths in the 15–24 age group. The most recent CDC data indicate that about one-third of all persons who completed suicide were positive for alcohol and about 20% were positive for drugs, including prescription medications and heroin. Methods of suicide are firearms (46%), suffocation (37%), and poisoning (8%). Fortunately, the majority of youth who attempt suicide do not complete it. Boys are more likely to die by suicide (84%) compared to girls (16%), but more girls attempt it. There are cultural differences in suicide attempters, with Native American/ Alaskan Native and Hispanic youth, especially Hispanic females, having higher rates of suicide attempts than either African American or white youth (CDC, 2007).

When combining the data in Fig. 13.2, 29% of the youth in the survey seriously considered suicide, 22.6% developed a plan, and 13.9% made an attempt. The notable pattern is that girls considered, planned, and attempted suicide at higher rates than boys. It is interesting that there was a larger difference between "considered" and "planned" for girls than for boys, with about 89% of boys who considered suicide developing a plan, compared to 72% for girls. Thus, boys who considered attempting suicide were more likely than girls to develop a plan. Of the girls who

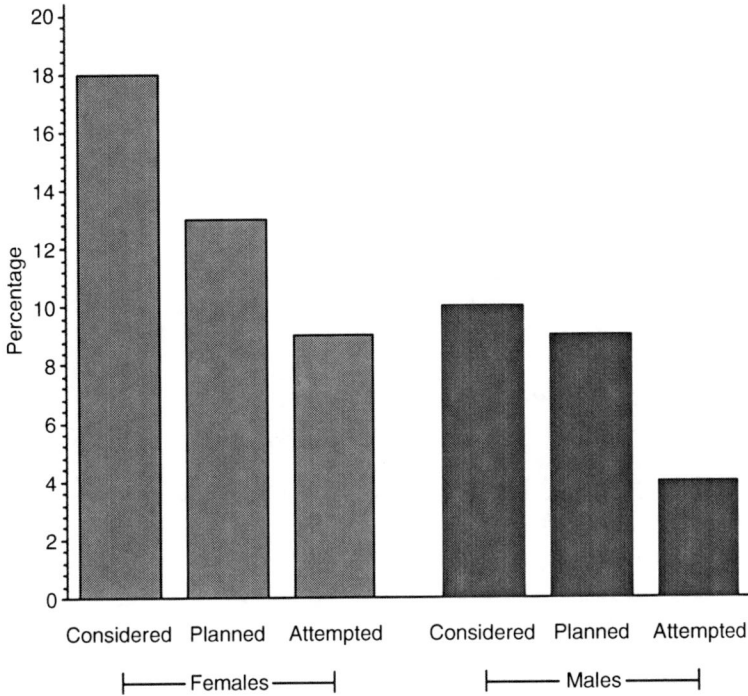

Fig. 13.2 National suicide statistics at a glance. Percentage (percentages weighted to be nationally representative) of US high school students reporting considering, planning, or attempting suicide in the past 12 months, by sex, USA, 2007. Among high school students in the USA, females were more likely to report having considered, planned, and attempted suicide compared to males (considered suicide: 18.7% versus 10.3%, planned suicide: 13.4% versus 9.2%, and attempted suicide: 9.3% versus 4.6%, respectively) in 2007. (*Source:* http://www.cdc.gov/violenceprevention/suicide/statistics/youth_risk.html. In the public domain)

planned to attempt suicide, about 69% followed through with an attempt, compared to 50% of boys. The data also show that girls were more likely to attempt suicide than boys at about a 2:1 ratio. For girls, approximately half of those who considered attempting suicide in fact made an attempt, and boys were similar at about 45%; thus, approximately half of adolescents who seriously considered suicide made an attempt within the 12 months prior to the survey. Firearms were the primary method for boys (56%), while poisoning was the primary method for girls (40.3%). The data show that between one-fourth and one-third of the youth considered suicide, suggesting that they found their lives to be so difficult, distressed, and painful that an option was to kill themselves. From a developmental psychopathology perspective, the data suggest that these youth had reached a point of helplessness and hopelessness and that their vulnerability was high and their resilience was low at some point during the preceding 12 months. Moreover, these data indicate that, compared to boys, being female is a risk factor for suicidal ideation, planning, and attempts. Although the data do not suggest reasons for these differences, they likely are due to a combination of genetic, biological, and environmental factors.

Risk Factors

The CDC identifies the following risk factors for suicide attempts:

- History of previous suicide attempts
- Family history of suicide
- History of depression or other mental illness
- Alcohol or drug abuse
- Stressful life event or loss
- Easy access to lethal methods
- Exposure to the suicidal behavior of others
- Incarceration
- Family history of child maltreatment
- Feelings of hopelessness
- Impulsive or aggressive tendencies
- Cultural and religious beliefs (e.g., belief that suicide is noble resolution of a personal dilemma)
- Local epidemics of suicide
- Isolation, a feeling of being cut off from other people
- Barriers to accessing mental health treatment
- Physical illness
- Unwillingness to seek help because of the stigma attached to mental health and substance abuse disorders or to suicidal thoughts

Psychological autopsy studies have found that these and other variables are risk factors for suicide. Moskos, Olson, Halbern, Keller, and Gray (2005) found that adolescents with a mood disorder and substance abuse disorder were the most common diagnoses in children who were more likely to die by suicide. Similarly, Shaffer et al. (1996) found that mood disorders alone or in combination with substance abuse or conduct disorder were associated with a higher rate of suicide. Anxiety disorders and mood disorders with onset prior to age 13 have been found to be associated with multiple nonlethal suicide attempts (Pfeffer et al., 1993). Consistent with the CDC data, some studies have found that previous suicidal attempts are significant predictors of future attempts (e.g., Borowsky, Ireland, & Resnick, 2001; Joiner et al., 2005).

Protective Factors

Relatively little is known about specific protective factors against suicide. However, the CDC provides a list of broad protective factors that lessen the risk of suicidal behavior:

- Effective clinical care for mental, physical, and substance abuse disorders
- Easy access to a variety of clinical interventions and support for help seeking

- Family and community support (connectedness)
- Support from ongoing medical and mental health care relationships
- Skills in problem solving, conflict resolution, and nonviolent ways of handling disputes
- Cultural and religious beliefs that discourage suicide and support instincts for self-preservation

Prevention

Prevention of suicide is a complex process that requires early identification of children and youth at risk for self-harm. The American Academy of Child and Adolescent Psychiatry has published practice parameters for prevention of suicide in young people (Shaffer & Pfeffer, 2001). These parameters are:

1. Establishment of crisis hotlines for children and youth in suicidal crisis
2. Reduction in the accessibility or availability of suicidal means (e.g., guns, substances, licit, or illicit drugs)
3. Training people who have frequent interactions with children to recognize the signs of suicidal behavior so that referrals to mental health professionals can be made, for example, parents, teachers, peers
4. Screening adolescents in the 15–19-year age group, which is the highest risk range for suicide attempts

In addition to these recommendations, children who have been identified as being at risk through screening or referral may be treated by many of the therapeutic, SEL, and CBT methods described in this chapter and in Chap. 11. Because depression is strongly associated with suicidal ideation and behavior, addressing the cognitive, behavioral, and physiological symptoms may alter a depressive trajectory and reduce suicidal risk. Of course, a child or adolescent who is actively suicidal should be treated immediately, and therapeutic or preventive methods can be used after the current crisis is resolved to the point where self-harm does not appear likely.

Universal prevention may help to reduce the likelihood of suicide, although the evidence regarding education of students is mixed. For example, classes developed for high school students regarding risk and suicidal behavior have not been found to increase the likelihood of adolescents seeking help (Shaffer, Garland, Vieland, Underwood, & Busner, 1991) and may be associated with increased distress in youth who have a history of suicidal ideation and behavior (Shaffer et al., 1990). Thus, programs in schools and other settings that intend to address suicidal behavior should screen the participants for suicidal ideation and behavior before implementation of the curriculum. Students who show these patterns should be referred for additional evaluation or consultation before proceeding with a prevention program. Adolescents who are not currently depressed but are at risk for depression may benefit from programs such as *Coping with Stress* (CWS; Clarke et al., 1995,

2001) and the *POD-TEAMS* program (Garber et al., 2009). For adolescents who are in an active depressive episode, the *Adolescent Coping with Depression* course (*CWD-A*; Clarke et al., 1999; Lewinsohn, Clarke, Hops, & Andrews, 1990) may be indicated. All of these programs have received research support for effectiveness. (The *CWS* and *CWD-A* programs may be obtained at http://www.kpchr.org/public/acwd/acwd.html).

Conclusion

As has been discussed in this chapter, prevention from a developmental psychopathology perspective has goals of (a) prevention of the onset of mental health problems or disorders when none existed originally, (b) prevention of the worsening of current problems or disorders in terms of symptom severity and intensity, (c) prevention of one disorder from evolving into another disorder, or (d) prevention of the onset of comorbid disorders. Thus, prevention is intervention and intervention is prevention. This chapter has attempted to review some of the current literature and describe practices that may be applied at universal, selective, and indicated levels. A focus on addressing the potential impact of risk factors and the enhancement of protective factors from a preventive perspective will hopefully accomplish several goals: (a) prevent the suffering that is often associated with anxiety and depression, (b) alleviate the symptoms that exist, (c) reduce the likelihood of the development of disorders, and (d) keep children and youth on positive developmental trajectories. It is usually easier and more effective to prevent disorders and their complications than it is to treat them, and children and adolescents deserve our best efforts to minimize their problems and enhance their future outcomes through prevention programs.

Part V
Legal Issues

Chapter 14
Legal Issues in Educating Anxious and Depressed Children

Apart from the family, school arguably is the most influential aspect of a child's life, and success or failure can have a significant effect on long-term social and psychological outcomes. In Chap. 12, school-based interventions were discussed within a problem-solving and tier intervention approach, which work well for the majority of students. When problems associated with anxiety and depression interfere with school performance to a significant degree, special attention and interventions may be necessary. Although many of the assessment and intervention methods discussed in earlier chapters could be used in the schools, often schools are not designed, equipped, or staffed to provide "traditional" therapeutic services. Rather, the goals of public schools include educating children academically and socially and help those who need extra assistance to make progress despite their apparent disabilities. In situations where special education services are needed to address problems associated with anxiety and depression, there are some laws and procedures that may apply.

The primary avenue for providing special education services in the public schools is the *Individuals with Disabilities Education Improvement Act of 2004* (IDEIA/IDEA; 20 U.S.C. § 1400 *et seq.*), which provides some funding to assist states for educating children with disabilities. The IDEA began as the *Education for All Handicapped Children's Act of 1975* (P.L. 94-142) and has undergone revisions and amendments since its enactment. The law sets forth requirements about how children with disabilities are to be identified, evaluated, and educated to the maximum extent appropriate with their peers in public school settings. The IDEA does not apply to private schools, which do not receive federal and state funding to educate students with disabilities. (Private school students with disabilities may be entitled to some services from the public schools, but the services are provided to the students and no assistance is given directly to the private schools in materials, personnel, services, or facilities.) Some key concepts are important in providing special education services to children with disabilities:

Eligibility for special education services—refers to children who have an identified disability, meet eligibility criteria, and who need special education services to progress in school.

T.J. Huberty, *Anxiety and Depression in Children and Adolescents: Assessment, Intervention, and Prevention*, DOI 10.1007/978-1-4614-3110-7_14, © Springer Science+Business Media, LLC 2012

Free Appropriate Public Education (FAPE)—requires that public schools provide an education that is considered appropriate for a child with a disability at no cost to the parents.

Least Restrictive Environment (LRE)—students who have been determined to be eligible for special education services are to be educated in the least restrictive environment possible and with their typical age peers to the extent feasible. For some children, an LRE might be the general education classroom, but for others, an LRE would be a residential treatment facility. The LRE is not immutable and can change depending on the current needs of the child.

Individualized Education Program (IEP)—students who are found eligible for special education must have an IEP that outlines their needs, eligibility, type and extent of disability, present levels of performance, goals, objectives/benchmarks, general description of instruction methods, methods of evaluation of progress, and timelines for achievement of objectives.

Continuum of services—refers to the range of services that may be available to a student with special needs; the continuum is related to the degree of restrictiveness necessary to meet the student's educational needs. Restrictiveness is characterized by the nature and intensity of the services that are needed and by the degree to which students are able to interact with typical age peers. In general, the continuum of services in order of least to most restrictive is:

- *General education classroom with no special services or support needed*—for students who do not have an identified disability or for those who have a disability or diagnosis but do not need special education services to progress in school (e.g., mild cases of ADHD that does not interfere with behavior or learning).
- *General education classroom with consultation services provided to instructional staff*—specialists and consultants provide consultative services to teachers and aides in the general education classroom who have the primary responsibility to implement the recommendations.
- *General education classroom with consultation or instruction provided to the student*—specialists and consultants provide direct services to the child in the general education classroom.
- *Part-time/"pull out" special education services*—a child may be "pulled out" of the classroom to meet with a teacher or other professional to receive some direct instruction or services for a relatively brief period of time. Examples of this level of service include speech therapy services for 20–30 minutes once or twice a week, counseling sessions with a school psychologist, or physical therapy sessions.
- *Part-time/resource special education services*—a student spends a specific amount of time per week receiving direct special education services in a separate classroom, such as one or two hours per day for reading and mathematics instruction. These services typically are represented as a specific percentage of time of the instructional day, for example, 25%.
- *Full-time special education services*—a student spends all or nearly all of instructional time in a separate setting, such as classrooms for children with significant emotional and behavioral problems that cannot be effectively addressed in a

general education or a part-time/resource classroom. The student may attend other classes or activities that are not core subject areas, such as art or music instruction and physical education.

- *Full-time special education services in a school-sponsored program*—a separate setting or facility recognized as distinct from the general education setting. In these settings, students receive educational instruction, but there is greater focus on addressing emotional and behavioral problems through various intervention approaches, such as milieu therapy, counseling and therapy, and behavior management.
- *Homebound instruction*—student receives instruction for a few hours per week by licensed teachers or specialists provided by the school. Typically, these services are provided to students who cannot attend school due to illness, severe behavioral or emotional problems, suspension or expulsion for violations of school policy, or are considered disruptive or dangerous to others. The amount of direct instruction is significantly less than what would be provided in the school setting, however, with a typical range of about 5–10 hours per week. Homebound students do not attend school for other activities, such as physical education or other non-core subjects, unless specified in the IEP. In some cases, such as for suspension or expulsion for bringing a weapon to school, they may be prohibited from attending other school-sponsored activities that occur during instructional time.
- *Day treatment programs*—community-based program where the student attends during the day and returns home in the evenings and weekends. These settings are often community-based mental health settings or hospitals where the focus is on addressing emotional and behavioral problems, although instruction is provided to help maintain and advance academic skills. These settings may include those that are often referred to as "partial hospitalization" programs where psychotherapy, medications, and more intensive psychological and psychiatric services are provided.
- *Short-term inpatient hospitalization*—for students whose emotional and behavioral problems represent a danger to self or others and their needs are more therapeutic in nature and cannot be met in other settings. The primary emphasis is on mental health issues, although some educational instruction is provided. Most often, these services occur as a result of a crisis situation and do not exceed 30 days. Psychotherapy, milieu therapy, psychiatric consultation, and medication management are typical services provided to children and youth.
- *Residential placement*—a student's emotional, behavioral, and developmental needs are of such significance that they cannot be met satisfactorily in any of the other elements of the continuum of services. Although there is great emphasis on the student's psychological and developmental needs, an identified educational component is included where instruction is provided for several hours per week. Placement in these settings typically is for several months or longer, depending on the student's needs. These programs provide intensive psychotherapy, activity therapy, milieu therapy, psychoeducation, family therapy, psychiatric consultation, medication management, and related services.

| Continuum of Special Education Services | | | |

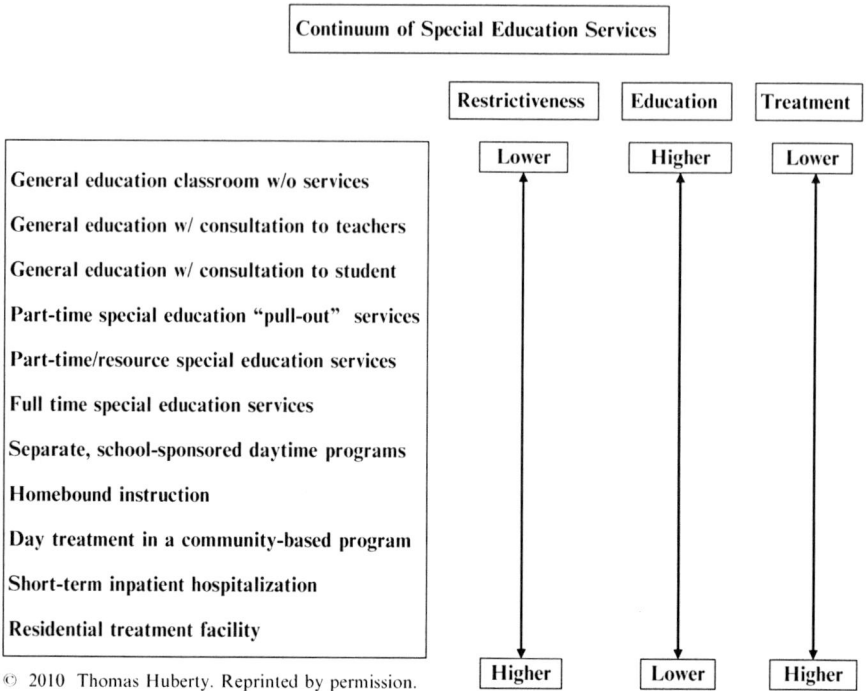

© 2010 Thomas Huberty. Reprinted by permission.

Fig. 14.1 Continuum of special education services

Depending on the level of restrictiveness, the emphasis on educational and thera-peutic services and interventions varies. With increased restrictiveness, there is greater emphasis on interventions for emotional, behavioral, and developmental needs, although the child continues to receive educational services to make aca-demic progress. If the child is placed out of the school setting, the IEP typically is revised to address these needs, but academic goals, objectives/benchmarks, and instruction must be included. Figure 14.1 provides a visual representation of the relationships among the continuum of services, level of restrictiveness, and the rela-tive emphasis on academic and emotional/behavioral interventions at each level.

The level of restrictiveness of homebound instruction (HI) is placed in the eighth position in the continuum, which is arguable, depending on how it is implemented for an individual student. Most often, HI services are provided due to the child's inability to attend school for medical or psychological reasons or because of sus-pension or expulsion for misbehavior, such as bringing weapons or illegal drugs to school. Children with high levels of externalizing behavior may not be manageable at school and may be placed in HI as an interim alternative educational setting until a more appropriate option is determined. Children who are highly anxious or severely depressed may be unable to attend school and receive HI until the symp-toms moderate sufficiently to permit attendance. In the interim, HI is provided with an emphasis on academic objectives to help the child progress toward meeting IEP goals, but relatively little attention is given to emotional/behavioral needs. Thus, HI can be considered to be restrictive because it removes the student from being near peers, where group instruction and socialization are provided and it emphasizes academic needs. However, HI typically does not involve high levels of psychological services, although a plan may be developed and implemented to provide a gradual transition back to school that becomes part of the IEP. Most schools consider expulsion or suspension as a disciplinary procedure that will have a positive effect on reducing future misbehavior, although the value of the practice has limited support for efficacy. Therefore, the placement of HI in the continuum of services for a specific child is variable, depending on individual circumstances. Also, HI could be provided in conjunction with any of the general placement options reference in Fig. 14.1.

Emotional Disturbance Category in the IDEA

Eligibility for special education services for anxious and depressed children most often is determined under the IDEA category of "Emotional Disturbance (ED)." Individual states may use different labels and criteria, but they must comply with federal requirements when evaluating and determining eligibility for special education services. Although the IDEA does not require that a student be labeled as ED or any other disability, most schools identify children with emotional and behavioral problems under the ED category or the corresponding state terminology and criteria. The IDEA definition and criteria for ED are presented at 34 CFR § 300.8(c)(4):

(i) *Emotional Disturbance* means a condition exhibiting one or more of the following characteristics over a long period of time and to a marked degree that adversely affects a child's educational performance:

    (A) An inability to learn that is not explained by intellectual, sensory, or health factors

    (B) An inability to build or maintain satisfactory interpersonal relationships with peers and teachers

    (C) Inappropriate types of behaviors or feelings under normal circumstances

    (D) A general pervasive mood of unhappiness or depression

    (E) A tendency to develop physical symptoms or fears associated with personal or school problems

(ii) Emotional disturbance includes schizophrenia. The term does not apply to children who are socially maladjusted, unless it is determined that they have an emotional disturbance.

The federal definition of ED has been a source of controversy for several years for many reasons including the following: (a) many of the terms are not defined or operationalized, (b) there is no guidance to differentiate children who have ED from those who do not have the condition, (c) it has been questioned if "educational performance" applies only to academic performance or if it includes social, emotional, and behavioral performance, (d) difficulty differentiating characteristics of ED from those of typical children who may show some similar behaviors but would not be considered to have an ED, (e) if terms such as "inability" are meant to imply a total inability or if they are relative to what might be expected of the child or same-age peers, and (f) what differentiates "socially maladjusted" from ED. These difficulties with the definition increase the likelihood that what is considered to be ED can vary considerably from clinician to clinician, school to school, and state to state. Arguments and positions to change or replace the definition have been advanced over several years, but the definition has remained unchanged since 1975 (Merrell, 2003). Thus, schools must determine eligibility for ED and provide appropriate services based on state definitions, which most often use the federal definition, perhaps with slight modifications.

DSM-IV Diagnoses vs. Educational Classification

Although psychologists and psychiatrists use the DSM-IV as a classification system for mental disorders, the IDEA does not require its use in the public schools. The DSM-IV requires specific differential diagnosis from among over 300 possible categories, but educational classifications for special education services do not require such fine discriminations. Rather, educational classifications such as ED are dichotomous in nature, i.e., they require a "yes" or "no" decision to indicate whether a child meets eligibility criteria to receive special education services. Under the IDEA, schools are not required to accept DSM-IV diagnoses to determine eligibility for special education services, and having a diagnosis does not assure that a child will receive services if there are no educational needs. It is not uncommon for a child to receive a psychological or psychiatric evaluation from a mental health professional or physician that is presented to the school as evidence that a child needs special education services. Although this information may be helpful, there must nevertheless be evidence that the child has educational needs. For example, a child who has a depressive disorder that is well managed with medication and psychotherapy and is doing well academically and socially at school may not be eligible for special education services because there are no educational needs. *Thus, DSM-IV diagnoses are neither necessary nor sufficient to determine eligibility for special education services.* Although DSM-IV diagnoses have significant value in clinical contexts, they have little relevance to educational needs and planning, due to their polythetic nature, comorbidity, and lack of specificity about associations with school problems. Ultimately, the IEP Team that includes the parents has the collective responsibility to assure that all evaluations, procedures, and identification methods are appropriately considered in determining eligibility for special education services. Thus, eligibility is based upon educational needs, not on a label or diagnosis.

Evaluations in Special Education

The IDEA contains requirements for evaluating a child who may be eligible for special education services, although it does not specify what measures or procedures are to be used, such as specific tests, rating scales, or observation methods. The law assumes that the professionals with the appropriate training and expertise are the qualified persons to determine the assessment methods and procedures, with the input of the IEP Team. State laws may have specific requirements about what types of tests are to be used, such as intelligence/cognitive ability or achievement tests, but typically do not mandate the specific measures to be used. In some states, for example, a cognitive ability test may be required in determining whether a child has an emotional disturbance, but other states do not have such a mandate. In Indiana, a cognitive ability test is not required to establish eligibility for children with an emotional disability but may be done if it is considered to provide useful information.

The law is clear that in conducting the evaluation, the public agency must:

(1) Use a variety of assessment tools and strategies to gather relevant functional, developmental, and academic information about the child, including information provided by the parent, that may assist in determining:

    (i) Whether the child is a child with a disability under § 300.8

    (ii) The content of the child's IEP, including information related to enabling the child to be involved in and progress in the general education curriculum (or for a preschool child, to participate in appropriate activities) (34 CFR § 300.304(b))

This requirement is consistent with the multimethod approach discussed in Chap. 7 and helps to assure that the child receives a complete, thorough evaluation that addresses all areas of suspected disability. The evaluative data derived from the assessment determine the child's "present levels of performance" (PLP) that are used to help determine eligibility and to develop an appropriate educational program. In the case of a child who has been referred for academic problems, PLP usually includes current level of performance and instructional level. In situations where behavior is the primary focus, PLP may be data such as attention to task, frequency of disruptiveness, level of anxiety or depression, or noncompliance.

A provision regarding a "sole criterion" in the IDEA is related to determining eligibility for special education services. The IDEA stipulates that a public agency (i.e., public school) is "…not to use any single measure or assessment as the sole criterion for determining whether a child is a child with a disability and for determining an appropriate educational program for the child" (34 CFR § 300.304(b)(2)). Thus, if a single score on a measure, a single psychiatric or psychological diagnosis, or other single index is used to determine whether a child has an emotional disturbance, it would not be consistent with this provision of the IDEA. An example of the "sole criterion" provision would be basing a determination of eligibility for special education services for a suspected mental or intellectual disability on a single IQ test score. Other factors, such as adaptive behavior and academic performance, must also be assessed and considered in making an eligibility determination.

For many years, it has been common practice to compare scores on intelligence tests and standardized achievement tests to and determine whether there is a significant discrepancy between them. If a specific difference did not exist between the scores, such as 18 standard score points, the child would not be found eligible as a student with a specific learning disability (SLD), despite any other available data. The author has presided over several due process hearings where such discrepancy formulas have been used by schools and challenged by parents whose children have not been found eligible as a student with a SLD. In cases where the discrepancy was found to be the sole criterion to determine eligibility, the school was found to have violated the sole criterion provision of the IDEA.

Another example in the behavioral domain is where parents provide documentation from a physician or mental health professional to a public school that their child has Attention Deficit/Hyperactivity Disorder (ADHD) and request special education services. Because ADHD is a psychiatric/psychological diagnosis, the IDEA does not require its acceptance to determine eligibility for special education services. Similarly, acceptance of a formal DSM-IV diagnosis from a physician or mental health provider alone to determine eligibility is a violation of the sole criterion provision. A school is required to consider such information, but the IEP Team is not required to accept it and cannot base its determination of eligibility on a diagnosis alone. The school is required to conduct a complete educational evaluation that would include assessment of academic, emotional, behavioral, and developmental needs to supplement the external information.

Another form of evaluation may occur with an independent educational evaluation (IEE), which is to be conducted by a professional who is not an employee of the public school district or service agency of the student and who does not have a personal or professional interest in the case. A parent is permitted to obtain an IEE and present the results to the school for consideration in determining a child's eligibility for special education services or when educational planning is conducted. A school must consider the information but is not required to accept the findings in lieu of its own evaluation. Alternatively, a parent may ask the school to pay for an IEE. If the school consents to pay for an IEE, it must consider the information but is not required to accept all of the findings for determining eligibility or for developing an educational plan. A parent may ask for an IEE, but the school can assert that its evaluation is appropriate and refuse the request. A school also has the right to conduct its own evaluation before consenting to paying for an IEE. If the parent nevertheless wants an IEE, he or she can request a due process hearing to determine whether the school should pay for an IEE or ask for reimbursement for an IEE completed at parent expense. If an IEE is ordered by an impartial/independent hearing officer (IHO), it is paid for by the school, and the evaluation report would be included in the exhibits for a due process hearing.

IEEs obtained by parents must be considered by schools if they meet agency criteria, which are those that the LEA uses when it conducts its own evaluation, including the qualifications of the examiner and the location where the evaluation will be performed (34 CFR § 300.502). The evaluator must be qualified by nature of license or certification according to the laws of a state, such as a school psychologist licensed by the state department of education or a psychologist licensed by the state board of psychology. A school may not impose conditions or timelines on the evaluation if being paid for at public expense, such as limiting it to a specific list of qualified evaluators, requiring that it not cost more than a specific amount, or that it must be done within an unreasonable period of time. The evaluation must be done in the same manner that the school would use in conducting its own evaluation. Failure of an independent evaluator to comply with this requirement could result in the evaluation not being fully considered or the school not being required to pay for all or part of it. The author has presided over hearings where a school has put restrictions on how an IEE is to be conducted, attempted to impose limits on cost, or used personnel who do not work in the child's local school but who work in other district schools. Cost may be considered in providing IEEs but may not be used as a basis for denying an IEE by a qualified evaluator. Such practices do not meet the intent or the spirit of the law with regard to being "independent" and are not permitted.

A school may ask parents why they disagree with its evaluation but cannot require an explanation or unreasonably delay approving the evaluation or filing a due process request to determine if its evaluation is appropriate (34 CFR § 300.502(4)). If a school denies a parent's request for an IEE and an IHO finds that its evaluation is appropriate, the parent is nevertheless entitled to obtain an IEE, but not at public expense (34 CFR § 300.502(4)).

Ultimately, it is the local school district's responsibility to assure that proper evaluation has been conducted, either through its own personnel or from external mental health, education, or other professionals. In all cases, the information used to determine whether a child has a disability and needs special education services must be obtained in compliance with federal and state laws, either from the school's personnel or from external sources.

Functional Behavioral Assessment

The IDEA also contains provisions that require a school to complete a functional behavioral assessment (FBA) when a child who has a disability is to be disciplined for a behavior that may not be characteristic of his or her disability, such as fighting or possession of drugs. In these cases, the school is to conduct a *manifestation determination* to establish whether the misbehavior is a manifestation of the child's disability (34 CFR § 300.530(e)). A required component of a manifestation determination is that the school conduct an FBA (34 CFR § 300.530(d)(1)(ii); 34 CFR § 300.530(f)(1)(i)) to help establish if the behavior is a function of the disability. The IDEA does not define FBA or specify the methods, procedures, or instruments used to gather the information. After completion of the FBA, the IEP Team is to determine whether the behavior is a manifestation of the child's disability and, if so, must develop a behavioral intervention plan (BIP) to address the behaviors.

Because the IDEA does not define FBA or specify how it is to be conducted, the school is responsible for conducting the assessment in a manner consistent with accepted practices, most often from the psychological assessment literature. FBA is based on principles of behavioral psychology that assume that behaviors serve an intended purpose or function to accomplish specific outcomes. By focusing on the antecedents and consequences of the behavior, the intended function may be determined and an intervention plan developed to alter the behavior. Behaviors may have one of several functions or purposes: power, revenge, escape, avoidance, attention, or a combination of several purposes. FBA is a component of a problem-solving model where the focus is to identify a problem, develop possible interventions, select interventions to be used, implement the interventions, and evaluate their effectiveness (Huberty, 2008). The data from the assessment are gathered in frequency, intensity, or duration of the behavior but may include other information such as behavioral history and standardized behavior rating scales. It is beyond the scope of this chapter to describe the components of FBA in detail, but typically they include:

- Systematic, structured observations across settings and time intervals
- Functional behavioral interviews with teachers, parents, and the child
- Completion of behavior setting checklists that include where the behaviors occur and do not occur, day of the week, the time of day, and variability across settings
- Determination of antecedents or possible "triggers" of the behavior
- Determination of consequences of the behavior, i.e., what happens after the behavior occurs that may affect the likelihood of recurrence

The IDEA requires that an FBA be conducted in cases of manifestation determination, but it may be conducted at other times and could be necessary when information is needed to establish current behaviors, revise an IEP, or develop a BIP. When an FBA is conducted as required by the IDEA, a BIP is to be developed to address the behaviors. An IHO may order that an FBA be conducted as part of a due process hearing, either on his/her own initiative or at the request of a parent or school.

Apart from being a requirement of the IDEA, FBA principles and procedures are considered to be effective assessment methods that lead to interventions, are scientifically based, and have substantial support in the research literature. Research has shown that interventions developed through an FBA process are more effective than those that do not use a functional approach to assessment (Ingram, Lewis-Palmer, & Sugai, 2005). Because the information obtained from an FBA is based upon observed behavior and interviews, it is more readily translated into a BIP. FBAs are required when a child who is receiving special education services is being considered for suspension or expulsion to determine whether misbehavior is a manifestation of the disability. The author has presided over hearings where a parent alleges that a necessary FBA was not conducted and the school has offered a defense that FBAs are only required in cases of manifestation determination. Although FBAs are required in these situations, they may also be required at other times when a child's behavior suggests that changes to an existing IEP or a change in placement are being considered.

Behavior Intervention Plans

As with FBAs, the IDEA does not specify how BIPs are to be constructed or the methods used to address problematic behaviors. Typically, BIPs contain four components: (a) identification of appropriate replacement behaviors, (b) instruction of the replacement behaviors, (c) adaptations and modifications to strengthen or reinforce the probability that the desired replacement behavior will occur and that the undesired behaviors will dissipate, and (d) a plan to systematically monitor and evaluate the effectiveness of the program (Crone & Horner, 2003; Umbreit, Ferro, Liaupsin, & Lane, 2007). In the school setting, a BIP is developed by a team of professionals in collaboration with the parents to address the behaviors that are the most problematic and cause the most impairment. A BIP is not a therapeutic intervention in the traditional sense of altering a child's psychological functioning. Rather, it focuses on changing environmental circumstances that lead to positive behavior change. An effective BIP will also change how other people react and the consequences that occur for appropriate behavior. For children who have significant emotional and behavioral problems, additional services may be needed, such as psychotherapy or family therapy. Typical components of BIPs include:

- Self-monitoring programs
- Reinforcement of appropriate, desired behaviors
- Lack of reinforcement of negative, inappropriate behaviors
- Social skills training
- Increased teacher attention
- Ongoing monitoring of progress on the development of appropriate behaviors
- Positive involvement with peers and others

Individualized Education Programs

The key element in a child's special education services is the Individualized Education Program (IEP) that contains several components:

(1) A statement of the child's present levels of academic achievement and functional performance including

    (i) How the child's disability affects the child's involvement and progress in the general education curriculum (i.e., the same curriculum as for nondisabled children) or

    (ii) For preschool children, as appropriate, how the disability affects the child's participation in appropriate activities

(2) (i) A statement of measurable annual goals, including academic and functional goals designed to

    (A) Meet the child's needs that result from the child's disability to enable the child to be involved in and make progress in the general education curriculum and

    (B) Meet each of the child's other educational needs that result from the child's disability

  (ii) For children with disabilities who take alternate assessments aligned to alternate achievement standards, a description of benchmarks or short-term objectives

(3) A description of:

  (i) How the child's progress toward meeting the annual goals described in paragraph (2) of this section will be measured

  (ii) When periodic reports on the progress the child is making toward meeting the annual goals (such as through the use of quarterly or other periodic reports, concurrent with the issuance of report cards) will be provided

(4) A statement of the special education and related services and supplementary aids and services, based on peer-reviewed research to the extent practicable, to be provided to the child, or on behalf of the child, and a statement of the program modifications or supports for school personnel that will be provided to enable the child:

  (i) To advance appropriately toward attaining the annual goals

  (ii) To be involved in and make progress in the general education curriculum in accordance with paragraph (a)(1) of this section and to participate in extracurricular and other nonacademic activities

  (iii) To be educated and participate with other children with disabilities and nondisabled children in the activities described in this section

(5) An explanation of the extent, if any, to which the child will not participate with nondisabled children in the regular class and in the activities described in paragraph (a)(4) of this section

(6) (i) A statement of any individual appropriate accommodations that are necessary to measure the academic achievement and functional performance of the child on State and districtwide assessments consistent with Section 612(a)(16) of the Act

  (ii) If the IEP Team determines that the child must take an alternate assessment instead of a particular regular State or districtwide assessment of student achievement, a statement of why:

    (A) The child cannot participate in the regular assessment

    (B) The particular alternate assessment selected is appropriate for the child

(7) The projected date for the beginning of the services and modifications described in paragraph (a)(4) of this section, and the anticipated frequency, location, and duration of those services and modifications (34 CFR § 300.320)

This description provides direction regarding what is to be included in the IEP but leaves specific provisions to the IEP Team, such as instructional methods, materials, and how progress is to be measured and monitored while the child receives services. In general, the school retains the right and responsibility to determine the methods of instruction and the materials to be used. Parents may express their preferences on these matters, but schools ultimately determine instructional methods, unless the methods are not appropriate for the student. Disagreements between parents and schools about instructional methods and materials often are issues in due process hearings. In a major decision by the US Supreme Court, it was determined that public schools are not required to provide the "best" education or to comply with parents' requests to provide specific methodologies, but must offer and deliver a program that has the potential to confer educational benefit (*Board of Education v. Rowley, 458 U. S. 176 (1982)*).

Implications for Anxious and Depressed Students

Eligibility

Anxious and depressed students who are eligible for special education services will most often be classified under "Emotional Disturbance" or its individual state variations. The criteria in the federal definition describe some of the characteristics of anxious and depressed students, with two specifically addressing anxiety (a tendency to develop physical symptoms or fears associated with personal or school problems) and depression (a general pervasive mood of unhappiness or depression). It is not uncommon for anxious and depressed children to exhibit "inappropriate behavior under normal circumstances," such as anxious children who have shown extreme social anxiety that interferes with activities such as volunteering in class, giving oral presentations, or relating with other students. Similarly, depressed children can show behaviors that could be interpreted to meet this criterion, such as withdrawal, irritability, and failure to complete assignments. Both anxious and depressed children tend to have difficulties developing and maintaining relationships with others, which could meet that criterion. Most anxious and depressed children do not have significant cognitive delays or health and sensory issues that would meet the first criterion. Although the behaviors to be considered are not limited to the five criteria, they are often the primary ones considered because they are stated in the definition. All of these examples are consistent with the notion of "educational performance" in the ED definition that includes both academic and nonacademic performance.

The criterion that children who are "...socially maladjusted, unless it is determined that they have an emotional disturbance" is challenging because they are difficult to differentiate as they relate to problems with educational performance. This issue has been debated over many years and remains an area of uncertainty and controversy. In the late 1980s and early 1990s, this criterion was interpreted by some to mean that social maladjustment (SM) was equivalent to a DSM-III-R diagnosis of conduct disorder (Slenkovich, 1992a, b). Consequently, children who had a conduct disorder were considered not to be ED but socially maladjusted, and they were not eligible for special education services. Children who are identified as ED are more difficult to suspend or expel from school for misbehavior (Merrell, 2003), and there may be reluctance by some schools to identify children who have behavioral problems as ED to avoid this issue. Adopting such an approach likely would be a violation of the sole criterion provision, even if other information was collected but disregarded in the determination of eligibility for special education services.

Another approach to addressing the issue of SM vs. ED has been to consider the internalizing–externalizing dimension, where children whose behaviors were primarily internalizing would be seen as ED and those with primarily externalizing problems would correspond with the SM designation. Walker (cited in Kauffman, 1997) advocated consideration of this approach to help distinguish between emotional and behavioral disorders for purposes of addressing the SM vs. ED issue. There is some evidence to support such a consideration in that internalizing patterns are seen as emotional or "overcontrolled" and externalizing behaviors as behavioral or "undercontrolled" patterns (Achenbach & Rescorla, 2001). Although this approach does have some empirical support and some intuitive value, it has the potential to be a variation of the sole criterion problem associated with using DSM diagnoses alone without adequate consideration of other information. Moreover, there is considerable correlation between internalizing and externalizing patterns with an average correlation among all the forms of the *Child Behavior Checklist* of about 0.53 (Achenbach & Rescorla). Thus, many children with internalizing patterns will show externalizing behaviors (e.g., irritability, temper outbursts), and those with primarily externalizing patterns will show internalizing behaviors (e.g., withdrawal, depressive mood). It is common for children showing each dimension to also have similar behaviors, such as inattention and social skill deficits. Consequently, although the internalizing and externalizing dimensions offer some guidance in helping to identify ED and SM children, they are not sufficiently distinct to differentiate the two conditions to determine special education eligibility. If eligibility were to be determined only on the basis of a high or low score on an internalizing or externalizing scale, it would be a violation of the sole criterion provision as well as not being consistent with the multimethod approach advocated in comprehensive clinical assessment.

Illustrative Court Cases

Several court cases have addressed the issue of emotional disturbance vs. SM where the issue of "educational performance" has been the pivotal point in the decision-making process. IHOs, review panels/officers, and courts have viewed these cases in different ways, although each one had unique circumstances.

Mars Area School District v. Laurie L., 827 A. 2d 1249 (Pa. Cmwlth, 2003)

This case (to be discussed in more depth below with regard to the role of the evaluation process) addressed whether a 15-year-old boy with behavioral problems was emotionally disturbed or socially maladjusted. The court concluded that, although the student had behavioral problems, his academic achievement in terms of grades and other performance indicators were not impaired. Because his "educational performance" was based on academic criteria, he was considered "socially maladjusted" and therefore was not eligible for special education services.

Mr. I. v. Maine School Administrative Dist. No. 55, 480 F.3d 1 (1st Cir. 2007)

This case heard by the US Court of Appeals, First Circuit, concerned a girl in Maine who had excelled academically in the fourth grade, but began showing signs of sadness and anxiety. Her grades declined from "high honors" to "honors," but she remained in public school until the sixth grade, when she began being truant, inflicting self-injury, and had increasing problems with peers. She also attempted suicide and was hospitalized and instructed to remain out of school for two days. A neuropsychological evaluation was conducted with a conclusion of a diagnosis of Asperger's syndrome and adjustment disorder with depressed mood. The school did not determine her to be eligible for special education because her condition had not been shown to be to a "marked degree" or to have existed "over a long period of time." She was determined to be eligible under Section 504 (to be described below) with services that included close supervision, tutoring, and social skills training. The parents requested a due process hearing, where an IHO found that the student successfully took tests, completed homework and assignments, and was not a behavior problem in class. The IHO concluded that neither federal nor state law required the school "to provide special education services to address what is essentially a mental health issue" and ruled that she was not eligible for special education services.

The parents appealed the decision to a federal district court that appointed a magistrate judge who found that the mental health episode was too brief to meet eligibility criteria for special education services. The federal district court overturned the ruling, finding instead that the student's condition "…did adversely affect her educational performance as Maine defines that term…[,]" and that the events preceding her suicide attempt were not isolated and constituted a pattern. Because the school agreed to provide accommodations to the student under Section 504, it met the definition of "special education" under state and federal law. The school asserted that eligibility for special education required a negative impact on educational performance, which was interpreted as academic areas only. The court concluded that the Maine regulations stated that "educational performance" included academic and nonacademic functioning, and that the regulations had "an expansive notion of educational performance" that included consideration of both areas. The court rejected the IHO's conclusion that a child was not eligible for special education services if there were no academic needs, finding that the IDEA supports the conclusion that educational performance was not limited to grades and other academic indicators.

A.E. v. Westport Board of Educ., 463 F.Supp.2d 208 (D. Conn., 2006)

Although the primary issue in this dispute focused on parents' disagreements with the evaluation, IEP, and private school vs. public school placement, the issue of whether eligibility for special education services is limited to academic areas was embedded in the case. The student was a boy who had no academic difficulties in elementary school, but began demonstrating more behavioral problems over subsequent years. The parent rejected a school evaluation but agreed to a neuropsychological evaluation by an independent psychologist, who found that the student had a serious emotional disturbance. The school accepted the evaluation and concluded that he was eligible for special education services, placing him in the district's middle school for sixth grade. He achieved well, but the parents wanted placement in a private school and rejected the IEP. The court found that the public school placement was appropriate, including behavior management practices, and upheld the IHO's ruling in favor of the school. This case indicated that the school and the court focused on nonacademic areas as primary considerations in determining eligibility for special education services.

Board of Educ. of Montgomery County, Maryland v. S. G., 230 Fed. Appx. 330 (4th Cir. 2007)

The student was described as "bright, motivated, sociable, well-organized," and a successful student prior to fifth grade, when behavioral problems emerged including stealing, suicidal ideation, disturbing writing samples, and difficulty with completing assignments and organization. In the sixth grade, the problems worsened to include daytime enuresis, "violent and hypersexual writings," memory problems, self-injurious behavior, and hearing voices. She was diagnosed with a psychotic disorder and was hospitalized multiple times, as well as missing several days of school. Her academic performance declined in the sixth grade, although the parent asserted that her grades were "grossly inflated" because they were based on completed work and did not include incomplete or missed assignments. Teachers reported that, although the student was withdrawn in class, she had academic strengths. Consequently, the school did not find her eligible for special education services due to lack of "adverse educational impact," despite finding that she engaged in inappropriate behavior over a long time and to a marked degree.

The parent requested a due process hearing. The administrative law judge (ALJ) found that the school had committed a major violation of the IDEA by failing to find the student eligible for special education services. The ALJ ordered a therapeutic school placement. The school complied with the order but appealed the ruling to a federal district court, asserting that the ALJ did not give appropriate consideration to the school's witnesses and also committed procedural errors. The court did not find such errors, and the school appealed to the US Fourth Circuit Court of Appeals, which upheld the ALJ's decision, finding that the conclusions were legally sound and that the district court had properly considered them. The court also found that IHOs are not always required to defer to a school's experts. Importantly, the court found that being in a public middle school exacerbated the student's symptoms and contributed to hearing voices, "zoning out," and impetus to harm herself. The condition was considered not to be purely medical in nature and affected her ability to obtain an education. As a consequence, the court upheld the judgment. This case also indicates that academic areas do not need to be the sole or primary areas of "adverse educational performance" or impact for a student to be eligible for special education services as a child with an emotional disturbance.

Eschenasy v. New York City Dep't of Educ., 604 F. Supp. 2d 639 (S. D. N. Y. 2009)

This case involved a girl who showed high levels of externalizing behavior since entering public school, including stealing, drug use, sexual misbehavior, inappropriate attire, and body piercings and tattoos. She also engaged in self-injury by cutting herself, had a purging eating disorder, violated school conduct rules, struggled academically, and failed some classes. In 10th grade, she forged checks and was hospitalized. In the 11th grade, she used drugs, skipped classes, and was expelled for truancy. She had been diagnosed with a mood disorder and had taken a mood-stabilizing medication. She ran away from home and attempted suicide. Subsequently, her therapist recommended a residential therapeutic school. The parents requested a due process hearing, and the IHO found that the student was both "socially maladjusted" and "seriously emotionally disturbed." The school appealed the decision, and a state review officer (SRO) reversed the IHO, finding that the student was not emotionally disturbed but was socially maladjusted.

An appeal was made to a federal district court, which found that the state and federal definitions of emotional disturbance were the same. The court held that the student had a conduct disorder and that the state's definition of emotional disturbance did not apply to SM. The court also determined that the student had an emotional disturbance. The decision reversed the SROs ruling by finding that the student met the criteria for a "long period of time" and "to a marked degree." The court noted that the student had failing grades, had been expelled numerous times for misbehavior, and needed tutoring. She also improved academically in the residential program where her emotional problems were addressed. Thus, the court upheld the original IHO's decision of finding the student eligible for special education services as having an emotional disturbance, despite the high level of externalizing behavior. This case demonstrates how a student can have both internalizing and externalizing behaviors, which is a common occurrence. The co-occurrence of these behaviors often is difficult to differentiate and to determine which ones are the primary contributors to a child's academic and nonacademic performance.

K.M. v. Wappingers Central School District, 688 F. Supp.2d 282 (S.D. N. Y. 2010)

The student was a girl who had been diagnosed as having ADHD, GAD, Asperger's syndrome, pervasive developmental disorder (PDD), and dysgraphia during a five-year period from about the age of 7–12. At the age of 11, the school conducted an educational evaluation that included the *Wechsler Intelligence Scale for Children-III* (Wechsler, 1991). The results indicated the following: Verbal IQ = 96th percentile, Performance IQ = 34th percentile, Verbal Comprehension Index = 96th percentile, Perceptual Organization Index = 63rd percentile, Freedom from Distractibility = 98th percentile, and Processing Speed = 6th percentile. These results indicate that K.M. had superior verbal skills that would predict good school success and she did not show high levels of distractibility, but did have significantly lower ability in processing some information. About two months later, she was evaluated by a neuropsychologist upon referral by the school. The neuropsychologist found that the student had "…a clinically significant cognitive deficit in the 'domains of visual and aural attention and response inhibition, visuo-spatial processing and response speed'" (p. 8). She concluded that the student experienced anxiety that "… is secondary to [K.M.'s] increasing consciousness of the negative social and academic effects of her cognitive deficits" (p. 8). She was also diagnosed with a moderate language disability by a speech pathologist.

In sixth grade, she began weekly counseling sessions with a social worker who concluded that K.M. was demonstrating anxiety and depression that appeared to be a "residual effect" of her Asperger's syndrome and PDD. Later that year, she was seen for emergency psychiatric treatment for attention problems, debilitating anxiety, unstable mood, deficient interpersonal relationship, and "…assorted learning deficits contributing to persistent and progressive episodes of inconsolable agitation and lability" (p. 9).

The school's records indicated that she excelled academically from about second through sixth grades in the public school with some accommodations. During the sixth grade, her parents requested that K.M. be reevaluated and found to be eligible for special education services under the IDEA. The school recognized her emotional problems but did not find her eligible for special education because she was doing well academically and that the problems did not have an educational impact. Prior to starting the seventh grade, the parents again requested that she be found eligible for special education services under the IDEA, but the school again did not find her eligible, stating that the accommodation plan met her needs. K.M. continued to do well in the first quarter of seventh grade when her parents removed her from the public school and placed her in a private school where she continued to get high grades.

The parents requested a due process hearing, and the IHO recognized that the student had been achieving well, but also concluded that he could consider "adverse effect" on educational performance to include nonacademic areas "...including 'social development, physical development and management needs'" (p. 11). The IHO ruled that the student's problems interfered with "social discourse and social development" and that she needed continued special education services to benefit from her education and that the private school was an appropriate placement. Interestingly, the IHO allowed only partial reimbursement for the private school, based on the parents "overinvolvement" that included putting pressure on the student to excel and for removing the child from the public school on several days.

The school appealed the ruling to a SRO who reversed the IHO's decision, concluding that the student did not qualify for special educational services due to her high academic achievement and performance on standardized tests. The SRO concluded that, although her social and emotional problems were present, they were not "...adversely affecting her classroom performance, her ability to learn in class, to function in her classes or to continue in school, or her ability to benefit from regular education" (p. 12).

The parents appealed the SRO's decision to the federal district court of New York, which upheld the ruling. In the opinion, the court found that "educational performance" should be interpreted as applying only to academic performance and not to social or behavioral issues. Because neither the State of New York's regulations nor the IDEA define "educational performance," the court referred to similar cases within the Second Circuit, which also considered the term to mean academic performance, and not social or other nonacademic areas. Consequently, the student could not be considered to be eligible for special education services, because she had been achieving well academically, despite her social and interpersonal difficulties.

A.J. v. East Islip Union Free School District,
53 IDELR (E.D.N.Y. 2010)

In this case, the student was a kindergartener who was doing well academically but was having social and behavioral difficulties in the classroom and was diagnosed with Asperger's syndrome and ADHD by external professionals. Although Asperger's syndrome is on the autism spectrum and is a separate disability category in the IDEA and state regulations from Emotional Disturbance, the case is nevertheless instructive with regard to the issue of whether social, emotional, and behavioral problems constitute "educational performance."

A.J. was progressing well in the classroom but had some behavior problems that the teacher said were not much more than occur with typical children and that she could not address successfully. A special education teacher and a retired psychologist also testified that, although the student exhibited some inappropriate, hyperactive, and impulsive behavior, the teacher maintained control and no extra services were indicated. The educational evaluation conducted by the school psychologist indicated that the student "...does well academically [but] has difficulty socializing with peers" and also that the student had average ability. The school did not find the student eligible for special education services as a child with autism.

The student's parents requested a due process hearing, and the IHO found that A.J. was not eligible for special education services because he was achieving well academically and that his problems were not so severe that he needed services. The determination of "educational performance" was based on academic performance, which the IHO found was not negatively affected by the student's behavior, because he continued to perform well academically. Upon appeal by the parents, a SRO upheld the IHO's decision, concluding that "educational performance" referred only to academic performance, which was not affected by the student's behavior.

The parents appealed to the federal district court of New York, which upheld the decisions of the IHO and SRO. The court also addressed the question of "adverse affect" and whether a "severe" or "significant" effect must be demonstrated. The court concluded that severity qualifiers should not be added to "adverse effect" and that "...the term 'adversely affects' should be given its ordinary meaning." The reasoning of the court was similar to the *A.J. v. East Islip Union Free School District* case discussed above, which also originated in New York and where the court referred to similar cases within the Second Circuit.

Hansen v. Republic R-III School Dist., No. 10-1514, 2011 WL 181530 (8th Cir. 1/21/11)

In this case, the student had a history of making threats and poor performance in class and on standardized tests since entering the school district in the fifth grade. At the end of the fifth grade, the student's father asked for special education services, but the school did not find the student eligible for special education services, prompting a request for a due process hearing. The case was heard by a state review panel, who issued a one-paragraph ruling that the student did not qualify for special education services under the IDEA. Upon review by a federal district court, it was found that he had conduct and bipolar disorders and ADHD. There was an established record of him being suspended for making threats to classmates and teachers and making suicidal comments. Consequently, the court reversed the review panel, which was appealed by the school to the US Court of Appeals, Eighth Circuit. The school asserted that the student was "socially maladjusted" and did not have an emotional disturbance and did well with some teachers, rendering him ineligible for special education services. The court held that the student had suffered academically because of his bipolar disorder and that he could not build or maintain satisfactory interpersonal relationships. Therefore, he was found eligible for special education services as a student with an emotional disturbance. The court also found that he had a secondary disability of Other Health Impairment due to his ADHD that interfered with his ability to learn.

This case demonstrated that a student can have an emotional disturbance that affects both academic and social–behavioral functioning and results in eligibility for special education services. Although this student had externalizing, acting out problems, they were considered to be associated with an emotional disturbance that required special education services.

These cases are examples of how differences in interpretation of data, conceptualizations of "social maladjustment" and "emotional disturbance," the lack of specificity of the federal and state criteria, definitions of "educational performance," and specific circumstances can result in different outcomes at the administrative and judicial levels. As an IHO, the author has presided over cases where similar issues have arisen and has found them among the more difficult to adjudicate. In the majority of these cases, the central issue often is defining "educational performance," with some schools and adjudicators focusing solely on academic areas, while others consider nonacademic areas as well. The IDEA is clear that it does not limit the definition of "educational performance" to only academic areas, but it also does not define the term. Because a state cannot be more restrictive in its state law than is the federal law, denying eligibility for special education for emotional disturbance where a child is achieving well academically despite emotional and behavioral problems in the school setting is questionable. Individual states may have other statutes and regulations that address definitions of children with disabilities, emotional disturbance/disabilities, and provisions for providing services to children with emotional and behavioral problems. The reader is encouraged to become familiar with these laws in the respective state that may apply to definitions and services to these students.

Evaluations

The IDEA evaluation requirements listed above apply to children who are suspected or known to have anxiety and depression that affect academic and functional performance. The methods to be used are not specified, which leaves those decisions to the school, most often the school psychologist. In all hearings, the school's educational evaluations are included in the record and are often a focal point of evidence and testimony. In the author's experience, many of the evaluations are incomplete and often do not correspond with the multimethod approach described in Chap. 7. In the majority of cases where a child is being evaluated for anxiety and depression, the evaluation consists of a behavior rating scale completed by one or more teachers, a brief teacher interview, limited developmental history, and classroom observation. The evaluations often do not include an extensive clinical interview or developmental history, systematic input from parents, the use of self-report measures to assess anxious and depressive symptomatology, or multidimensional personality measures, where appropriate.

IEEs often include information only from the parents and child but are more likely to include self-report measures, clinical interviews, extensive developmental histories, and parent input. However, these evaluations often do not include contact with school personnel, school-based observations, or review of school records, performance, and social functioning. Because IEEs are completed in a minority of cases and school-based evaluations of anxious and depressed children may not comply with recommended best practices, these students may not receive thorough assessment.

The author presided over a due process hearing regarding the appropriate placement for a student with anxiety, depression, and health issues. The school completed an evaluation, most of which was conducted by the school psychologist. The evaluation was considered thorough, with the exception of little input from the parents. The student also was evaluated by an independent psychologist who did not have any contact with the school or obtain any information other than from the parents. The psychologist also used outdated tests, which was noted by the school psychologist during testimony. Further, the psychologist did not offer a viable rationale for failing to contact the school or for using outdated measures. Consequently, considerably more weight was given to the school's evaluation, which falls within the discretion of the trier of fact in a due process hearing. Although reimbursement for the IEE was not at issue in the hearing, failure to conduct evaluations that meet accepted professional standards and that do not comply with special education regulations may result in denial of reimbursement.

In *Mars Area School District v. Laurie L.,* 827 A. 2d 1249 (Pa. Cmwlth, 2003) discussed above, the IHO found that a 15-year-old student did not meet the definition of "emotional disturbance." His grades were average to above average through most of his school years, but behavioral problems resulted in referral for special education in the fifth grade, where he was found ineligible for services as an ED student. He was diagnosed with ADHD and oppositional defiant disorder (ODD), with possible depression to be ruled out. He was suspended several times for misbehavior and was reevaluated again in the sixth grade and found to be eligible for special education as a student with an emotional disturbance and other health impairments. It was determined that his behavior interfered with his learning and that of others due to problems with attention, completion of assignments, accepting adult direction, attention-seeking behavior, disruptive behavior, drastic mood changes, and placing blame on others for his behavior.

He was suspended multiple times for his misbehavior and placed in an alternative program. He was evaluated again by the school district using multiple tests, including an intelligence test, achievement tests, two behavior rating scales, observations, and a measure of visual-motor integration, visual perception, and motor coordination. Based in part on that evaluation, the student was determined to be socially maladjusted and not to have an emotional disturbance, thus not being eligible for special education. "It was determined at that time that recent testing revealed that [the student] had been inadequately and inappropriately identified as handicapped because he had no educational or academic needs that were not being met. Rather, his behavior met the description of a socially maladjusted youngster" (at 1,253). The student was evaluated by a private psychologist, who reviewed records, administered a depression scale and an incomplete sentence technique, the latter being a projective measure without a score or norms. He concluded that the student suffered from depression, ADHD, and ODD and did meet the criteria for Emotional Disturbance and Other Health Impairment.

During the administrative due process hearing, the IHO relied more on the school's evaluation, which he considered more thorough and comprehensive than the one completed by the private psychologist. He concluded that the student was not ED but had a conduct disorder and was socially maladjusted. The student appealed the decision to a state review panel, asserting that the hearing officer did not properly apply the definition of emotional disturbance. The panel found that the school failed to establish that, although the student's behaviors might be consistent with SM, the student did not meet definitional criteria for ED. The panel vacated the IHO's decision and remanded the case to the school to conduct a more thorough evaluation and, *sua sponte*, concluded that the school district made no reference to other health impairments that the student might have. The school appealed to the state court, which concluded that the review panel exceeded its authority and reviewed the case with regard to whether the student's constitutional rights were violated, if an error of law occurred, or if the findings of fact were supported by substantial evidence. The court found that the IHO's reliance on the school's evaluation rather than that of the private psychologist was not in error and that review panels are to defer to the credibility determinations of an IHO, unless there is evidence to the contrary. The court upheld the ruling of the hearing officer and reversed the decision of the review panel, concluding that the student was socially maladjusted and did not have an emotional disturbance.

These cases demonstrate how the weight given to a psychological or educational evaluation can have a significant impact on the determinations of a hearing officer, review panel, or court. Hearing officers have the discretion and responsibility to determine the credibility and probative value of documents, testimony, and witnesses. In these last two cases, the thoroughness of the school's evaluation was given substantially more weight, albeit for different reasons, with the private evaluation given less credence.

Functional Behavioral Assessment

FBA of internalizing problems is more challenging, due to their subjective nature, overcontrolled and withdrawn/inhibited characteristics, and that their intended outcomes typically are quite different from externalizing behaviors. For many, if not most, children with internalizing conditions, the goal or intended outcome of their behaviors is not for power, revenge, or control of situations but is attempts to avoid or escape situations that might trigger symptoms, such as

- Fear of negative evaluation
- Stress
- Feelings of humiliation or embarrassment

- Anticipation of failure
- Onset of physical symptoms or hyperarousal
- Increase in feelings of low self-esteem
- Appearing inadequate to others
- Onset of depressive mood
- Panic attacks
- Rejection or negative reactions from others

Nevertheless, FBAs can be completed with children who have internalizing problems. Many of the problems that anxious and depressed children experience are related to social competence and performance. Social problems can be of two types: (a) skill deficits or (b) performance deficits. *Skill deficits* refer to problems associated with the lack of skills to perform tasks. For example, an anxious child might not know how to initiate a conversation with a peer group and withdraw when in a group setting. *Performance deficits* occur when a child has a skill but is unable or unwilling to demonstrate it under some conditions. An anxious child might know the answer to test questions but become so anxious that he cannot give the correct answer. Thus, many FBAs and behavioral intervention programs (BIP) often are focused on social competence issues that may involve skill or performance deficits.

Not all behavioral issues of children with internalizing problems are based in social competence issues, however. Other problems include initiation of activities, task completion, public performances, and withdrawal. These kinds of deficits may be displayed in both academic and social situations, requiring an FBA to attempt to determine the antecedents and consequences of the behaviors that will inform the development of a BIP. In many cases, the antecedents of the behaviors may not be obvious because they often are internal and subjective, such as worry, inadequate emotion regulation, distorted thinking, and other cognitive processes. Table 14.1 provides a partial list of the behaviors and possible replacement behaviors that may be seen in anxious and depressed students.

Individualized Education Programs

Developing and implementing IEPs for anxious and depressed students can be challenging, due to the subjective nature and primarily covert symptomatology. In the author's experience as an IHO, some IEPs for anxious and depressed students were not well developed and did not meet legal requirements for six primary reasons: (a) the objectives were general and lacked a clear focus (e.g., "the student will show improved self-esteem"), (b) the objectives were not stated in behavioral terms, (c) the objectives were not readily measureable, (d) the instructional or intervention methods were not well defined, (e) the criteria for achievement of the objectives were not well stated, and (f) methods for evaluation of the objectives lacked specificity. Nevertheless, all of these potential shortcomings can be avoided if the assessment

Table 14.1 Partial list of functional and replacement behaviors of children with internalizing problems

Functional behaviors	Possible replacement behaviors
• Lack of initiation of social behavior	• Demonstrate appropriate initiation of behavior in groups or dyads
• Social withdrawal	• Increase social interaction with peers
• Failure to participate in class	• Increase voluntary participation
• Failure to respond to directives	• Respond appropriately to teacher directives
• Excessive perfectionistic behavior	• Child accepts less than perfect performance
• Does not complete tasks	• Increase percentage of task completion
• Does not complete tasks in a timely manner	• Increase rate or frequency of task completion
• Engages in "fidgety" or "nervous" behavior	• Replace behavior with purposeful and goal-directed behavior, such as completion of tasks
• High levels of physiological hyperarousal	• Reduce hyperarousal with relaxed behavior and lower physiological symptoms
• Does not seek assistance from others	• Seeks assistance from others in appropriate manner

and conceptualization of the student's problems are done properly. The following examples of IEP goals and objectives are provided to demonstrate how some areas might be addressed for anxious and depressed students in the school setting.

Example of Anxiety Interventions

This example of performance anxiety was chosen because it is a common problem in schools and is a frequent symptom of children with generalized anxiety disorder and social phobia/social anxiety disorder. Fear of negative evaluation (FNE) is a core feature of performance anxiety and is a contributory factor to lowered academic achievement in children and youth with anxiety disorders. The extreme anxiety associated with FNE is an example of the difficulty that anxious children have with regulating emotions in social and academic situations. Thus, an overall goal of regulating emotions could be included in an IEP, with objectives/benchmarks developed that address specific symptoms.

In the example provided in Table 14.2, the behavior is stated objectively in terms of giving an oral presentation, such as a speech or reading aloud. A functional assessment would be conducted to determine if there is a skill or performance deficit. In addition to the interventions listed, instruction for these deficits may be needed. Several methods of establishing criteria are presented that include establishing criteria that are reported by the child, as well as external criteria from someone who observes the performance, such as a teacher. The performance

Table 14.2 Example of IEP goals and objectives for anxiety

Objective/benchmark	Criterion to achieve objective	Timeline to achieve objective	Intervention methods	Evaluation methods
To increase the ability to give an oral presentation without a high level of impairing anxiety	Teacher ratings of 90% accuracy; student self-ratings of at least 8 on a 10-point scale of comfort in making an oral presentation; teacher ratings using the same scale; teacher checklist of anxiety-related behaviors with ratings of "4" or higher on a five-point scale	By the completion of the third oral presentation and maintenance in subsequent presentations	Student practices at home and with teacher, aide, or other "coach"; student is taught self-relaxation techniques; student develops a cognitive "script" to use before and during the presentation; teacher "cues" student if errors or anxiety becomes too high	Teacher grades and ratings of accuracy of presentation based on criteria; teacher ratings of anxiety-related behavior during presentation; student self-rating of comfort level on a 10-point scale with 10 being minimal anxiety and able to function well; uses same scale as the teacher

Goal: improve emotion regulation skills in classroom tasks

criteria would be developed based on the specific symptoms presented but should include both internal (child self-report/assessment) and external criteria that provide feedback about performance. The timeline to achieve the objective would be based on the frequency of the behavior or task, the severity of the symptoms, the complexity of the pattern (including consideration of comorbid factors), and other variables.

The intervention methods listed are examples of approaches that might be considered to treat performance anxiety. It would not be feasible or desirable to include a large number of strategies simultaneously. Using a problem-solving approach, a variety of intervention strategies should be developed, and one or two selected that are feasible, that are able to be implemented in the specific situations, and that have a reasonable likelihood of success. In the example, it is important for the child to be a participant in the intervention process, but it is also necessary for others to be involved, especially if the child is young. The evaluation methods for treating anxiety involve obtaining reports from the child and others. In Chap. 4, it was proposed that input from others, such as parents and teachers, helps children learn emotion regulation skills. In cases of performance anxiety, external feedback serves both regulatory and information roles so that when similar situations arise, the child will be better able to manage the associated emotions.

Finally, the examples provided likely would meet federal and state special education guidelines because the objectives are behaviorally stated, are measureable, and the intervention (instructional) methods are scientifically based. All of the interventions listed have been well established in the research literature as being efficacious or likely efficacious in treating anxiety symptoms and can be presented in due process hearings as defensible approaches. Evaluation methods such as behavioral observations and subjective self-ratings are common to many forms of behavioral and cognitive–behavioral therapy and have been shown to be useful for baseline assessment and assessment of effectiveness. Other methods could be included, such as standardized rating scales, although they may not be sufficiently sensitive to detect treatment change, especially over a short period of time.

Example of Depression Intervention

In this example, the frequent symptom of social interaction skills associated with depression is identified as an overall goal to be addressed, with a specific objective of initiating social interaction as the focus of an intervention. As with the anxiety example, the objective is behaviorally stated, a criterion for initial success is set along with a projected timeline, and interventions and evaluation methods are specified. The intervention methods would result from "brainstorming" about possible interventions, and those that are selected would be deemed to be feasible, implementable, and have a high likelihood of success. The evaluation and intervention methods are well established in professional practice and the research literature and would meet federal and state special education requirements (Table 14.3).

Table 14.3 Example of IEP goals and objectives for depressive symptoms

Objective/benchmark	Criterion to achieve objective	Timeline to achieve objective	Intervention methods	Evaluation methods
To increase frequency of initiation of social interaction	Increase frequency of initiation of interaction with others by 50%; postintervention ratings of at least "4" on a five-point scale by teacher and child	By the completion of the first grading period and maintained through the next grading period	Social skills instruction; modeling of appropriate social behavior; peer-mediated activities; pairing with a socially adept peer	Observational recording; teacher ratings, such as a scale of "1" to "5" or a standardized rating scale; self-ratings using similar approaches are to be included

Goal: improve social interaction skills

Section 504 of the Rehabilitation Act of 1973

In addition to the IDEA, schools are also required to comply with this law, which applies to certain persons with known or suspected disabilities, who had a history of disabilities, or who are considered to have disabling conditions. It predated the Education for All Handicapped Children's Act of 1975, which incorporated some of the language and provisions of Section 504 (29 U.S.C. § 794). Section 504, however, is not an education law that provides funds to states to educate children with disabilities. Rather, it is an antidiscrimination law that also applies to postsecondary educational settings, i.e., colleges and universities. It does not provide funding for services but requires that educational institutions assure due process for all persons and to prohibit discrimination of persons who have or are considered to have a disability. The law requires that a person has a disability or condition that substantially impairs a "major life activity," such as mobility, breathing, eating, hearing, or similar problems. With regard to public education, the major life activity affected is most often identified as "learning," with accommodations addressing both academic and nonacademic areas. Section 504 does not have the prescriptive requirements regarding evaluation, IEPs, review of progress, and other areas that are included in the IDEA.

It is not uncommon for children who have not been found eligible for special education under the IDEA to be found eligible under Section 504. If found eligible for Section 504, a "plan" is to be developed that contains modifications and accommodations that address the disability areas. A 504 plan does not have the same degree of precision and specific requirements as an IEP under the IDEA, but review and modifications are to be conducted as needed. This practice is controversial, however, because some authorities suggest that Section 504 has a higher standard for determining the presence of a disability than does the IDEA. Thus, finding a child eligible for Section 504 but not under the IDEA may be contrary to the notion that a disability exists that requires specialized services or accommodations. Zirkel (2003) has suggested that courts have taken such a narrow view of the Section 504 definition of a disability that finding a child eligible for services "…as an automatic fall-back in the wake of existing or not qualifying in the first place under the IDEA is clearly questionable." It is beyond the scope of this chapter to discuss Section 504 in depth, but it remains an avenue to provide educational services to children with disabilities, including those with anxiety and depression.

Implications for Psychoeducational Assessment

The challenges associated with the issue of SM vs. ED have implications for assessment by school personnel and by evaluators who conduct IEEs. The IDEA requirements that educational evaluations are to be based on multiple sources of information are consistent with the multimethod of assessment described in Chap. 7. As applied to assessment of emotional and behavioral problems that have implications for addressing the SM vs. ED issue, evaluations to determine eligibility should include a variety of methods to comply with the IDEA and best practices in assessment, i.e., the multimethod approach. Because determining if a child has an emotional disturbance cannot be conducted by using only one method, a multimethod approach is needed. Also, there is no one measure that accurately differentiates ED from SM, and the use of a single measure would violate the "sole criterion" prohibition of the IDEA. As an IHO/ALJ, the author has observed that the majority of assessments typically include observations in the school setting, the use of behavior rating scales, a developmental history, and limited observations are most often conducted. It is infrequent that self-report measures, such as anxiety and depression measures, are conducted as part of the evaluation. In the author's opinion, a comprehensive assessment should include the following components to comply with IDEA requirements and with best practice guidelines:

- Thorough developmental history
- Systematic observations across multiple school settings
- Clinical interview with child
- Parent interview
- Teacher interview
- Appropriate self-report measures (e.g., MASC, CDI-2, RCMAS-2, BYI-II)
- Behavior rating scales completed by child (as appropriate), parents, and teachers
- Multidimensional inventories, as appropriate

Not only will such assessments comply with IDEA requirements, but they also will provide comprehensive information upon which to (a) determine if a child requires special education services, (b) develop appropriate interventions, and (c) to create a baseline upon which evaluation of intervention programs can be made. Some state special education regulations may have specific requirements for conducting psychoeducational evaluations to determine eligibility for special education services as a child with an Emotional Disturbance, which should be followed, but can also be supplemented as suggested above. A comprehensive evaluation is also more defensible in a due process hearing or in a state or federal court and will be given strong consideration by an IHO/ALJ or judge.

When IEEs are conducted, the IDEA requires that the evaluation must be comparable to what a school would conduct. A DSM-IV diagnosis by itself is not sufficient, and reliance on such a diagnosis may violate the sole criterion provision of the IDEA. It is common for independent evaluators to rely solely on parent and child report and their own assessment methods. Most often, independent evaluators do not observe the child at school or talk with teachers, and they may not have sufficient understanding of a child's educational program to be able to offer relevant recommendations. A school is required to consider an IEE in determining eligibility for special education service, but is not required to accept it, although it can accept it in lieu of its own evaluation. A school is not required to consider an IEE if it does not meet public agency guidelines (34 CFR § 300.502(c)(1)). If a school accepts the evaluation in part or in total, it is responsible to assure that it complies with state and federal requirements. An incomplete IEE may be given less weight by an IHO/ALJ or court if it does not meet requirements, as was noted in some of the court cases cited above.

Assessment of anxiety and depression and their association with school functioning must comply with state and federal requirements, as well. Because of the subjective nature of the two disorders, a thorough evaluation is necessary to determine eligibility, conduct appropriate educational planning, and otherwise meet IDEA requirements. If a student is anxious or depressed and needs modifications or accommodations, the school is responsible to evaluate these problems and must assure that all relevant information is available and considered appropriately.

Concluding Comments

The interface between public education and disability law is a well-established relationship that is intended to assure that children with disabilities are provided a free appropriate public education. Children and youth with anxiety and depression may be considered for services as a student with an emotional disturbance, but differentiation from "social maladjustment" and whether nonacademic areas are included under "educational performance" remain central issues. The reader is encouraged to consult attorneys, state statutes and regulations, and administrative and judicial rulings in state or federal courts and to engage in multimethod assessment and intervention services that are as scientifically based as possible. The overall goal of special education law is to assure that children with disabilities receive an appropriate education to have the opportunity to progress in their program. Adherence to standards of professional practice and legal requirements will help to assure that appropriate services are provided to anxious and depressed students in the school setting, giving them a better chance of achieving successful outcomes and to follow a positive developmental trajectory.

Part VI
Appendices

Chapter 15
Appendices

Appendix A: Family and Developmental History

Date:_____

Child's Name:_____ DOB:_____ Age:_____ Sex: __M ___F
Home Address: _____
School: _____ Grade: _____ Teacher: _____
Family Physician/Pediatrician:_____ Address:_____
Last date child has seen Family Physician/Pediatrician: _____ Reason:_____
Referral Source: □ Self/Family □ Physician □ School □ Court □ Family Services
□ Community agency (specify):_____ □ Other (specify): _____

_____

Person(s) completing this form: □ Mother □ Father □ Stepmother □ Stepfather
□ Grandmother □ Grandfather □ Other caregiver (name): _____
□ Agency staff: (name) _____ □ Other:_____

PARENT INFORMATION:

Mother's Name: _____ Age:_____ Occupation:_____
Education: □ 9th grade or less □ 10th grade □ 11th grade □ H. S. Graduate □ Some college □ College
Graduate □ Post graduate work or degree □ Other:_____

Father's Name: _____ Age:_____ Occupation:_____
Education: □ 9th grade or less □ 10th grade □ 11th grade □ H. S. Graduate □ Some college □ College
Graduate □ Post Graduate work or degree □ Other:_____

Stepmother's Name: _____ Age: _____ Occupation:_____
Education: □ 9th grade or less □ 10th grade □ 11th grade □ H. S. Graduate □ Some college
□ College Graduate □ Post Graduate work or degree □ Other:_____

Stepfather's Name: _____ Age: _____ Occupation:_____
Education: □ 9th grade or less □ 10th grade □ 11th grade □ H. S. Graduate □ Some college
□ College Graduate □ Post Graduate work or degree □ Other:_____

T.J. Huberty, *Anxiety and Depression in Children and Adolescents:*
Assessment, Intervention, and Prevention, DOI 10.1007/978-1-4614-3110-7_15,
© Springer Science+Business Media, LLC 2012

Marital status of natural parents: □ Married □ Separated □ Divorced □ Remarried
If separated, age of child at time of separation: _____
If divorced, age of child at time of divorce: _____
If remarried, age of child at time when step-parent entered into the family: _____

If divorced, with whom does the child live most often? □ Mother □ Father □ Both about equally
If divorced, what is the custody arrangement? □ Mother □ Father □ Joint

Is either natural parent incarcerated? □ Yes □ No   If yes, which parent? □ Mother □ Father
If a natural parent is incarcerated, age of child at time of incarceration: _____

Is either natural parent deceased? □ Yes □ No   If yes, which parent? □ Mother □ Father
If a natural parent is deceased, when did it occur? _____
What were the circumstances of the death? _____

Is the child adopted? □ Yes □ No
If yes, does the child know that she or he is adopted? □ Yes □ No
How old was she or he when adopted? _____
When was she or he told of the adoption? _____
What was her/his reaction when knowing of the adoption? _____
Does medical or developmental information exist prior to the adoption? □ Yes □ No

CURRENT FAMILY CONSTELLATION:

List all persons living in the home:

Name	Sex	Relationship to Child	Age

List all significant persons living outside the home (e.g., grown siblings, half-siblings)

Name	Sex	Relationship to Child	Age

Primary language spoken in the home: □ English □ Spanish □ Chinese □ Other _____
Primary language used by child at home: □ English □ Spanish □ Chinese □ Other _____
Primary language used by child out of home: □ English □ Spanish □ Chinese □ Other _____

REASON FOR REFERRAL:

Why is the child being referred, i.e., what are the primary problems that concern you? Please be as specific as possible. _____

How long have the problems been present? _____

Has the child been seen for these problems before? □ Yes □ No □ Don't know

If yes, when? _____ Do you have copies of the information? □Yes □ No □ Don't know

Who provided the services? _____

What services were provided? _____

Why are you seeking help at this time? _____

If there is more than one problem, please state them as specifically as possible (e.g., hits others, withdraws, etc.) in the order of importance to you. For example, if you are concerned about hitting others, withdrawal, and not completing homework in that order, you would list them that way. Then, check the box that indicates how much the problem interferes with the child's social, personal, or academic functioning.

Behavior	Severe Problem	Moderate Problem	Mild Problem
1. _____	□	□	□
2. _____	□	□	□
3. _____	□	□	□
4. _____	□	□	□
5. _____	□	□	□

SOCIAL, BEHAVIORAL, AND EMOTIONAL PATTERNS

Below is a list of behaviors often seen in children. Please rate each one in terms of how often they occur using this scale: "3" = "Daily or almost daily", "2" = "Occasionally", or "1" = "Rarely" or "Never"

Behavior	Rating	Behavior	Rating	Behavior	Rating
Shy	_____	Clings to others	_____	Distractible	_____
Withdrawn	_____	Risky behavior	_____	Impulsive	_____
Aggressive	_____	Cries a lot	_____	Sleeping problems	_____
Fights with others	_____	Daydreams	_____	Stares a lot	_____
Physical complaints	_____	Temper tantrums	_____	Fearful	_____
Hyperactive	_____	Mood swings	_____	Runs away	_____
"Fidgety"	_____	Talks rapidly	_____	Talks about suicide	_____
Inattentive	_____	Talks softly	_____	Easily angered	_____
Low Self-Esteem	_____	Sulks	_____	Feelings easily hurt	_____
Anxious	_____	Wants own way	_____	Memory problems	_____
Depressed	_____	Low energy	_____	Social skills probs.	_____
Hurts others physically	_____	High energy	_____	Acts young for age	_____
Hurts others' feelings	_____	Seeks attention	_____	Easily frustrated	_____
Worries a lot	_____	Talkative	_____	Self-conscious	_____

| Injures self | _____ | Wets the bed | _____ | Pressured speech | _____ |
| Accident prone | _____ | Disobeys adults | _____ | Feels stressed | _____ |

Please explain or elaborate on any items that concern you or were rated as a "3". Use additional sheet if necessary.

_____
_____
_____
_____
_____
_____
_____
_____
_____

DEVELOPMENTAL HISTORY

Age of mother at pregnancy:_____   Was prenatal care provided? □ Yes □ No □ Don't know
If yes, when did prenatal care begin? _____ Was this a first pregnancy/ □ Yes □ No
Were there problems during the pregnancy? □ Yes □ No □ Don't know. *If yes, please describe* (e.g., bleeding, eclampsia, high blood pressure of mother, gestational diabetes, etc.) _____
_____

Did the mother do any of the following during the pregnancy?
□ Smoke cigarettes   □ first trimester   □ second trimester   □ third trimester
If yes, how many cigarettes per day? _____
_____

□ Drink alcohol   □ first trimester   □ second trimester   □ third trimester
If yes, what type and how much? _____
_____

□ Take drugs   □ first trimester   □ second trimester   □ third trimester
If yes, what drugs and how often? _____

Was the mother involved in any accidents or injured during the pregnancy? □ Yes □ No □ Don't know
If yes, describe the circumstances: _____
_____

Was the mother exposed to infectious diseases or toxins during pregnancy? □ Yes □ No □ Don't know
If yes, please describe and if there were problems with the pregnancy as a result. _____
_____

What type of delivery was it? □ Normal □ Induced □ Caesarean □ Don't know
If the delivery was induced or Caesarean, what was the reason? _____
_____
_____

Were there problems with the delivery, e.g., breech birth, umbilical cord around the neck, etc. □ Yes
□ No □ Don't know *If yes, please describe:* _____
_____
_____

Was the child premature? □ Yes □ No □ Don't know *If yes, how many weeks?*_____

Were there any problems right after birth, e.g., stopped breathing, fevers, seizures? □ Yes □ No □
Don't know *If yes, please describe:*_____
_____
_____

Did the child receive neonatal care? □ Yes □ No □ Don't know *If yes, what kind of care was given
and how long did it last?*_____
_____
_____

Child's birth weight: _____ lb. _____ oz. Length: _____ inches □ Don't know

Were any birth defects present? □ Yes □ No □ Don't know *If yes, please describe.* _____
_____
_____

DEVELOPMENTAL MILESTONES:

At what age did the child first show the following (put "U" if unknown or "N" if not yet shown):

Behavior	Age	Behavior	Age	Behavior	Age
Cognitive		**Fine Motor**		**Gross Motor**	
Knew basic colors	____	Used scissors well	____	Sat unsupported	____
Could count to 10	____	Fastened buttons	____	First rolled over	____
Knew basic shapes	____	Color w/in lines	____	First crawled	____
Knew body parts	____	Used pencil well	____	Pulled up to stand	____
Wrote first letters	____	Tied shoelaces	____	First stood alone	____
Read first words	____	Stacked 3 small blocks	____	Walked alone	____
Language		**Self-Help/Adaptive**		**Social**	
First babbled	____	When toilet trained	____	Fear of strangers	____
First used single words	____	Fed self	____	Separation anxiety	____
First said 2-3 word sentences	____	Drank from cup by self	____	Shared well	____
First Multi-word sentences	____	Undressed self	____	Played well w/	
Asked questions	____	Dressed self	____	others	____
Point to desired objects	____	Stayed dry at night	____	Stayed overnight	
Understood directions	____	Slept alone	____	at friend's house	____

INFANCY AND PRESCHOOL BEHAVIOR:

Feeding problems: □ Yes □ No □ Don't know *If yes, please describe.*_____
_____

Difficult to soothe: □ Yes □ No □ Don't know *If yes, please describe.*_____
_____

Temper tantrums: □ Yes □ No □ Don't know *If yes, please describe.* _____
_____

Liked to be held: □ Yes □ No □ Don't know *If no, please describe.*_____
_____

Excessive fears: □ Yes □ No □ Don't know *If yes, please describe.* _____
_____

Played well with others: □ Yes □ No □ Don't know *If no, please describe.* _____
_____

Sleep problems: □ Yes □ No □ Don't know *If yes, please describe.* _____
_____

Appetite problems: □ Yes □ No □ Don't know *If yes, please describe.* _____
_____

Self-injurious behavior (e. g., head banging, biting self) □ Yes □ No □ Don't know *If yes, please describe.* _____
_____

Delayed use of spoken language: □ Yes □ No □ Don't know *If yes, please describe.* _____
_____

Interested in other children: □ Yes □ No □ Don't know *If no, please describe.* _____
_____

Interested in objects, toys, etc. □ Yes □ No □ Don't know *If no, please describe.* _____
_____

CHILD'S MEDICAL HISTORY

Please check if the child has had any of the following and, if so, the approximate age, if known.

Illness/Problem	Age	Illness/Problem	Age	Illness/Problem	Age
□ Measles	___	□ Convulsions	___	□ Anemia	___
□ Mumps	___	□ Vision problems	___	□ Bleeding	___
□ Chicken Pox	___	□ Hearing problems	___	□ Fevers	___
□ Jaundice	___	□ Diabetes	___	□ Headaches	___
□ Hepatitis	___	□ Asthma	___	□ Gross Motor	___
□ Ear infections	___	□ Meningitis	___	□ Fine Motor	___
□ Head injury	___	□ Encephalitis	___	□ Seizures	___
□ Broken bone	___	□ Whooping cough	___	□ Epilepsy	___
□ Fainting	___	□ Allergies	___	□ Other	___

For items printed in italics, *please elaborate and describe if there were or currently are problems associated with them and what treatment was or is being provided, such as medications or therapy. Feel free to elaborate on any item and please explain if you checked "Other." _____*

_____
_____
_____
_____
_____
_____
_____
_____
_____

Has the child had any serious illnesses? □ Yes □ No □ Don't know *If yes, please describe.* _____
_____

Has the child had any operations? □ Yes □ No □ Don't know *If yes, please describe.* _____
_____

Has the child been hospitalized?   □ Yes □ No □ Don't know *If yes, please describe.*_____
_____

Has the child had any accidents? □ Yes □ No □ Don't know *If yes, please describe.* _____
_____

Is the child taking prescribed medications? □ Yes □ No □ Don't know *If yes, please list the medications, their purpose, and dosage.* _____
_____

EDUCATIONAL HISTORY

How well does your child do in the following school subjects?

Reading	□ Above Average	□ Average	□ Below Average	□ N/A
Math	□ Above Average	□ Average	□ Below Average	□ N/A
Writing	□ Above Average	□ Average	□ Below Average	□ N/A
English	□ Above Average	□ Average	□ Below Average	□ N/A
Science	□ Above Average	□ Average	□ Below Average	□ N/A

How hard does the child work in school?   □ Above Average □ Average □ Below Average □N/A
How easy is learning for the child?   □ Above Average □ Average □ Below Average □N/A

Has the child been retained in school? □ Yes □ No □ Don't know *If yes, what grade(s)?* _____
_____

What were the reasons for the retention(s)? _____
_____

Has the child received special education services? □ Yes □ No □ Don't know *If yes, in what grade(s)?* _____

If yes, what were the major problems? _____

Type of special education services:

- □ Autism Spectrum Disorder
- □ Emotional/Behavioral Disability
- □ Orthopedic Impairment
- □ Traumatic Brain Injury

- □ Cognitive/Intellectual Disability
- □ Hearing Impairment
- □ Other Health Impairment
- □ Vision Impairment

- □ Developmental Delay
- □ Learning Disability
- □ Speech/Language
- □ Other _____

FAMILY MEDICAL AND PSYCHOLOGICAL HISTORY

History of Natural Mother's Family:

If known, please check whether any of the following occurred in relatives of the natural mother's family, beginning with the natural mother and through grandparents and great grandparents.

	Relationship		*Relationship*
□ Alcoholism	_____	□ Hyperactivity	_____
□ Anxiety	_____	□ Learning Disorder	_____
□ Attention Deficit	_____	□ Manic Depression	_____
□ Autism	_____	□ Mental Retardation	_____
□ Bipolar Disorder	_____	□ Neurological D/O	_____
□ Conduct Disorder	_____	□ Schizophrenia	_____
□ Depression	_____	□ Seizure Disorder	_____
□ Develop. Delay	_____	□ Sleep Disorder	_____
□ Drug Abuse	_____	□ Suicide	_____
□ Eating Disorder	_____	□ Tic Disorder	_____
□ Epilepsy	_____	□ Tourette's Disorder	_____
□ Genetic Disorder	_____	□ Other _____	_____
□ Head Injury	_____	□ Other _____	_____

History of Natural Father's Family:

If known, please check whether any of the following occurred in relatives of the natural father's family, beginning with the natural father and through grandparents and great grandparents.

	Relationship		*Relationship*
□ Alcoholism	_____	□ Hyperactivity	_____
□ Anxiety	_____	□ Learning Disorder	_____
□ Attention Deficit	_____	□ Manic Depression	_____
□ Autism	_____	□ Mental Retardation	_____
□ Bipolar Disorder	_____	□ Neurological D/O	_____
□ Conduct Disorder	_____	□ Schizophrenia	_____
□ Depression	_____	□ Seizure Disorder	_____
□ Develop. Delay	_____	□ Sleep Disorder	_____
□ Drug Abuse	_____	□ Suicide	_____
□ Eating Disorder	_____	□ Tic Disorder	_____
□ Epilepsy	_____	□ Tourette's Disorder	_____
□ Genetic Disorder	_____	□ Other _____	_____

☐ Head Injury _____   ☐   Other _____   _____

CURRENT OR RECENT STRESSORS

Please check all stressors that are current or have occurred within the last 12 months.

☐ Abuse of child	☐ Death of grandfather	☐ Parent separated
☐ Assault on child	☐ Death of family pet	☐ Parent remarried
☐ Bullying of child	☐ Family moved	☐ Parent injured or ill
☐ Child changed schools	☐ Financial stress	☐ Parent lost job
☐ Death of mother	☐ Health problems	☐ Parent emotional problems
☐ Death of father	☐ Natural disaster	☐ School problems
☐ Death of sibling	☐ Parents divorced	☐ Other _____
☐ Death of grandmother	☐ Parent incarcerated	☐ Other _____

Please describe those stressors that you feel are or have been significantly related to your concerns.

_____
_____
_____
_____

BEHAVIOR MANAGEMENT TECHNIQUES

If appropriate, each parent is asked to report the behavior management techniques that she or he applies without discussing it with the other person, so that we can get an accurate perspective on child management. Please indicate how often you use the specific technique and if it works reasonably well.

Who is the primary disciplinarian? ☐ Mother/Stepmother   ☐ Father/Stepfather   ☐ Both equally

Mother/Stepmother:

				Effective?	
☐ Ignore the behavior	☐ Usually	☐ Sometimes	☐ Rarely/never	☐ Yes	☐ No
☐ Yell at her/him	☐ Usually	☐ Sometimes	☐ Rarely/never	☐ Yes	☐ No
☐ Spank her/him	☐ Usually	☐ Sometimes	☐ Rarely/never	☐ Yes	☐ No
☐ Send to room/isolate	☐ Usually	☐ Sometimes	☐ Rarely/never	☐ Yes	☐ No
☐ Reason with her/him	☐ Usually	☐ Sometimes	☐ Rarely/never	☐ Yes	☐ No
☐ Threaten w/ consequences	☐ Usually	☐ Sometimes	☐ Rarely/never	☐ Yes	☐ No
☐ Loss of privileges	☐ Usually	☐ Sometimes	☐ Rarely/never	☐ Yes	☐ No
☐ Redirect her/him	☐ Usually	☐ Sometimes	☐ Rarely/never	☐ Yes	☐ No
☐ Distract her/him	☐ Usually	☐ Sometimes	☐ Rarely/never	☐ Yes	☐ No
☐ Other _____	☐ Usually	☐ Sometimes	☐ Rarely/never	☐ Yes	☐ No
☐ Other _____	☐ Usually	☐ Sometimes	☐ Rarely/never	☐ Yes	☐ No

Please feel free to explain or elaborate. _____

_____

_____

Father/Stepfather:

				Effective?	
□ Ignore the behavior	□ Usually	□ Sometimes	□ Rarely/never	□ Yes	□ No
□ Yell at her/him	□ Usually	□ Sometimes	□ Rarely/never	□ Yes	□ No
□ Spank her/him	□ Usually	□ Sometimes	□ Rarely/never	□ Yes	□ No
□ Send to room/isolate	□ Usually	□ Sometimes	□ Rarely/never	□ Yes	□ No
□ Reason with her/him	□ Usually	□ Sometimes	□ Rarely/never	□ Yes	□ No
□ Threaten w/ consequences	□ Usually	□ Sometimes	□ Rarely/never	□ Yes	□ No
□ Loss of privileges	□ Usually	□ Sometimes	□ Rarely/never	□ Yes	□ No
□ Redirect her/him	□ Usually	□ Sometimes	□ Rarely/never	□ Yes	□ No
□ Distract her/him	□ Usually	□ Sometimes	□ Rarely/never	□ Yes	□ No
□ Other _____	□ Usually	□ Sometimes	□ Rarely/never	□ Yes	□ No
□ Other _____	□ Usually	□ Sometimes	□ Rarely/never	□ Yes	□ No

Please feel free to explain or elaborate. _____

_____

_____

CHILD'S ACTIVITIES AND RESPONSIBILITIES

□ Has hobbies	□ Is a member of a social or interest group
□ Plays organized sports	□ Dresses self and manages own clothing
□ Take care of own hygiene needs	□ Takes responsibility for homework
□ Has assigned chores	□ Completes tasks and chores in a timely manner
□ Plays a musical instrument	□ Other _____
□ Other_____	□ Other _____

Please elaborate on any of these items to give us an idea of interests, preferences, and responsibilities.

_____

_____

_____

_____

List some activities that you do as a family:

_____

_____

_____

_____

_____

ADDITIONAL COMMENTS THAT YOU FEEL ARE HELPFUL FOR US TO KNOW.

Thank you for taking the time to complete this form. The information is important to us as we work with you and your child.

CLINICIAN NOTES:

Appendix B: Mental Status Examination Form

Name:_____ DOB:_____ Date:_____

1. Appearance	□ Dress: □ Appropriate □ Disheveled □ Soiled/Torn * □ Hygiene: □ Good □ Fair □ Poor * □ Grooming: □ Good □ Fair □ Poor * □ Other (describe):_____ *
2. Attitude	□ Cooperative/Compliant □ Uncooperative/Noncompliant □ Calm □ Agitated/Hostile □ Other (describe):_____
3. Behavior	□ Psychomotor: □ Agitated □ Normal □ Slowed/sluggish □ Distractibility: □ High □ Moderate □ Mild □ Normal □ Other (describe):_____
4. Speech	□ Rate: □ Rapid □ Normal □ Slow □ Tone: □ Excessive/variable □ Normal □ Flat/Monotone □ Volume: □ Loud □ Normal □ Low □ Pressure: □ High □ Moderate □ Mild □ Normal □ Other (describe):_____
5. Affect	□ Reactivity: □ Over-reactive □ Normal □ Under-reactive □ Congruence: □ Congruent □ Non-congruent □ Lability: □ High □ Moderate □ Mild □ Normal □ Range: □ Variable □ Normal □ Flat □ Quality: □ Tearful □ Blunted □ Constricted □ Other (describe):_____
6. Mood	□ Manic □ Hypomanic □ Euthymic □ Dysthymic □ Depressed □ Elevation: □ High □ Moderate □ Mild □ Normal □ Anxious: □ High □ Moderate □ Mild □ Normal □ Irritability: □ High □ Moderate □ Mild □ Normal □ Other (describe):_____
7. Thought Processes	□ Organization: □ Good □ Fair □ Poor □ Goal directed: □ Good □ Fair □ Poor □ Tangential: □ Normal □ Impaired _____ □ Amount: □ Normal □ Impaired _____ □ Capacity/IQ: □ Above Average □ Average □ Below Average □ General Information: □ Calculation □ Abstraction □ Comprehension □ Other (describe):_____

8. Thought Content	□ Suicidal ideation: □ Yes □ No
	If yes: □ Active □ Passive
	If active, evaluate for presence of: □ Plan: □ Yes □ No
	                                                          □ Intent: □ Yes □ No
	                                                          □ Means: □ Yes □ No

	□ Homicidal ideation: □ Yes □ No
	If yes: □ **Active** □ **Passive**
	If active, evaluate for presence of: □ Plan: □ Yes □ No
	                                       □ Intent: □ Yes □ No
	                                       □ Means: □ Yes □ No
	                                       □ Target: □ Yes □ No
	If target person(s) identified, specify:_____
	□ Delusions present: □ Yes □ No
	If yes, describe:_____
	_____
	□ Obsessions/compulsions present: □ Yes □ No
	If yes, describe:_____
	_____
	□ Phobias present: □ Yes □ No
	If yes, describe:_____
	_____
	□ Other (describe):_____

9. Perception/Sensation	□ Hallucinations present: □ Yes □ No If yes, specify: □ Auditory □ Visual □ Kinesthetic □ Olfactory □ Gustatory Describe:_____ □ Other (describe):_____
10. Orientation	□ Orientation x 3: □ Time □ Place □ Person If impaired, describe:_____ □ Other (describe):_____
11. Memory/Concentration	□ Short-term memory: □ Good □ Fair □ Poor □ Long-term memory: □ Good □ Fair □ Poor □ Concentration: □ Good □ Fair □ Poor □ Attention span: □ Good □ Fair □ Poor □ Other (describe):_____
12. Insight/Judgment	□ Level: □ Good □ Fair □ Poor □ Other (describe):_____

* If present in children and youth, evaluate for quality of adult caregiving and supervision.

Notes:

Clinician's Signature:_____

Appendix C: Cognitive–Behavioral Therapy Case Conceptualization Worksheet for Children and Adolescents

Name:_____ Age:_____ Date:_____
Male:___ Female:___ Parents' Names:_____
Reason for Referral:_____
_____

Specific problems identified (add as necessary):

1. _____

   Behavioral antecedents: _____
   _____

   Behavioral consequences: _____
   _____

2. _____

   Behavioral antecedents: _____
   _____

   Behavioral consequences: _____
   _____

3. _____

   Behavioral antecedents: _____
   _____

   Behavioral consequences: _____
   _____

4. _____

   Behavioral antecedents: _____
   _____

   Behavioral consequences: _____
   _____

5. _____

   Behavioral antecedents: _____
   _____

   Behavioral consequences: _____
   _____

Protective factors: _____
_____
_____

Risk factors: _____
_____
_____

Assessment Results: _____
_____
_____
_____

Contributory or maintaining stimuli or circumstances: _____
_____
_____

Historical considerations: _____
_____
_____

Developmental considerations: _____
_____
_____

Genetic/biological considerations: _____
_____
_____

Cultural considerations: _____
_____
_____

Family considerations: _____
_____
_____

Social/environmental considerations: _____
_____
_____

School/academic considerations: _____
_____
_____

Assessment of family, social, and school resources: _____

_____

_____

_____

Provisional case conceptualization: _____

_____

_____

_____

_____

_____

_____

_____

Treatment plan: _____

_____

_____

_____

_____

_____

_____

_____

Treatment goals (add as necessary):
Cognitive

1. _____
2. _____
3. _____
4. _____
5. _____

Behavioral

1. _____
2. _____
3. _____
4. _____
5. _____

Affective

1. _____
2. _____
3. _____
4. _____
5. _____

Factors that may facilitate treatment: _____
_____
_____
_____

Factors that may impede treatment: _____
_____
_____
_____

Tentative treatment timeline: _____
_____

Methods to evaluate effectiveness: _____
_____
_____
_____

Criteria to determine effectiveness: _____
_____
_____
_____

Comments/Notes: _____
_____
_____
_____
_____
_____

Appendix D: Common Medications Used to Treat Anxiety Disorders

Group	Generic name	Trade name	Common side effects	Disorder treated
Selective serotonin reuptake inhibitors (SSRIs)	Fluoxetine Citalopram Sertraline Paroxetine Escitalopram	Prozac® Celexa® Zoloft® Paxil® Lexapro®	Headaches, nausea, agitation, sleeplessness, drowsiness, sexual problems (SSRIs are often preferred due to generally mild side effects that dissipate rather quickly)	Panic disorder, OCD, PTSD, social phobia
Serotonin and norepinephrine reuptake inhibitors (SNRIs)	Venlafaxine	Effexor®	Similar to SSRIs	GAD
Dopamine agents	Buproprion	Wellbutrin®	Appetite changes, nervousness, weight loss, constipation, headache, nausea, sleeping problems, dizziness, drowsiness, dry mouth	GAD
Tricyclics (TCAs)	Amytriptaline Clomipramine Imipramine Protriptaline Desipramine	Elavil® Anafranil® Tofranil® Vivactil® Norpramin®	Dry mouth, constipation, drowsiness (some TCAs may be prescribed for insomnia), dizziness, increased appetite, weight gain (perhaps significant), blurry vision, changes in sexual function	Panic disorder, GAD, OCD
Anti-anxiety medications (benzodiazepines)	Lorazepam Alprazolam Diazepam	Ativan® Xanax® Valium®	Drowsiness, dizziness, upset stomach, blurred vision, headache, confusion, grogginess, nightmares	Panic disorder Panic disorder, GAD GAD
Anti-anxiety medications (piperazine and azapirone classes)	Buspirone	Buspar®	Dizziness, headaches, nausea, nervousness, lightheadedness, excitement, trouble sleeping	GAD
Anticonvulsants	Klonazepam	Klonopin®	Drowsiness, fatigue, sedation, anorexia, irritability, confusion, headache, nausea, lethargy	Social phobia, GAD

(continued)

Group	Generic name	Trade name	Common side effects	Disorder treated
Monoamine oxidase inhibitors (MAOIs)	Phenalzine Tranylcypromine Isocarboxazid	Nardil® Parnate® Marplan®	Drowsiness, constipation, nausea, diarrhea, stomach upset, fatigue, dry mouth, dizziness, low blood pressure, lightheadedness, low urine output, decreased sexual function, sleep disturbances, muscle twitching, weight gain, blurred vision, headache, increased appetite, restlessness, shakiness, trembling, weakness, increased sweating; can have negative interactions with certain foods that contain high levels of tyramine, e.g., wines, cheeses, pickled foods, and chocolate*	Antidepressants also used to treat anxiety symptoms
Beta blockers	Propranolol	Inderal®	Fatigue, cold hands, dizziness, weakness; contraindicated in persons with asthma or diabetes	Helps control physical symptoms of anxiety, e.g., trembling, sweating

Source: http://www.nimh.nih.gov/health/publications/mental-health-medications/complete-index.shtml#pub5 (except as noted below). In the public domain
**Source*: http://www.mayoclinic.com/health/maois/MH00072
Note. Many side effects of some these medications dissipate within a few days after beginning the regimen. Medications may be combined with anti-depressants and other medications to treat anxiety symptoms

Appendix E: Mood Monitoring Form

Mood	Day/Time	What I Was Doing	How I Felt*	What I Did	How It Worked**

*Rate on a scale of 1–10 of the intensity of the mood, with "1"="Low Intensity" to "10"="High Intensity"

**Rate on a scale of 1–10 in how well what I did worked to cope with the intensity of the mood, with "1"="Did not Work" to "10"="Worked Extremely Well"

Appendix F: Common Medications Used to Treat Mood Disorders

Group	Generic name	Trade name	Common side effects	Disorder treated
Selective serotonin reuptake inhibitors (SSRIs)	Fluoxetine Citalopram Sertraline Paroxetine Escitalopram Fluvoxamine	Prozac® Celexa® Zoloft® Paxil® Lexapro® Luvox®	Headaches, nausea, agitation, sleeplessness, drowsiness, sexual problems (SSRIs are often preferred due to generally mild side effects that dissipate rather quickly)	Unipolar depression/ major depressive disorder
Serotonin and norepineph-rine reuptake inhibitors (SNRIs)	Venlafaxine Duloxetine	Effexor® Cymbalta®	Similar to SSRIs	Unipolar depression/ major depressive disorder
Dopamine agents	Buproprion	Wellbutrin®	Appetite changes, nervousness, weight loss, constipation, headache, nausea, sleeping problems, dizziness, drowsiness, dry mouth	Unipolar depression/ major depressive disorder
Tricyclics (TCAs)	Amytriptaline Clomipramine Imipramine Protriptaline Desipramine	Elavil® Anafranil® Tofranil® Vivactil® Norpramin®	Dry mouth, constipation, drowsiness (some TCAs may be prescribed for insomnia), dizziness, increased appetite, weight gain (perhaps significant), blurry vision, changes in sexual function	Unipolar depression/ major depressive disorder
Monoamine oxidase inhibitors (MAOIs)	Phenalzine Tranylcy promine Isocarboxazid	Nardil® Parnate® Marplan	Drowsiness, constipation, nausea, diarrhea, stomach upset, fatigue, dry mouth, dizziness, low blood pressure, lightheadedness, low urine output, decreased sexual function, sleep disturbances, muscle twitching, weight gain, blurred vision, headache, increased appetite, restlessness, shakiness, trembling, weakness, increased sweating; can have negative interactions with certain foods that contain high levels of tyramine, e.g., wines, cheeses, pickled foods, and chocolate*	Unipolar depression/ major depressive disorder

(continued)

Group	Generic name	Trade name	Common side effects	Disorder treated
Mood stabilizers	Lithium	Lithobid®	Loss of coordination, excessive thirst, frequent urination, blackouts, seizures, slurred speech, heart reactions (rapid, slow, or irregular rate or pounding), hallucinations, vision changes, itching, rash, swelling of the eyes, face, lips, tongue, throat, hands, feet, ankles, or lower legs	Bipolar disorder
Anticonvulsants (used as mood stabilizers)	Valproic acid Carbamapezine Lamotrigine Oxcarbazepine	Depakote® Tegretol® Lamictal® Trileptal®	Drowsiness, fatigue, sedation, anorexia, irritability, confusion, headache, nausea, lethargy	Bipolar disorder
Antipsychotics (used as mood stabilizers)	Olanzapine Aripripazole Risperidone Ziprasidone Clozapine Quetiapine	Zyprexa® Abilify® Risperdal® Geodon® Clorazil® Seroquel®	Drowsiness, dizziness when changing positions, blurred vision, rapid heart rate, sunlight sensitivity, skin rashes, menstrual problems in women, rigidity, tremors, restlessness; long-term use can lead to tardive dyskinesia	Bipolar disorder

Source: http://www.nimh.nih.gov/health/publications/mental-health-medications/complete-index. shtml#pub5 (except as noted below). In the public domain
*Source: http://www.mayoclinic.com/health/maois/MH00072
Note. Many side effects of some these medications dissipate within a few days after beginning the regimen. Medications may be combined with anti-anxiety and other medications to treat depressive symptoms

References

A. E. v. Westport Board of Educ., No. 3:05cv705 (SRU), 2006 WL 3455096 (D. Conn. 11/19/06).

A. J. v. East Islip Union Free School District, 53 IDELR (E.D.N.Y. 2010).

Abe, J. A., & Izard, C. E. (1999). The developmental function of emotions: An analysis in terms of differential emotions theory. *Cognition and Emotion, 13*, 523–549.

Abela, J. R. Z., & Taylor, G. (2003). Specific vulnerability to depressive mood reactions in school-children: The moderating role of self-esteem. *Journal of Clinical Child and Adolescent Psychology, 32*, 408–418.

Abela, J. R. Z., Zinck, S., Kryger, S., Zilber, I., & Hankin, B. L. (2009). Contagious depression: Negative attachment cognitions as a moderator of the temporal association between parental depression and child depression. *Journal of Clinical Child and Adolescent Psychology, 38*, 16–26.

Abela, J. R. A., Zuroff, D. C., Ho, R., Adams, P., & Hankin, B. I. (2006). Excessive reassurance seeking, hassles, and depressive symptoms in children of affectively-ill parents: A multi-wave longitudinal study. *Journal of Abnormal Child Psychology, 34*, 171–187.

Abramson, L. Y., Seligman, M. E. P., & Teasdale, J. D. (1978). Learned helpless in humans: Critique and reformulation. *Journal of Abnormal Psychology, 87*, 49–74.

Achenbach, T. (1982). *Developmental psychopathology* (2nd ed.). New York: Wiley.

Achenbach, T. (1991). *Manual for the child behavior checklist and 1991 child behavior profile.* Burlington, VT: University of Vermont, Department of Psychiatry.

Achenbach, T. (1993). *Empirically based taxonomy: How to use syndromes and profile types derived from the CBCL/4-16, TRF, and YSR.* Burlington, VT: University of Vermont, Department of Psychiatry.

Achenbach, T. M., Howell, C. T., McConaughey, S. H., & Stanger, C. (1995). Six-year predictors of problems in a national sample of children and youth: I. Cross-informant syndromes. *Journal of the American Academy of Child and Adolescent Psychiatry, 34*, 335–347.

Achenbach, T. M., McConaughey, S. H., & Howell, C. T. (1987). Child/adolescent behavioral and emotional problems: Implications of cross-informant correlations for situational specificity. *Psychological Bulletin, 101*, 213–232.

Achenbach, T., & Rescorla, I. A. (2001). *Manual for the ASEBA school-age forms and profiles.* Burlington, VT: University of Vermont, Research Center for Children, Youth, & Families.

Adelman, H. S., & Taylor, L. (2010). *Mental health in schools: Engaging learners, preventing problems, and improving schools.* Thousand Oaks, CA: Corwin Press.

Albano, A. M., Causey, D., & Carter, B. (2001). Fear and anxiety in children. In C. E. Walker & M. C. Roberts (Eds.), *Handbook of clinical child psychology* (3rd ed., pp. 291–316). New York: Wiley.

American Psychiatric Association. (1952). *Diagnostic and statistical manual of mental disorders.* Washington, DC: Author.

T.J. Huberty, *Anxiety and Depression in Children and Adolescents: Assessment, Intervention, and Prevention*, DOI 10.1007/978-1-4614-3110-7,
© Springer Science+Business Media, LLC 2012

American Psychiatric Association. (1968). *Diagnostic and statistical manual of mental disorders-* (2nd ed.). Washington, DC: Author.

American Psychiatric Association. (1980). *Diagnostic and statistical manual of mental disorders-* (3rd ed.). Washington, DC: Author.

American Psychiatric Association. (1987). *Diagnostic and statistical manual of mental disorders-* (3rd ed., rev.). Washington, DC: Author.

American Psychiatric Association. (1994). *Diagnostic and statistical manual of mental disorders-* (4th ed.). Washington, DC: Author.

American Psychiatric Association. (2000). *Diagnostic and statistical manual of mental disorders-* (4th ed., text rev.). Washington, DC: Author.

Angold, A., Costello, E. J., & Erkanli, A. (1999a). Comorbidity. *Journal of Child Psychology and Psychiatry and Allied Disciplines, 40*, 57–87.

Angold, A., Costello, E. J., Erkanli, A., & Worthman, C. M. (1999b). Pubertal changes in hormones of adolescent girls. *Psychological Medicine, 29*, 1043–1053.

Angold, A., Costello, E. J., & Worthman, C. M. (1998). Puberty and depression: The roles of age, pubertal status, and pubertal timing. *Psychological Medicine, 28*, 51–61.

Arsenio, W. F., & Lemerise, E. A. (2004). Aggression and moral development: Integrating social information processing and moral domain models. *Child Development, 75*, 897–1002.

Assistance to states for the education of children with disabilities and preschool grants for children with disabilities: Final rule. 34 C.F.R. § 300 *et. seq.*

Avenevoli, S., Stolar, J., Li, J., Dierker, L., & Merikangas, K. R. (2001). Comorbidity of depression in children and adolescents: Models and evidence from a prospective high-risk family study. *Biological Psychiatry, 49*, 1071–1081.

Baer, L. (1994). Factor analysis of symptom subtypes of obsessive compulsive disorder and their relation to personality and tic disorders. *Journal of Clinical Psychiatry, 55*, 18–23.

Ballenger, J. C., Carek, D. J., Steele, J. J., & Cornish-McTighe, D. (1989). Three cases of panic disorder with agoraphobia. *American Journal of Psychiatry, 146*, 922–924.

Barkley, R. A. (2004). Attention-deficit hyperactivity disorder and self-regulation: Taking an evolutionary perspective on executive functioning. In E. J. Mash & R. A. Barkley (Eds.), *Child psychopathology* (2nd ed., pp. 75–143). New York: Guilford.

Barlow, D. H. (1988). *Anxiety and its disorders: The nature and treatment of anxiety and panic.* New York: Guilford.

Barlow, D. H. (2002). *Anxiety and its disorders: The nature and treatment of anxiety and panic* (2nd ed.). New York: Guilford.

Barlow, D. H., Gorman, J. M., Shear, M. K., & Woods, S. W. (2000). Cognitive-behavioral therapy, imipramine, or their combination: A randomized controlled trial. *Journal of the American Medical Association, 283*, 2529–2536.

Barlow, D. H., & Seidner, A. L. (1983). Treatment of adolescent agoraphobics: Effects on parent-adolescent relations. *Behaviour Research and Therapy, 21*, 519–526.

Barnish, A. J., & Kendall, P. C. (2005). Should parents be co-clients for cognitive-behavioral therapy for anxious youth? *Journal of Clinical Child and Adolescent Psychology, 34*, 569–581.

Barrett, P. M., Lowry-Webster, H., & Turner, C. (2000a). *FRIENDS program for children: Parents' supplement.* Brisbane: Australian Academic Press.

Barrett, P. M., Lowry-Webster, H., & Turner, C. (2000b). *FRIENDS program for children: Group leaders manual.* Brisbane: Australian Academic Press.

Barrett, P. M., Lowry-Webster, H., & Turner, C. (2000c). *FRIENDS program for children: Participants workbook.* Brisbane: Australian Academic Press.

Barrett, P. M., Lowry-Webster, H., & Turner, C. (2000d). *FRIENDS program for youth: Group leaders manual.* Brisbane: Australian Academic Press.

Barrett, P. M., Lowry-Webster, H., & Turner, C. (2000e). *FRIENDS program for youth: Parents' supplement.* Brisbane: Australian Academic Press.

Barrett, P. M., Lowry-Webster, H., & Turner, C. (2000f). *FRIENDS program for youth: Participants workbook.* Brisbane: Australian Academic Press.

Barrett, P. M., Rapee, R. M., Dadds, M. R., & Ryan, S. M. (1996). Family enhancement of cognitive style in anxious and aggressive children: Threat bias and the fear effect. *Journal of Abnormal Child Psychology, 24*, 187–203.

Barrett, P. M., Sonderegger, R., & Sonderegger, N. L. (2001). Evaluation of an anxiety-prevention and positive-coping program (FRIENDS) for children and adolescents of non-English-speaking background. *Behaviour Change, 18*, 78–91.

Barrett, P. M., & Turner, C. M. (2001). Prevention of anxiety symptoms in primary school children: Preliminary results from a universal trial. *British Journal of Clinical Psychology, 40*, 399–410.

Baumrind, D. (1991). Parenting styles and adolescent development. In R. M. Lerner, A. C. Peterson, & J. Brooks-Gunn (Eds.), *Encyclopedia of adolescence* (Vol. 11, pp. 746–758). New York: Guilford.

Beardslee, W. R., Versage, E. M., & Gladstone, T. R. G. (1998). Children of affectively ill parents: A review of the last 10 years. *Journal of the American Academy of Child and Adolescent Psychiatry, 37*, 1134–1141.

Beck, A. T. (1967). *Depression: Clinical, experimental, and theoretical aspects*. New York: Hoeber.

Beck, A. T. (1976). *Cognitive therapy and the emotional disorders*. New York: International Universities Press.

Beck, A. T. (1987). Cognitive models of depression. *Journal of Cognitive Psychotherapy, 1*, 5–37.

Beck, A. T. (1993). *Beck hopelessness scale*. New York: Harcourt.

Beck, J. S., Beck, A. T., & Jolly, J. B. (2005). *Beck youth inventories* (2nd ed.). Bloomington, MN: Pearson Assessments.

Beck, A. T., Rush, A. J., Shaw, B. F., & Emery, C. (1979). *Cognitive therapy of depression*. New York: Guilford.

Beck, A. T., Steer, R. A., & Brown, G. K. (1996). *Beck depression inventory-II (BDI-II)*. New York: Harcourt Brace.

Beck, A. T., Ward, C. H., Mendelson, M., Mock, J., & Erbaugh, J. (1961). An inventory for measuring depression. *Archives of General Psychiatry, 4*, 561–571.

Beevers, C. G., Rohde, P., Stice, E., & Nolen-Hoeksema, S. (2007). Recovery from major depressive disorder among female adolescents: A prospective test of the scar hypothesis. *Journal of Consulting and Clinical Psychology, 75*, 888–900.

Beidel, D. (1988). Psychophysiological assessment of anxious emotional states in children. *Journal of Abnormal Psychology, 97*, 80–82.

Beidel, D. C., Turner, S. M., & Fink, C. M. (1996). Assessment of childhood social phobia: Construct, convergent, and discriminative validity of the social phobia and anxiety inventory for children (SPAI-C). *Psychological Assessment, 8*, 235–240.

Beidel, D. C., Turner, S. M., & Morris, T. L. (1999). Psychopathology of social phobia. *Journal of the American Academy of Child and Adolescent Psychiatry, 26*, 643–650.

Bellodi, L., Sciuto, G., Diaferia, G., Ronchi, P., & Smeraldi, E. (1992). Psychiatric disorders in the families of patients with obsessive compulsive disorder. *Psychiatry Research, 32*, 814–834.

Berg, C. J., Rapoport, J. L., & Flament, M. (1986). The Leyton obsessional inventory-child version. *Journal of the American Academy of Child and Adolescent Psychiatry, 25*, 85–91.

Berg, C. J., Whitaker, A., Davies, M., Flament, M. F., & Rapoport, J. L. (1988). The survey form of the Leyton obsessional inventory-child version: Norms from an epidemiological study. *Journal of the American Academy of Child and Adolescent Psychiatry, 27*, 759–763.

Berndt, D. J., & Kaiser, C. F. (1996). *Multiscore depression inventory for children*. Los Angeles, CA: Western Psychological Services.

Bernstein, G. A., Borchardt, C. M., Perwien, A. R., Crosby, R. D., Kushner, M. G., Thuras, P. D., et al. (2000). Imipramine plus cognitive-behavioral therapy in the treatment of school refusal. *Journal of the American Academy of Child and Adolescent Psychiatry, 39*, 276–283.

Biederman, J. (1998). Resolved: Mania is mistaken for ADHD in prepubertal children. *Journal of the American Academy of Child and Adolescent Psychiatry, 37*, 1091–1093.

Biederman, J., Faraone, S. V., Hirshfeld-Becker, D. R., Friedman, D., Robin, J. A., & Rosenbaum, J. F. (2001). Patterns of psychopathology and dysfunction in high-risk children of parents with panic disorder and major depression. *American Journal of Psychiatry, 158,* 49–57.

Biederman, J., Faraone, S. V., Mick, E., Wozniak, J., Chen, L., Ouelette, C., et al. (1996). Attention-deficit hyperactivity disorder and juvenile mania: An overlooked comorbidity? *Journal of the American Academy of Child and Adolescent Psychiatry, 35,* 997–1008.

Biederman, J., Hirshfeld-Becker, D. R., Rosenbaum, J. F., Herot, C., Friedman, D., Snidman, N., et al. (2001). Further evidence of association between behavioral inhibition and social anxiety in children. *American Journal of Psychiatry, 158,* 1673–1679.

Biederman, J., Newcorn, J., & Sprich, S. (1991). Comorbidity of attention deficit hyperactivity disorder with conduct, depressive, anxiety, and other disorders. *American Journal of Psychiatry, 148,* 565–577.

Biederman, J., Petty, C. R., Monuteaux, M. C., Evans, M., Parcell, T., Faraone, S. V., & Wozniak, J. (2009). The child behavior checklist-pediatric bipolar disorder profile predicts a subsequent diagnosis of bipolar disorder and associated impairments in ADHD youth growing up: A longitudinal analysis. *Journal of Clinical Psychiatry, 70,* 732–740.

Biederman, J., Rosenbaum, J. F., Chaloff, J., & Kagan, J. (1995). Behavioral inhibition as a risk factor for anxiety disorders. In J. S. March (Ed.), *Anxiety disorders in children and adolescents* (pp. 61–81). New York: Guilford.

Biederman, J., Rosenbaum, J. F., Hirshfeld, D. R., Faraone, S. V., Bolduc, E. A., Gersten, M., Meminger, S. R., Kagan, J., Snidman, N., & Reznick, J. S. (1990). Psychiatric correlates of behavioral inhibition in young children with and without psychiatric disorders. *Archives of General Psychiatry, 47,* 21–26.

Birmaher, B., Arbelaez, C., & Brent, D. (2002). Course and outcome of child and adolescent major depressive disorder. *Child and Adolescent Psychiatry Clinics of North America, 11,* 619–637.

Birmaher, B., & Ollendick, T. H. (2004). Childhood onset panic disorder. In T. H. Ollendick & J. S. March (Eds.), *Phobic and anxiety disorders in children and adolescents: A clinician's guide to effective psychosocial and pharmacological interventions* (pp. 306–333). New York: Oxford University Press.

Birmaher, B., Ryan, N. D., Williamson, D. E., Brent, D. A., Kaufman, J., Dahl, R. E., Perel, J., & Nelson, B. (1996). Childhood and adolescent depression: A review of the past 10 years. Part I. *Journal of the American Academy of Child and Adolescent Psychiatry, 35,* 1427–1439.

Birmaher, B., Waterman, G. S., Ryan, N., Cully, M., Balach, L., Ingram, J., et al. (1994). Fluoxetine for childhood anxiety disorders. *Journal of the American Academy of Child and Adolescent Psychiatry, 33,* 993–999.

Birmhaer, B., Khetarpal, S., Brent, D., Cully, M., Balach, L., Kaufman, J., & Neer, S. M. (1997). The screen for child anxiety related emotional disorders (SCARED): Scale construction and psychometric characteristics. *Journal of the American Academy of Child and Adolescent Psychiatry, 36,* 545–553.

Black, B., & Uhde, T. W. (1995). Psychiatric characteristics of children with selective mutism: A pilot study. *Journal of the American Academy of Child and Adolescent Psychiatry, 34,* 847–856.

Blair, C. (2002). School readiness: Integrating cognition and emotion in a neurobiological conceptualization of children's functioning at school entry. *American Psychologist, 53,* 111–127.

Blatt, S. J., & Homman, E. (1992). Parent-child interaction in the etiology of dependent and self-critical depression. *Clinical Psychology Review, 12,* 47–91.

Board of Educ. of Montgomery County, Maryland v. S. G., 230 Fed. Appx. 330 (4th Cir. 2007).

Board of Education v. Rowley, 458 U. S. 176 (1982).

Bolton, D., Eley, T. C., O'Connor, T. G., Perrin, S., Rabe-Hesketh, S., Rijsdijk, F., et al. (2006). Prevalence and genetic and environmental influences on anxiety disorders in 6-year-old twins. *Psychological Medicine, 36,* 335–344.

Borkovec, T. D., & Hu, S. (1990). The effect of worry on cardiovascular response. *Behaviour Research and Therapy, 28,* 69–73.

Borowsky, I. W., Ireland, M., & Resnick, M. D. (2001). Adolescent suicide attempts: Associations with psychological functioning. *Pediatrics, 107,* 485–493.

Bracken, B. (1992). *Multidimensional self-concept scale*. Austin, TX: PRO-ED.

Bradley, S. J., & Hood, J. (1993). Psychiatrically referred adolescents with panic attacks: Presenting symptoms, stressors, and comorbidity. *Journal of the American Academy of Child and Adolescent Psychiatry, 32*, 826–829.

Brendgen, M., Wanner, B., Morin, A. J. S., & Vitaro, F. (2005). Relations with parents and with peers, temperament, and trajectories of depressed mood during early adolescence. *Journal of Abnormal Child Psychology, 33*, 579–594.

Brent, D. A. (2006). Glad for what TADS adds, but many TADS grads still sad. *Journal of the American Academy of Child and Adolescent Psychiatry, 45*, 1461–1464.

Briere, J. N. (1996). *Trauma symptom checklist for children. Manual*. Odessa, FL: Psychological Assessment Resources.

Brown, T. A., DiNardo, P. A., Lehman, C. L., & Campbell, L. A. (2001). Reliability of DSM-IV anxiety and mood disorders: Implications for classification of emotional disorders. *Journal of Abnormal Psychology, 110*, 49–58.

Bruner, J. (1986). *Actual minds, possible worlds*. New York: Plenum Press.

Brunwasser, S. M., Gillham, J. E., & Kim, E. S. (2009). A meta-analytic review of the Penn Resiliency Program's effect on depressive symptoms. *Journal of Clinical and Consulting Psychology, 77*, 1042–1054.

Burge, D., Hammen, C., Davila, J., Daley, S. E., Paley, R., Lindberg, N., et al. (1997). The relationship between attachment cognitions and psychological adjustment in late adolescent women. *Development and Psychopathology, 9*, 151–167.

Burhans, K. K., & Dweck, C. S. (1995). Helplessness in early childhood: The role of contingent self-worth. *Child Development, 66*, 1719–1738.

Burke, K. C., Burke, J. D., Reger, D. A., & Rae, D. S. (1990). Age at onset of selected mental disorders in five community populations. *Archives of General Psychiatry, 47*, 511–518.

Butcher, J. N., Graham, J. R., Archer, R. P., Ben-Porath, Y. S., Tellegen, A., & Dahlstrom, W. G. (1992). *Minnesota multiphasic personality inventory—2*. Minneapolis, MN: University of Minnesota Press.

Butcher, J. N., Williams, C. L., Graham, J. R., Archer, R. P., Tellegen, A., Ben-Porath, Y. S., & Kaemer, B. (1992). *Minnesota multiphasic personality inventory-adolescent*. Minneapolis, MN: University of Minnesota Press.

Butler, E. A., Lee, T. L., & Gross, J. J. (2007). Emotion regulation and culture: Are the social consequences of emotion suppression culture-specific? *Emotion, 7*, 30–48.

Campbell, S. B. (1986). Developmental issues in childhood anxiety. In R. Gittleman (Ed.), *Anxiety disorders of childhood* (pp. 24–57). New York: Guilford.

Cantwell, D. P. (1996). Classification of child and adolescent psychopathology. *Journal of Child Psychology and Psychiatry, 37*, 3–12.

Capara, G. V., Barbaranelli, C., Pastorelli, C., Bandura, A., & Zimbardo, P. G. (2000). Prosocial foundations of children's academic achievement. *Psychological Science, 11*, 302–306.

Cartwright-Hatton, S. C., Roberts, P., Chitsabesan, C., Fothergill, C., & Harrington, R. (2004). Systematic reviews of the efficacy of cognitive behaviour therapies for childhood and adolescent anxiety disorders. *British Journal of Clinical Psychology, 43*, 421–436.

Caspi, A. (2000). The child is father of the man: Personality continuities from childhood to adulthood. *Journal of Personality and Social Psychology, 78*, 158–172.

Caspi, A., Henry, B., McGee, R. O., Moffitt, T. E., & Silva, P. A. (1995). Temperamental origins of child and adolescent behavior problems: From age three to age fifteen. *Child Development, 66*, 55–68.

Catalano, R. F., Hawkins, J. D., Ryan, J. A. M., Lonczak, H. S., & Hawkins, J. D. (2002). Positive youth development in the United States: Research findings on evaluations of positive youth development programs. *Prevention and Treatment, 5(1)*, 15. Retrieved 15 July 2010 from http://psycnet.apa.org/journals/pre/5/1/15a/.

Centers for Disease Control (2007). *National suicide statistics at a glance*. Retrieved 18 July 2010 from http://www.cdc.gov/violenceprevention/suicide/statistics/youth_risk.html.

Chambless, D. L., & Ollendick, T. H. (2000). Empirically supported psychological interventions: Controversies and evidence. *Annual Review of Psychology, 52*, 685–716.

Chaplin, T. M., & Cole, P. M. (2005). The role of emotion regulation in the development of psychopathology. In B. L. Hankin & J. R. Z. Abela (Eds.), *Development of psychopathology* (pp. 49–74). Thousand Oaks, CA: Sage.

Chen, X., Rubin, K. H., & Li, Z. Y. (1995). Social functioning and adjustment in Chinese children: A longitudinal study. *Developmental Psychology, 31*, 531–539.

Chorpita, B. F. (2002). The tripartite model and dimensions of anxiety and depression: An examination of structure in a large school sample. *Journal of Abnormal Child Psychology, 107*, 177–190.

Chorpita, B. F., Albano, A. M., & Barlow, D. H. (1996). Cognitive processing in children: Relation to anxiety and family influences. *Journal of Clinical Child Psychology, 25*, 170–176.

Chorpita, B. F., & Barlow, D. H. (1998). The development of anxiety: The role of control in the early environment. *Psychological Bulletin, 124*, 3–21.

Chorpita, B. F., Brown, T. A., & Barlow, D. H. (1998). Perceived control as a mediator of family environment in etiological models of childhood anxiety. *Behavior Therapy, 29*, 457–476.

Cichetti, D., & Cohen, D. (Eds.). (1995). *Developmental psychopathology: Vol. 1. Theory and methods.* New York: Wiley.

Cichetti, D., & Rogosch, F. A. (1996). Equifinality and multifinalilty in developmental psychopathology. *Development and Psychopathology, 8*, 597–600.

Cichetti, D., & Sroufe, I. A. (2000). Reflecting on the past and planning for the future of developmental psychopathology. *Development and Psychopathology, 12*, 255–550.

Cichetti, D., Toth, S., & Bush, M. (1988). Developmental psychopathology and incompetence in childhood: Suggestions for intervention. In B. B. Lahey & A. E. Kazdin (Eds.), *Advances in clinical child psychology* (Vol. II) (pp. 1–77). New York: Plenum

Clark, R., Anderson, N. B., Clark, V. R., & Williams, D. R. (1999). Racism as a stressor for African Americans: A biopsychosocial model. *American Psychologist, 54*, 805–816.

Clark, L. A., & Watson, D. (1991). Tripartite model of anxiety and depression: Psychometric evidence and taxonomic implications. *Journal of Abnormal Psychology, 100*, 316–336.

Clarke, A. T. (2006). Coping with interpersonal stress and psychosocial health among children and adolescents: A meta-analysis. *Journal of Youth and Adolescence, 35*, 11–24.

Clarke, G., Hawkins, W., Murphy, M., Sheeber, L., Lewinsohn, P., & Seely, J. (1995). Targeted prevention of unipolar depressive disorder in an at-risk sample of high school adolescents: A randomized trial of a group cognitive intervention. *Journal of the American Academy of Child and Adolescent Psychiatry, 34*, 312–321.

Clarke, G., Hops, H., Lewinsohn, P. M., Andrew, J., & Williams, J. (1992). Cognitive-behavioral treatment of adolescent depression: Prediction of outcome. *Behavior Therapy, 23*, 341–354.

Clarke, G. N., Hornbrook, M., Lynch, F., Polen, M., Gale, J., Beardslee, W., O'Connor, E., & Seeley, R. (2001). A randomized trial of a group cognitive intervention for preventing depression in adolescent offspring of depressed parents. *Archives of General Psychiatry, 58*, 1127–1134.

Clarke, G. N., & Lewinsohn, P. M. (1995). *The adolescent coping with stress class.* Leader manual. Available at http://www.kpchr.org/research/public/acwd/acwd.html#downloads.

Clarke, G. N., Lewinsohn, P. M., Rohde, P., Hops, H., & Seeley, J. R. (1999). Cognitive-behavioral treatment of adolescent depression: Efficacy of acute group treatment and booster sessions. *Journal of the American Academy of Child and Adolescent Psychiatry, 38*, 272–279.

Cobham, V. E., Dadds, M. R., & Spence, S. H. (1998). The role of parental anxiety in the treatment of childhood anxiety. *Journal of Consulting and Clinical Psychology, 67*, 583–589.

Cohen, P. (1999). Personality development in childhood: Old and new findings. In C. R. Cloninger (Ed.), *Personality and psychopathology* (pp. 101–127). Washington, DC: American Psychiatric Press.

Cohen, J. A. (2001). Pharmacologic treatment of traumatized children. *Trauma, Violence, and Abuse, 2*, 255–171.

Cohn, J. F., Matias, R., Tronick, E., Connell, D., & Lyons-Ruth, K. (1986). Face-to-face interactions of depressed interactions of depressed mothers and their infants. In E. Z. Tronick &

T. Field (Eds.), *New directions for child development: Maternal depression and infant disturbance* (Vol. 31–46). San Francisco: Jossey-Bass.

Coie, J., & Koeppl, G. (1990). Adapting intervention to the problems of aggressive and rejected disruptive children. In S. Asher & J. Coie (Eds.), *Peer rejection in childhood* (pp. 309–337). New York: Cambridge University Press.

Cole, D. A. (1991). Preliminary support for a competency-based model of depression in children. *Journal of Abnormal Psychology, 100,* 181–190.

Cole, P. M., Martin, S. E., & Dennis, T. A. (2004). Emotion regulation as a scientific construct: Methodological challenges and directions for child development research. *Child Development, 75,* 317–333.

Cole, D. A., Martin, J. M., & Powers, B. (1997). A competency-based model of child depression: A longitudinal study of peer, parent, teacher, and self-evaluations. *Journal of Child Psychology and Psychiatry, 18,* 505–514.

Cole, D. A., Martin, S. E., Powers, B., & Truglio, R. (1996). Modeling causal relations between academic and social competence and depression: A multitrait-multimethod longitudinal study of children. *Journal of Abnormal Psychology, 105,* 258–270.

Cole, D. A., Peeke, L. G., Martin, J. M., Truglio, R., & Ceroczyski, D. (1998). A longitudinal look at the relation between depression and anxiety in children and adolescents. *Journal of Consulting and Clinical Psychology, 66,* 451–460.

Cole, D. A., Tram, J. M., Martin, L. M., Hoffman, I. B., Ruiz, M. D., Jasquez, F. M., et al. (2002). Individual differences in the emergence of depressive symptoms in children and adolescents: A longitudinal investigation of parent and child reports. *Journal of Abnormal Psychology, 111,* 156–165.

Collaborative for Academic and Social Emotional Learning (CASEL). (1994). http://www.casel.org.

Compton, S. N., March, J. S., Brent, D., Albano, A. H., Weersing, V., & Curry, J. (2004). Cognitive-behavioral psychotherapy for anxiety and depressive disorders in children and adolescents: An evidence-based medicine review. *Journal of the American Academy of Child and Adolescent Psychiatry, 43,* 930–959.

Conduct Problems Prevention Research Group. (1999). Initial impact of the Fast Track prevention trial for conduct problems: II. Classroom effects. *Journal of Consulting and Clinical Psychology, 67,* 648–657.

Cooper, P. J., & Goodyear, I. (1993). A community study of depression in adolescent girls: I. Estimates of symptom and syndrome prevalence. *British Journal of Psychiatry, 163,* 369–374.

Costello, E. J., & Angold, A. (1995a). Epidemiology. In J. S. March (Ed.), *Anxiety disorders in children and adolescents* (pp. 109–124). New York: Guilford.

Costello, E. J., & Angold, A. (1995b). Epidemiology. In J. S. March (Ed.), *Anxiety disorders in children and adolescents* (pp. 109–124). New York: Guilford.

Costello, E. J., Angold, A., Burns, B. J., Stangl, D. K., Tweed, D. L., Erkanli, A., & Wortham, C. M. (1996). The Great Smoky Mountain Study of Youth: Goals, design, methods, and the prevalence of DSM-III-R disorders. *Archives of General Psychiatry, 53,* 1129–1136.

Costello, E. J., Costello, A. J., Edelbrock, C., Burns, B. J., Dulcan, M. K., Brent, D. A., et al. (1988). Psychiatric disorders in pediatric primary care: Prevalence and risk factors. *Archives of General Psychiatry, 45,* 1107–1116.

Costello, E. J., Egger, H. L., & Angold, A. (2004). The developmental epidemiology of anxiety disorders. In T. H. Ollendick & J. S. March (Eds.), *Phobic and anxiety disorders in children and adolescents: A clinician's guide to effective psychosocial and pharmacological interventions* (pp. 61–91). New York: Oxford University Press.

Costello, E. J., Egger, H. L., & Angold, A. (2005). 10-Year research update review: The epidemiology of child and adolescent psychiatric disorders: I. Method and public health burden. *Journal of the American Academy of Child and Adolescent Psychiatry, 44,* 972–986.

Costello, E. J., Erkanli, A., & Angold, A. (2006). Is there an epidemic of child or adolescent depression? *Journal of Child Psychology and Psychiatry, 47,* 1265–1271.

Costello, E. J., Mustillo, S., Erkanli, A., Keeler, G., & Angold, A. (2003). Prevalence and development of psychiatric disorders in childhood and adolescence. *Archives of General Psychiatry, 60,* 837–844.

Costello, E. J., Stouthamer-Loever, M., & DeRosier, M. (1993). Continuity and change in psychopathology from childhood and adolescence. Paper presented at the Annual Meeting of the Society for Research in Child and Adolescent Psychopathology, Santa Fe, New Mexico.

Coyne, M., Simonsen, B., & Fagella-Luby, M. (2008). Cooperating initiatives: Supporting behavioral and academic improvement through a systems approach. *Teaching Exceptional Children, 40,* 54–59.

Craighead, W. E., Smucker, M. R., Craighead, L. W., & Hardi, S. S. (1998). Factor analysis of the Children's depression inventory in a community sample. *Psychological Assessment, 10,* 156–165.

Craske, M. G., & Barlow, D. H. (1988). A review of the relationship between panic and avoidance. *Clinical Psychology Review, 8,* 667–685.

Crick, N. R., & Bigbee, M. A. (1998). Relational and overt forms of peer victimization: A multi-informant approach. *Journal of Consulting and Clinical Psychology, 66,* 337–347.

Crone, D. A., & Horner, R. H. (2003). *Building positive behavior support systems in schools. Functional behavior assessment.* New York: Guilford.

Cutuli, J. J., Chaplin, T. M., Gillham, J. E., Reivich, K. R., & Seligman, M. E. P. (2006). Preventing co-occurring depression symptoms in adolescents with conduct problems: The Penn Resiliency Program. *Annals of the New York Academy of Sciences, 1094,* 282–286.

Dadds, M. R., Holland, D. E., Laurens, K. R., Mullins, M., Barrett, P. M., & Spence, S. H. (1999). Early intervention and prevention of anxiety disorders in children: Results at 2-year follow-up. *Journal of Consulting and Clinical Psychology, 67,* 145–150.

Dadds, M. R., Spence, S. H., Holland, D. E., Barrett, P. M., & Laurens, K. R. (1997). Prevention and early intervention for anxiety disorders: A controlled trial. *Journal of Consulting and Clinical Psychology, 65,* 627–635.

Dalgleish, T., Moradi, A. R., Taghavi, M. R., Neshat-Doost, H. T., & Yule, W. (2001). An experimental investigation of hypervigilance for threat in children and adolescents with post-traumatic stress disorder. *Psychological Medicine, 3,* 541–547.

Dashiff, C. J. (1995). Understanding separation anxiety disorder. *Journal of Child and Adolescent Psychiatric Nursing, 8,* 27–38.

Davidson, R. J. (1994). Asymmetric brain function, affective style, and psychopathology: The role of early experience and plasticity. *Development and Psychopathology, 6,* 741–758.

Davidson, R. J., Putnam, K. M., & Larson, C. L. (2000). Dysfunction in the neural circuitry of emotion regulation: A possible prelude to violence. *Science, 289,* 591–594.

Davis, B., Sheeber, L., Hops, H., & Tildesley, E. (2000). Adolescent responses to depressive parental behaviors in problem-solving interactions: Implications for depressive symptoms. *Journal of Abnormal Child Psychology, 28,* 451–465.

Dodge, K., & Petit, G. (2003). A biopsychosocial model of the development of chronic conduct problems in adolescence. *Developmental Psychology, 39,* 349–371.

Dummitt, E. S., Klein, R. G., Tancer, N. K., Asche, B., Martin, J., & Fairbanks, J. A. (1997). Systematic assessment of 50 children with selective mutism. *Journal of the American Academy of Child and Adolescent Psychiatry, 36,* 653–660.

Durbin, C. M., & Shafir, D. M. (2008). Emotion regulation and risk for depression. In J. R. Z. Abela & B. L. Hankin (Eds.), *Handbook of depression in children and adolescents* (pp. 149–176). New York: Guilford.

Eaves, I. J., Silberg, J., Meyer, J. M., Maes, H. H., Simonoff, E., Pickles, A., et al. (1997). Genetics and developmental psychopathology: 2. The main effects of genes and environment on behavioral problems in the Virginia Twin study of adolescent behavioral development. *Journal of Child Psychology and Psychiatry, 38,* 965–980.

Eisen, J. L., Goodman, W. K., Keller, M. B., Warshaw, B. G., DeMarco, L. M., Luce, D. D., et al. (1999). Patterns of remission and relapse in obsessive-compulsive disorder: A 2-year prospective study. *Journal of Clinical Psychiatry, 60,* 346–351.

Eisenberg, N., Gershoff, E. T., Fabes, R. A., Shepard, S. A., Cumberland, A. J., Losoya, S. H., et al. (2001). Mothers' emotional expressivity and children's behavior problems and social competence: Mediation through children's regulation. *Developmental Psychology, 37*, 475–490.

Eisenberg, N., Spinrad, T. L., Fabes, R. A., Reiser, M., Cumberland, A., Shepard, S. A., et al. (2004). The relation of effortful control and impulsivity to children's resiliency and adjustment. *Child Development, 75*, 25–46.

Eisenberg, N., Valiente, C., Morris, A. S., Cumberland, A., Reiser, M., et al. (2003). Longitudinal relations among parental emotional expressivity, children's regulation, and quality of socioemotional functioning. *Developmental Psychology, 39*, 3–19.

Eley, T. C. (2001). Contributions of behavioral genetics research: Quantifying genetic, shared environmental and nonshared environmental influences. In M. W. Vasey & M. R. Dadds (Eds.), *The developmental psychopathology of anxiety* (pp. 45–59). New York: Oxford University Press.

Elias, M. J., Parker, S., & Rosenblatt, J. L. (2006). Building educational opportunity. In S. Goldstein & R. B. Brooks (Eds.), *Handbook of resilience in children* (pp. 315–336). New York: Springer.

Ellis, A. (1962). *Reason and emotion in psychotherapy*. New York: Lyle Stewart.

Emslie, G. J., Bush, A. J., Weinberg, W. A., Kowactch, B. A., Hughes, C. W., Carmody, T., & Rintelmann, J. (1997). A double-blind randomized, placebo-controlled trial of fluoxetine in children and adolescents with depression. *Archives of General Psychiatry, 54*, 1031–1037.

Emslie, G. J., Helligenstein, J. H., Wagner, K. D., Hoog, S. L., Ernest, D. E., Brown, E., et al. (2002). Fluoxetine for acute treatment of depression in children and adolescents: A placebo-controlled randomized clinical trial. *Journal of the American Academy of Child and Adolescent Psychiatry, 41*, 1205–1215.

Erchul, W. P. (1992). On dominance, cooperation, teamwork, and collaboration in school-based consultation. *Journal of Educational and Psychological Consultation, 3*, 363–366.

Erchul, W. P. (1999). Two steps forward, one step back: Collaboration in school-based consultation. *Journal of School Psychology, 37*, 191–203.

Eschenasy v. New York City Dep't of Educ., 604 F. Supp. 2d 639 (S. D. N. Y. 2009).

Essau, C. A., Conradt, J., & Petermann, F. (2000). Frequency, comorbidity, and psychosocial impairment of specific phobias in adolescents. *Journal of Clinical Child Psychology, 29*, 221–231.

Evans, G. W., & English, K. (2002). The environment of poverty: Multiple stressor exposure, psychophysiological stress, and socioemotional adjustment. *Child Development, 73*, 1238–1248.

Faedda, G., Baldessarini, R., Suppes, T., Tondo, L., Becker, I., & Lipschitz, D. (1995). Pediatric-onset bipolar disorder: A neglected clinical and public health problem. *Harvard Review of Psychiatry, 3*, 171–195.

Fairbanks, J. M., Pine, D., Tancer, N. K., Dummit, E. S., III, Kentgen, L. M., Ashce, B. K., et al. (1997). Open fluoxetine treatment of mixed anxiety disorders in children and adolescents. *Journal of the American Academy of Child and Adolescent Psychiatry, 7*, 17–29.

Faraone, S. V., Biederman, J., Mennin, D., Wozniak, J., & Spencer, T. (1997). Attention-deficit hyperactivity disorder with bipolar disorder: A familial subtype? *Journal of the American Academy of Child and Adolescent Psychiatry, 36*, 1378–1387.

Field, T., Healy, B., Goldstein, S., & Guthertz, M. (1990). Behavior-state matching and synchrony in mother-infant interactions of nondepressed vs. depressed dyads. *Psychology, 26*, 7–14.

Fleming, J. E., Offord, D. R., & Boyle, M. H. (1989). Prevalence of childhood and adolescent depression in the community—Ontario Child Health Study. *British Journal of Psychiatry, 155*, 647–654.

Fletcher, K. E. (2003). Childhood posttraumatic stress disorder. In E. J. Mash & R. A. Barkley (Eds.), *Child psychopathology* (3rd ed., pp. 330–371). New York: Guilford.

Foa, E. B., & Kozak, M. J. (1986). Emotional processing of fear: Exposure to corrective information. *Psychological Bulletin, 90*, 21–35.

Foley, D. L., Rowe, R., Maes, H., Silberg, J., Eaves, L., & Pickles, A. (2008). The relationship between separation anxiety and impairment. *Journal of Anxiety Disorders, 22*, 635–641.

Folsetin, M. F., Folstein, S. E., White, T., & Messer, M. A. (2010). *Mini mental state examination-2 (MSSE-2)*. Lutz, FL: Professional Assessment Resources.

Fordham, K., & Stevenson-Hinde, J. (1999). Shyness, friendship quality, and adjustment during middle childhood. *Journal of Child Psychology and Psychiatry, 40*, 757–768.

Forehand, R., Brody, G. H., Long, N., & Fauber, R. (1988). The interactive influence of adolescent and maternal depression on adolescent social and cognitive functioning. *Cognitive Therapy and Research, 12*, 341–350.

Fornesca, A. C., Yule, C., & Erol, N. (1994). Cross cultural issues. In T. H. Ollendick, N. J. King, & W. Yule (Eds.), *International handbook of phobic and anxiety disorders in children and adolescents* (pp. 67–84). New York: Plenum.

Francis, G., Last, C. G., & Strauss, C. C. (1987). Expression of separation anxiety disorder: The roles of age and gender. *Child Psychiatry and Human Development, 18*, 82–89.

Freud, S. (1955). Analysis of a phobia in a five-year-old boy. In J. Strachey (Ed. & Trans.), *The standard edition of the complete psychological works of Sigmund Freud* (Vol. 10), (pp. 3–149). London: Hogarth. (Original work published 1909).

Frey, A. J., Lingo, A., & Nelson, C. M. (2010). Implementing positive behavior support in elementary schools. In M. R. Shinn & H. M. Walker (Eds.), *Interventions for achievement and behavior problems in a three-tier model including RTI* (pp. 397–433). Bethesda, MD: National Association of School Psychologists.

Frick, P. J., Kamphaus, R. W., Lahey, B. B., Christ, M. A. G., Hart, E. L., & Tannenbaum, T. E. (1991). Academic underachievement and the disruptive behavior disorders. *Journal of Consulting and Clinical Psychology, 59*, 289–294.

Friedberg, R. D., & McClure, J. M. (2002). *Clinical practice of cognitive therapy with children and adolescents: The nuts and bolts*. New York: Guilford.

Garbarino, J. (1997). Growing up in a socially toxic environment. In D. Cichetti & S. L. Toth (Eds.), *Rochester symposium on developmental psychopathology—developmental perspectives on trauma: Theory, research, and intervention* (Vol. 8, pp. 141–154). Rochester, NY: Rochester University Press.

Garber, J., Clarke, G. N., Weersing, V. R., Beardslee, W. R., Brent, D. A., Gladstone, T. R., DeBar, L. L., Lynch, F. L., D'Angelo, E., Hollon, S. D., Shamseddeen, W., & Iyengar, S. (2009). Prevention of depression in at-risk adolescents: A randomized controlled trial. *Journal of the American Medical Association, 301*, 2215–24.

Garber, J., & Flynn, C. (1998). Origins of depressive cognitive style. In D. K. Routh & R. J. DeRubeis (Eds.), *The science of clinical psychology: Accomplishments and future directions* (pp. 53–93). Washington, DC: American Psychological Association.

Garber, J., Keiley, M. K., & Martin, N. C. (2002). Developmental trajectories of adolescents' depressive symptoms: Predictors of change. *Journal of Consulting and Clinical Psychology, 70*, 79–95.

Garnefski, N., Legerstee, J., Kraaij, V. V., Van Den Kommer, T., & Teerds, J. (2002). Cognitive coping strategies and symptoms of depression and anxiety: A comparison between adolescents and adults. *Journal of Adolescence, 25*, 603–611.

Garrison, C. A., Jackson, K. L., Marsteller, F., McKeown, R., & Addy, C. (1990). A longitudinal study of depressive symptomatology in young adolescents. *Journal of the American Academy of Child and Adolescent Psychiatry, 29*, 581–585.

Geller, D. A., Biederman, J., Faraone, S. V., Bellodre, C. A., Kim, G. S., Hagermoser, L., Cradock, K., Frazier, J., & Coffey, B. J. (2001). Disentangling chronological age from age of onset in children and adolescents with obsessive-compulsive disorder. *International Journal of Neuropsychopharmacology, 4*, 169–178.

Geller, D. A., Hoag, S. L., Heiligenstein, J. H., Ricardi, R. K., Tamura, R., Kluzynski, S., et al. (2001). Fluoxetine treatment for obsessive-compulsive disorder in children and adolescents: A placebo-controlled clinical trial. *Journal of the American Academy of Child and Adolescent Psychiatry, 40*, 773–779.

Gerlsma, C., Emmellkamp, P. M. G., & Arrindell, W. A. (1990). Anxiety, depression, and perception of early parenting: A meta-analysis. *Clinical Psychology Review, 10*, 251–277.

Gibb, B. E., Wheeler, R., Alloy, L. B., & Abramson, L. Y. (2001). Emotional, physical, and sexual maltreatment in childhood versus adolescence and personality dysfunction in young adulthood. *Journal of Personality Disorders, 15*, 505–511.

Gillham, J. E., Jaycox, L. H., Reivich, K. J., Seligman, M. E. P., & Silver, T. (1990). *The Penn Resiliency Program*. Philadelphia: University of Pennsylvania. Unpublished manual.

Gillham, J. E., & Reivich, K. J. (1999). Prevention of depressive symptoms in school children: A research update. *Psychological Science, 10*, 461–462.

Gillham, J. E., Reivich, K. J., Freres, D. R., Chaplin, T. M., Shatté, A. J., Samuels, B., et al. (2006). School-based prevention of depression and anxiety symptoms in early adolescence: A pilot of a parent intervention component. *School Psychology Quarterly, 21*, 323–348.

Gillham, J. E., Reivich, K. J., Jaycox, L. H., & Seligman, M. E. P. (1995). Preventing depressive symptoms in schoolchildren: Two-year follow-up. *Psychological Science, 6*, 343–353.

Ginsburg, G. S., & Walkup, J. T. (2004). Treatment of specific phobias. In T. H. Ollendick & J. S. March (Eds.), *Phobic and anxiety disorders in children and adolescents: A clinician's guide to effective psychosocial and pharmacological interventions*. New York: Oxford University Press.

Gittleman-Klein, R., & Klein, D. F. (1971). Controlled imipramine treatment of school phobia. *Archives of General Psychiatry, 2*, 204–207.

Goldsmith, H. H., Pollak, S. D., & Davidson, R. J. (2009). Developmental neuroscience perspectives on emotion regulation. *Child Development Perspectives, 2*, 132–140.

Goodman, W. K., Price, L. H., & Rasmussen, S. A. (1989a). The Yale-Brown obsessive compulsive scale I: Development, use and reliability. *Archives of General Psychiatry, 46*, 1006–1011.

Goodman, W. K., Price, L. H., & Rasmussen, S. A. (1989b). The Yale-Brown obsessive compulsive scale, II: Validity. *Archives of General Psychiatry, 46*, 1012–1016.

Goodman, S. H., Schwab-Stone, M., Lahey, B. B., Shaffer, D., & Jensen, P. S. (2000). Major depression and dysthymia in children and adolescents: Discriminant validity and differential consequences in a community sample. *Journal of the American Academy of Child and Adolescent Psychiatry, 39*, 761–770.

Gould, M. S., Shaffer, D., & Greenberg, T. (2003). The epidemiology of youth suicide. In R. A. King & A. Apter (Eds.), *Suicide in children and adolescents* (pp. 1–40). Cambridge, UK: Cambridge University Press.

Gray, J. A. (1982). *The neuropsychology of anxiety*. New York: Oxford University Press.

Gray, J. A., & McNaughton, N. (2000). *The neuropsychology of anxiety*. New York: Oxford University Press.

Greenburg, M. T., Weissberg, R. P., Utne O'Brien, M., Zins, J. E., Redericks, L., Resnik, H., et al. (2003). Enhancing school-based prevention and youth development through coordinated social, emotional, and academic learning. *American Psychologist, 58*, 466–474.

Greene, J. P., & Winters, M. A. (2005). *Public high school graduation and college-readiness rates: 1991–2002*. (Education Working Paper N.8). New York: Manhattan Institute for Policy Research.

Gregory, A. M., & Eley, T. C. (2007). Genetic influences on anxiety in children: What we've learned and where we're heading. *Clinical Child and Family Psychiatry, 10*, 199–212.

Gresham, F. (2010). Evidence-based social skills interventions: Empirical foundations for instructional approaches. In M. R. Shinn & H. M. Walker (Eds.), *Interventions for achievement and behavior problems in a three-tier model including RTI* (pp. 337–362). Bethesda, MD: National Association of School Psychologists.

Gresham, F., & Elliott, S. N. (1990). *Social skills rating system*. Circle Pines, MN: American Guidance Service.

Gresham, F., & Elliott, S. N. (2008). *Social skills improvement system*. San Antonio, TX: Pearson.

Gross, J. J., & Levenson, R. W. (1997). Hiding feelings: The acute effects of inhibiting negative and positive emotion. *Journal of Abnormal Psychology, 106*, 95–103.

Gross, J. J., & Thompson, R. A. (2007). Emotion regulation: Conceptual foundations. In J. J. Gross (Ed.), *Handbook of emotion regulation* (pp. 3–24). New York: Guilford.

Gullone, E., & King, N. J. (1992). Psychometric evaluation of a revised fear survey schedule for children and adolescents. *Journal of Child Psychology and Psychiatry and Allied Disciplines, 33*, 987–998.

Gullone, E., & Lane, B. (2002). The fear survey schedule for children-II: A validity examination across response format and instruction type. *Clinical Psychology and Psychotherapy, 9*, 55–67.

Gutkin, T. B. (1996). Patterns of consultant and consultee verbalization: Examining communication leadership during initial consultation interviews. *Journal of School Psychology, 34*, 199–219.

Gutkin, T. B. (1999). Collaborative versus directive/nondirective/expert school-based consultation: Reviewing and resolving a false dichotomy. *Journal of School Psychology, 37*, 161–190.

Haines, B. A., Metalksy, G. I., Cardamone, A. L., & Joiner, T. E. (1999). Interpersonal and cognitive pathways into the origins of attributional style: A developmental perspective. In T. E. Joiner & J. Coyne (Eds.), *The interactional nature of depression* (pp. 65–82). Washington, DC: American Psychological Association.

Hammen, C. L., Burge, D., Daley, S. E., Davila, J., Paley, B., & Rudolph, K. D. (1995). Interpersonal attachment cognitions and prediction of symptomatic responses to interpersonal stress. *Journal of Abnormal Psychology, 104*, 436–443.

Han, S. S., & Weiss, B. (2005). Sustainability of teacher implementation of school-based mental health programs. *Journal of Abnormal Child Psychology, 33*, 665–679.

Hankin, B. L., Abramson, L. Y., Moffitt, T. E., Silva, P. A., McGee, R., & Angell, K. E. (1998). Development of depression from preadolescence to young adulthood: Emerging gender differences in a 10-year longitudinal study. *Journal of Abnormal Psychology, 107*, 128–140.

Hansen v. Republic R-III School Dist., No. 10-1514, 2011 WL 181530 (8th Cir. 1/21/11).

Hariri, A. R., & Forbes, E. E. (2007). Genetics of emotion regulation. In J. J. Gross (Ed.), *Handbook of emotion regulation* (pp. 110–132). New York: Guilford.

Harlacher, J. E., & Merrell, K. W. (2010). Social and emotional learning as a universal level of student support: Evaluating the follow-up effect of strong kids on social and emotional outcomes. *Journal of Applied School Psychology, 26*, 212–229.

Harrington, R., Fudge, H., Rutter, M., Pickles, A., & Hill, J. (1990). Adult outcomes of child and adolescent depression: I. Psychiatric status. *Archives of General Psychiatry, 47*, 465–473.

Harris, A. M., & Reid, J. B. (1981). The consistency of a class of coercive child behaviors across school settings for individual subjects. *Journal of Abnormal Child Psychology, 9*, 219–227.

Harter, S. (1985). *Self-perception profile for children.* Denver, CO: University of Denver Department of Psychology.

Harter, S. (1988). *Self-perception profile for adolescents.* Denver, CO: University of Denver Department of Psychology.

Haynes, N. M., Ben-Avie, M., & Ensign, J. (2003). *How social and emotional development add up: Getting results in math and science education.* New York: Teachers College Press.

Hayward, C., Gotlib, I., Schraedley, P. K., & Litt, I. F. (1999). Ethnic differences in the association between pubertal status and symptoms of depression in adolescent girls. *Journal of Adolescent Health, 25*, 142–149.

Hayward, C., Killen, J. D., Hammer, L. D., Litt, I. F., Wilson, D. M., Simmonds, B., et al. (1992). Pubertal stage and panic attack history in sixth-and seventh-grade girls. *American Journal of Psychiatry, 149*, 1239–1243.

Hayward, C., Killen, J. D., Kraemer, H. C., & Taylor, C. B. (2000). Predictors of panic attacks in adolescents. *Journal of the American Academy of Child and Adolescent Psychiatry, 39*, 207–214.

Heimberg, R. G., Hope, D. A., Dodge, C. S., & Becker, R. E. (1990). DSM-III-R subtypes of social phobia: Comparison of generalized social phobics and public speaking phobics. *Journal of Nervous and Mental Diseases, 178*, 172–179.

Helm, C., Owens, M. J., Plotsky, P. M., & Nemeroff, C. B. (1997). Persistent changes in corticotrophin-releasing factor systems due to early life stress: Relationship to the pathophysiology of major depression and post-traumatic stress disorder. *Psychopharmacology Bulletin, 33*, 185–192.

Henriques, G., Beck, A. T., & Brown, G. K. (2003). Cognitive therapy for adolescent and young adult suicide attempters. *American Behavioral Scientist, 46,* 1258–1268.

Hetema, J. M., Neale, M. C., & Kendler, K. S. (2001). A review and meta-analysis of the genetic epidemiology of anxiety disorders. *American Journal of Psychiatry, 158,* 1568–1578.

Hinshaw, S. P., Lahey, B. B., & Hart, E. L. (1993). Issues of taxonomy and comorbidity in the development of conduct disorder. *Development and Psychopathology, 5,* 31–49.

Hinshaw, S. P., & Lee, S. S. (2003). Conduct and oppositional defiant disorders. In E. J. Mash & R. A. Barkley (Eds.), *Child psychopathology* (2nd ed.), (pp. 144–199).

Hirschfield, R. M. A. (1996). Placebo response in the treatment of panic disorder. *Bulletin of the Menninger Clinic, 60,* A76–A86.

Hoagwood, K., & Jensen, P. (1997). Developmental psychopathology and the notion of culture. *Applied Developmental Science, 1,* 108–112.

Hoagwood, K., & Johnson, J. (2003). School psychology: A public health framework. *Journal of School Psychology, 41,* 3–21.

Hoehn-Saric, R., Hazlett, R. L., & McLeod, D. R. (1993). Generalized anxiety disorder with early and late onset of anxiety symptoms. *Comprehensive Psychiatry, 34,* 291–298.

Hoffman, K. B., Cole, D. A., Martin, J. M., Tram, J., & Serocaynski, A. D. (2000). Are discrepancies between self- and others' appraisals of competence predictive of reflective or depressive symptoms in children and adolescents: A longitudinal study, part H. *Journal of Abnormal Psychology, 109,* 651–662.

Horowitz, A. V., Widom, C. S., Mclaughlin, J., & White, H. R. (2001). The impact of childhood abuse and neglect on adult mental health: A prospective study. *Journal of Health and Social Behavior, 42,* 184–201.

Houk, J. L., & Lewandowski, L. J. (1996). Consultant verbal control and consultee perceptions. *Journal of Educational and Psychological Consultation, 7,* 107–118.

Hovey, J. D., & King, C. A. (1996). Acculturative stress, depression, and suicidal ideation among immigrant and second-generation Latino adolescents. *Journal of the American Academy of Child and Adolescent Psychiatry, 35,* 1183–1192.

Howard, B., Chu, B. C., Krain, A. L., Marrs-Garcia, M. A., & Kendall, P. C. (2000). *Cognitive-behavioral family therapy for anxious children: Therapist manual* (2nd ed.). Ardmore, PA: Workbook Publishing.

Howard, B. L., & Kendall, P. C. (1996). Cognitive-behavioral family therapy for anxiety-disordered children: A multiple-baseline evaluation. *Cognitive Therapy and Research, 20,* 423–443.

Howse, R., Calkins, S., Anastopolous, A., Keane, S., & Shelton, T. (2003). Regulatory contributors to children's academic achievement. *Early Education and Development, 14,* 101–119.

Huberty, T. J. (2008). Best practices in school-based interventions for anxiety and depression. In A. Thomas & J. Grimes (Eds.), *Best practices in school psychology-V* (pp. 1473–1486). Bethesda, MD: National Association of School Psychologists.

Huberty, T. J. (2009). Interventions for internalizing disorders. In A. Akin-Little, S. G. Little, M. A. Bray, & T. J. Kehle (Eds.), *Behavioral interventions in schools: Evidence-based positive strategies* (pp. 281–296). Washington, DC: American Psychological Association.

Huberty, T. J., Austin, J. K., Huster, G. A., & Dunn, D. (2000). Relations of change in condition severity and school self-concept to change in achievement-related behavior in children with asthma or epilepsy. *Journal of School Psychology, 38,* 259–276.

Hudson, J. L., & Rapee, R. M. (2001). Parent-child interactions and anxiety disorders: An observational study. *Behaviour Research and Therapy, 39,* 1411–1427.

Hughes, J., Cavell, T., & Jackson, T. (1999). Influence of the teacher-student relationship on childhood conduct problems: A prospective study. *Journal of Clinical Child Psychology, 28,* 173–184.

Ialongo, N., Edelsohn, G., Werthamer-Larson, L., Crockett, L., & Kellam, S. G. (1996). A further look at the prognostic power of young children's reports of depressed mood and feelings. *Child Development, 72,* 736–747.

Individuals with Disabilities Education Improvement Act of 2004, 20 U.S.C. § 1400 *et. seq.*

Ingolsdby, E. M., Shaw, D. S., Owens, E. B., & Winslow, D. B. (1999). A longitudinal study of interparental conflict, emotional and behavioral reactivity, and preschoolers' adjustment problems among low-income families. *Journal of Abnormal Child Psychology, 27,* 343–356.

Ingram, K., Lewis-Palmer, T., & Sugai, G. (2005). Function-based intervention planning: Comparing the effectiveness of FBA function-based and non-function-based intervention plans. *Journal of Positive Behavior Interventions, 7*, 224–236.

Ingram, R. E., & Luxton, D. D. (2005). Vulnerability-stress models. In B. L. Hankin & J. R. Z. Abela (Eds.), *Development of psychopathology: A vulnerability-stress perspective* (pp. 32–46). Thousand Oaks, CA: Sage.

Ingram, R. E., Miranda, J., & Segal, Z. V. (1998). *Cognitive vulnerability to depression*. New York: Guilford.

Ingram, R. E., & Price, J. M. (Eds.). (2001). *Vulnerability to psychopathology: Risk across the lifespan*. New York: Guilford.

Institute of Medicine (IOM). (1994). *Reducing risks for mental disorders: Frontiers for preventive intervention research*. Washington, DC: National Academy Press.

Ivanova, M. Y., Achenbach, T. M., Dumenci, L., Rescorla, I. A., Almquist, F., Bilenberg, F., et al. (2007). Testing the 8-syndrome structure of the CBCL in 30 societies. *Journal of Clinical Child and Adolescent Psychiatry, 36*, 405–417.

Ivanova, M. Y., Achenbach, T. M., Rescorla, L. A., Dumenci, L., Almquist, F., et al. (2007). The generalizability of the Youth Self-Report syndrome structure in 23 societies. *Journal of Consulting and Clinical Psychology, 75*, 729–738.

Jacobson, N. S., Martell, C. R., & Dimidjian, S. (2001). Behavioral activation therapy for depression: Returning to contextual roots. *Clinical Psychology: Science and Practice, 8*, 255–270.

Jang, K. L., Livesley, W. J., & Vernon, P. A. (1996). Heritability of the big five personality dimensions and their facets: A twin study. *Journal of Personality, 64*, 577–591.

Jaycox, L. H., Reivich, K. J., Gillham, J., & Seligman, M. E. P. (1994). Prevention of depressive symptoms in school children. *Behaviour Research and Therapy, 32*, 801–816.

John, O. P., & Gross, J. J. (2004). Healthy and unhealthy emotion regulation: Personality processes. *Journal of Personality, 72*, 1301–1333.

Johnson, J. G., Cohen, P., Skodol, A. E., Oldham, J. M., Kasen, S., & Brook, J. (2001). Association of maladaptive parental behavior with psychiatric disorder among parents and their offspring. *Archives of General Psychiatry, 58*, 453–460.

Joiner, T. E., Catanzaro, S. J., & Laurent, J. (1996). Tripartite structure of positive and negative affect, depression, and anxiety in child and adolescent psychiatric inpatients. *Journal of Abnormal Psychology, 105*, 401–409.

Joiner, T. E., Conwell, Y., Fitzpatrick, K. K., Witte, T. K., Schmidt, N. B., Berlim, M. T., et al. (2005). Four studies on how past and current suicidality rates even when "everything but the kitchen sink" is covaried. *Journal of Abnormal Psychology, 114*, 291–303.

Joiner, T. E., Coyne, J. C., & Blalock, J. (1999). On the interpersonal nature of depression: Overview and synthesis. In T. E. Joiner & J. C. Coyne (Eds.), *The interactional nature of depression* (pp. 3–19). Washington, DC: American Psychological Association.

Joiner, T. E., & Metalsky, G. I. (2001). Excessive reassurance seeking: Delineating a risk factor involved in the development of depressive symptoms. *Psychological Science, 12*, 371–378.

Jones, S. M., Brown, J. L., Hoglund, W. L. G., & Aber, J. L. (2010). A school-randomized clinical trial of an integrated social-emotional learning and literacy intervention: Impacts after 1 school year. *Journal of Clinical and Consulting Psychology, 79*, 829–842.

K. M. v. Wappingers Central School District, 688 F.Supp.2d 282 (S.D. N. Y. 2010).

Kagan, J. (1989). Temperamental contributions to social behavior. *American Psychologist, 44*, 446–674.

Kagan, J., Reznick, J. S., & Snidman, N. (1987). The physiology and psychology of behavioral inhibition. *Child Development, 60*, 838–845.

Kagan, J., Reznick, J. S., & Snidman, N. (1988). Biological bases of childhood shyness. *Science, 249*, 167–171.

Kam, C., Greenberg, M., & Walls, C. (2003). Examining the role of implementation quality in school-based prevention using the PATHS curriculum. *Prevention Science, 4*, 55–63.

Kashani, J. H., Burbach, D. J., & Rosenberg, T. K. (1988). Perception of family conflict resolution and depressive symptomatology in adolescents. *Journal of the American Academy of Child and Adolescent Psychiatry, 27*, 42–48.

Kashani, J. H., & Carlson, G. A. (1987). Seriously depressed preschoolers. *American Journal of Psychiatry, 144*, 348–350.

Kashani, J. H., McGee, R. O., Clarkson, S. E., Anderson, J. C., Walton, L. A., Williams, S., et al. (1983). Depression in a sample of 9-year-old children. *Archives of General Psychiatry, 40*, 1217–1223.

Kaslow, N. J., Deering, C. G., & Racusin, G. B. (1994). Depressed children and their families. *Clinical Psychology Review, 14*, 39–59.

Kaslow, N. J., & Rehm, L. P. (1991). Childhood depression. In T. J. Kratochwill & R. J. Morris (Eds.), *The practice of child therapy* (2nd ed., pp. 43–75). New York: Pergamon.

Kaslow, N. J., & Thompson, M. (1998). Applying the criteria for empirically supported treatments to studies of psychosocial interventions for child and adolescent depression. *Journal of Clinical Child Psychology, 27*, 146–155.

Katschnig, H., & Ameing, M. (1994). The long-term course of panic disorder. In B. E. Wolfe & J. D. Maser (Eds.), *Treatment of panic disorder: A consensus development conference* (pp. 73–81). Washington, DC: American Psychiatric Press.

Katz, J., Beach, S. R. H., & Joiner, T. E. (1999). Contagious depression in dating couples. *Journal of Social and Clinical Psychology, 18*, 1–13.

Kauffman, J. M. (1997). *Characteristics of emotional and behavioral disorders of children and youth* (6th ed.). Columbus, OH: Merrill/Prentice Hall.

Kaufman, J. (1991). Depressive disorders in maltreated children. *Journal of the American Academy of Child and Adolescent Psychiatry, 30*, 257–265.

Kazdin, A. E. (1989a). Childhood depression. In E. J. Mash & R. A. Barkley (Eds.), *Treatment of childhood disorders* (pp. 135–166). New York: Guilford.

Kazdin, A. E. (1989b). Identifying depression in children: A comparison of alternative selection criteria. *Journal of Abnormal Child Psychology, 17*, 437–454.

Kazdin, A. E., Rodgers, A., & Colbus, D. (1986). The hopelessness scale for children: Psychometric characteristics and concurrent validity. *Journal of Consulting and Clinical Psychology, 54*, 241–245.

Kazdin, A. E., & Weisz, J. R. (1998). Identifying and developing empirically supported child and adolescents. *Journal of Consulting and Clinical Psychology, 66*, 19–36.

Keane, E. M., Dick, R. W., Bechtold, D. W., & Manson, S. M. (1996). Predictive and concurrent validity of the suicidal ideation questionnaire among American Indian adolescents. *Journal of Abnormal Child Psychology, 24*, 735–747.

Keenan, K., & Hipwell, A. E. (2005). Preadolescent clues to understanding depression in girls. *Clinical Child and Family Psychology Review, 8*, 89–105.

Keller, M. B., Ryan, N. D., Strober, M., Klein, D. N., Arnow, B., Dunner, D. L., et al. (2001). Efficacy of paroxetine in the treatment of adolescent major depression: A randomized, controlled trial. *Journal of the American Academy of Child and Adolescent Psychiatry, 40*, 762–772.

Kendall, P. C. (1984). Cognitive-behavioral self-control therapy for children. *Journal of Child Psychology and Psychiatry and Allied Disciplines, 25*, 173–179.

Kendall, P. C. (1992). *Anxiety disorders in youth: Cognitive-behavioral interventions*. New York: Allyn & Bacon.

Kendall, P. C. (1994). Treating anxiety disorders in youth: Results of a randomized clinical trial. *Journal of Consulting and Clinical Psychology, 62*, 100–110.

Kendall, P. C. (2008). *Camp cope-a-lot*. Ardmore, PA: Workbook Publishing.

Kendall, P. C., Flannery-Schroeder, E., Panichelli-Mindel, S., Southam-Gerow, M., Henin, A., & Warman, M. (1997). Therapy for youth with anxiety disorders: A second randomized clinical trial. *Journal of Consulting and Clinical Psychology, 65*, 366–380.

Kendall, P. C., & Hedtke, K. A. (2006). *Coping cat workbook* (2nd ed.). Ardmore, PA: Workbook Publishing.

Kendall, P. C., & Hollon, S. D. (1979). *Cognitive-behavioral interventions: Theory, research, and procedures*. New York: Academic Press.

Kendall, P. C., Hudson, J., Gosch, E., Flannery-Schroeder, E., & Suveg, C. (2008). Child and family therapy for anxiety-disordered youth: Results of a randomized clinical trial. *Journal of Consulting and Clinical Psychology, 76*, 282–297.

Kendall, P. C., & Ronan, K. R. (1990). Assessment of children's anxieties, fears, and phobias: Cognitive-behavioral model and methods. In C. R. Reynolds & R. W. Kamphaus (Eds.), *Handbook of psychological and educational assessment of children* (pp. 223–244). New York: Guilford.

Kendler, K. S., Gardner, C. O., & Prescott, C. A. (2003). Personality and the experience of environmental adversity. *Psychological Medicine, 33*, 1193–1202.

Kendler, K. S., Karbowski, L. M., & Prescott, C. A. (1999). Fears and phobias: Reliability and heritability. *Psychological Medicine, 29*, 539–553.

Kendler, K. S., Neale, M. C., Kessler, R. C., Heath, A. C., & Eaves, L. J. (1992). Major depression and generalized anxiety disorder: Same genes, (partly) different environments? *Archives of General Psychiatry, 49*, 716–722.

Kerig, P. K., & Wenar, C. (2005). *Developmental psychopathology* (5th ed.). Boston: McGraw-Hill.

Kessler, R. C., Anenevoli, S., & Merikangas, K. R. (2001). Mood disorders in children and adolescents: An epidemiologic perspective. *Biological Psychiatry, 49*, 1002–1014.

Kessler, R., Berglund, P., Demler, O., Jin, R., & Walters, E. (2005). Lifetime prevalence and age-of-onset distributions of DSM-IV disorders in the National Comorbidity Survey Replication. *Archives of General Psychiatry, 62*, 593–602.

Kessler, R. C., McGonagle, K., Swartz, M., Blazer, D., & Nelson, C. (1993). Sex and depression in the National Comorbidity Survey: I. Lifetime prevalence, chronicity, and recurrence. *Journal of Affective Disorders, 29*, 85–96.

Kessler, R. C., McGonagle, K., Zhao, S., Nelson, C. B., Hughes, M., Eshleman, S., Wittchen, H. U., & Kendler, K. S. (1994). Lifetime and 12-month prevalence of DSM-III-R psychiatric disorders in the United States. *Archives of General Psychiatry, 51*, 8–19.

Kessler, R. C., & Walters, E. E. (1998). Epidemiology of DSM-III-R major depression and minor depression among adolescents and young adults in the National Comorbidity Survey. *Depression and Anxiety, 7*, 3–14.

Kilpatrick, D. G., Saunders, B. E., Resnick, H. S., & Smith, D. W. (1995). *The National Survey of Adolescents: Preliminary findings on lifetime prevalence of traumatic events and mental health correlates*. Charleston: Medical University of South Carolina: National Crime Victims Research and Treatment Center.

Kim, J., & Cichetti, D. (2004). A process model of mother-child problems in maltreated and non-maltreated children. *Journal of Abnormal Child Psychology, 32*, 341–354.

Kim-Cohen, J., Caspi, A., Moffit, T. E., Harington, H. L., Milne, B. J., & Poulton, R. (2003). Prior juvenile diagnoses in adults with mental disorder: Developmental follow-back of a prospective-longitudinal cohort. *Archives of General Psychiatry, 60*, 709–717.

Klein, R. G., Koplewicz, H. S., & Kanner, A. (1992). Imipramine treatment of children with separation anxiety disorder. *Journal of the American Academy of Child and Adolescent Psychiatry, 31*, 21–28.

Klein, R. G., & Pine, D. S. (2002). Anxiety disorders. In M. Rutter, E. Taylor, & L. Hersov (Eds.), *Child and adolescent psychiatry: Modern approaches* (4th ed., pp. 486–509). London: Blackwell.

Kopp, C. B. (1989). Regulation of distresses and negative emotion: A developmental view. *Developmental Psychology, 25*, 343–354.

Kovacs, M. (1990). Comorbid anxiety disorders in childhood-onset depression. In J. D. Maser & C. R. Cloninger (Eds.), *Comorbidity of mood and anxiety disorders* (pp. 272–281). Washington, DC: American Psychiatric Press.

Kovacs, M. (1992). *Children's depression inventory*. North Tonawanda, NY: Multi-Health Systems.

Kovacs, M. (2010). *Children's depression inventory-2*. North Tonawanda, NY: Multi-Health Systems.

Kovacs, M., Gastonis, C., Paulauskas, L. L., & Richards, C. (1989). Depressive disorders in childhood: IV. A longitudinal study of comorbidity with and without risk for anxiety disorders. *Archives of General Psychiatry, 46*, 776–782.

Kraemer, H. C., Stice, E., Kazdin, A., Offord, D., & Kupfer, D. (2001). How do risk factors work together? Mediators, moderators, and independent, overlapping, and proxy risk factors. *American Journal of Psychiatry, 158*, 848–856.

Kronenberger, W. G., & Meyer, R. G. (2001). *The child clinician's handbook* (2nd ed.). Boston: Allyn & Bacon.

Lachar, D., & Gruber, C. P. (1995a). *Personality inventory for youth: Technical guide*. Lutz, FL: Psychological Assessment Resources.

Lachar, D., & Gruber, C. P. (1995b). *Personality inventory for youth: Administration and interpretation guide*. Lutz, FL: Psychological Assessment Resources.

Lachar, D., & Gruber, C. P. (2001). *Personality inventory for children-second edition*. North Tonawanda, NY: Multi-Health Systems.

Lachar, D., Wingenfeld, S. A., Kline, R. B., & Gruber, C. P. (2000). *Student behavior survey*. North Tonawanda, NY: Multi-Health Systems.

LaFreniere, P. J., & Capuano, F. (1997). Preventive intervention as means of clarifying direction of efforts in socialization: Anxious-withdrawn preschoolers' case. *Development and Psychopathology, 9*, 551–564.

LaGreca, A. M., & Harrison, M. (2005). Adolescent peer relations, friendships, and romantic relationships: Do they predict social anxiety and depression? *Journal of Clinical Child and Adolescent Psychology, 36*, 49–61.

LaGreca, A. M., & Stone, W. L. (1993). Social anxiety scale for children-revised: Factor structure and concurrent validity. *Journal of Clinical Child Psychology, 22*, 17–27.

Lapalme, M., Hodgins, S., & LaRoche, C. (1997). Children of parents with bipolar disorder: A meta-analysis of risk for mental disorders. *Canadian Journal of Psychiatry, 42*, 623–631.

Last, C. G., Hersen, M., Kazdin, A., Orvaschel, H., & Perrin, S. (1991). Anxiety disorders in children and their families. *Archives of General Psychiatry, 48*, 928–934.

Last, C. G., Perrin, S., Hersen, M., & Kazdin, A. E. (1992). DSM-III-R anxiety disorders in children: Sociodemographic and clinical characteristics. *Journal of the American Academy of Child and Adolescent Psychiatry, 31*, 1070–1076.

Last, C. G., & Strauss, C. C. (1989). Obsessive-compulsive disorder in childhood. *Journal of Anxiety Disorders, 3*, 87–95.

Last, C. G., Strauss, C. C., & Francis, G. (1987). Comorbidity among childhood anxiety disorders. *Journal of Nervous and Mental Disease, 175*, 726–730.

Laurent, J., Catanzaro, S. J., Joiner, T. E., Rudolph, K. D., Potter, K. I., Lambert, S., et al. (1999). A measure of positive and negative affect for children: Scale development and preliminary validation. *Psychological Assessment, 11*, 326–338.

LeBuffe, P. A., Shapiro, V. B., & Naglieri, J. A. (2009). *Devereux student strengths assessment*. Lewisville, NC: Kaplan Press.

Lefkowitz, M. M., & Burton, N. (1978). Childhood depression: A critique of the concept. *Psychological Bulletin, 85*, 716–726.

Leonard, H. L., Goldberger, E. L., Raporport, J. L., Cheslow, D. L., & Swedo, S. E. (1990). Childhood rituals: Normal development or obsessive compulsive symptoms? *Journal of the American Academy of Child and Adolescent Psychiatry, 29*, 17–23.

Lewinshohn, P. M. (1974). A behavioral approach to depression. In R. Friedman & M. Katz (Eds.), *The psychology of depression: Contemporary theory and research* (pp. 157–185). Washington, DC: Winston-Wiley.

Lewinshohn, P. M., Hops, H., Roberts, R. E., Seely, J. R., & Andrews, J. A. (1993). Adolescent psychopathology: I. Prevalence and incidence of depression and other DSM-III-R disorders in high school students. *Journal of Abnormal Psychology, 102*, 133–144.

Lewinshohn, P. M., Klein, D. N., & Seeley, J. R. (1995). Bipolar disorders in a community sample of older adolescents: Prevalence, phenomenology, comorbidity, and course. *Journal of the American Academy of Child and Adolescent Psychiatry, 34*, 454–463.

Lewinshohn, P. M., Steinmetz, J. L., Larson, D. W., & Franklin, J. (1981). Depression-related cognitions: Antecedent or consequence? *Journal of Abnormal Psychology, 90*, 213–219.

Lewinsohn, P. M., Clarke, G. N., Hops, H., & Andrews, J. (1990). Cognitive-behavioral group treatment of depression in adolescents. *Behavior Therapy, 21*, 385–401.

Lewinsohn, P. M., Gotlib, I. H., Lewinsohn, M., Seeley, J. R., & Allen, N. B. (1998). Gender differences in anxiety disorders and anxiety symptoms in adolescents. *Journal of Abnormal Psychology, 102*, 133–144.

Lewis, M. (1990). Models of developmental psychopathology. In M. Lewis & S. Miller (Eds.), *Handbook of developmental psychopathology* (pp. 15–28). New York: Plenum Press.

Lewis, M. (2000). Toward a development of psychopathology. In A. J. Sameroff, M. Lewis, & S. M. Miller (Eds.), *Handbook of developmental psychopathology* (2nd ed., pp. 3–22). New York: Kluwer Academic/Plenum.

Lewis, M. D., & Stieben, J. (2004). Emotion regulation in the brain: Conceptual issues and directions for developmental research. *Child Development, 75*, 371–376.

Li, H., & Zhang, Y. (2008). Factors predicting Chinese adolescents' anxieties, fears and depression. *School Psychology International, 29*, 376–384.

Liss, M., Fein, D., Allen, D., Dunn, M., Feinstein, C., Morris, R., Waterhouse, L., & Rapin, I. (2001). Executive functioning in high-functioning children with autism. *Journal of Child Psychology and Psychiatry, 42*, 261–270.

Lonigan, C. J., Carey, M., & Finch, A. J. (1994). Anxiety and depression in children: Negative affectivity and the utility of self-reports. *Journal of Consulting and Clinical Psychology, 62*, 1000–1008.

Lonigan, C. J., Elbert, J. C., & Johnson, S. B. (1998). Empirically supported psychosocial interventions for children: An overview. *Journal of Clinical Child Psychology, 27*, 138–145.

Lonigan, C. J., & Phillips, B. M. (2001). Temperamental influences on the development of anxiety disorders. In M. W. Vasey & M. R. Dadds (Eds.), *The developmental psychopathology of anxiety*. New York: Oxford University Press.

Lonigan, C. J., Vasey, M. W., Phillips, B. M., & Hazen, R. A. (2004). Temperament, anxiety, and the processing of threat-relevant stimuli. *Journal of Clinical Child and Adolescent Psychology, 33*, 8–20.

Lopez, S. R., & Guarnaccia, P. J. J. (2000). Cultural psychopathology: Uncovering the social world of mental illness. In S. T. Fiske, D. L. Schachter, & C. Zahn-Waxler (Eds.), *Annual review of psychology* (Vol. 51, pp. 571–598). Palo Alto, CA: Annual Reviews.

Lorber, M. F. (2004). Psychophysiology of aggression, psychopathy, and conduct problems: a meta-analysis. *Psychological Bulletin, 130*, 531–552.

Lovejoy, M. C., Graczyk, P. A., O'Hare, E., & Neuman, G. (2000). Maternal depression and parenting behavior: A meta-analytic review. *Clinical Psychology Review, 20*, 561–592.

Lowry-Webster, H. M., Barrett, P. M., & Dadds, M. R. (2001). A universal trial of anxiety and depressive symptomatology in childhood: Preliminary data from an Australian trial. *Behaviour Change, 18*, 36–50.

Luthar, S. S., Cichetti, D., & Becker, B. (2000). The concept of resilience: A critical evaluation and guidelines for future work. *Child Development, 71*, 543–562.

Lyon, G. R. (1996). Learning disabilities. *Special Education for Students with Disabilities, 6*, 54–76.

MacLeod, C., Rutherford, E., Campbell, L., Ebsworthy, G., & Holker, L. (2002). Selective attention and emotional vulnerability: Assessing the causal basis of their association through the manipulation of attentional bias. *Journal of Abnormal Psychology, 111*, 107–123.

Macmillan, S., Szeszko, P. R., Moore, G. J., Madden, R., Lorch, E., Ivey, J., et al. (2003). Increased amygdala/hippocampal volume ratio associated with severity of anxiety in pediatric major depression. *Journal of Child and Adolescent Psychopharmacology, 13*, 65–73.

Maggini, C., Ampollini, P., Garibaldi, S., Cella, P. L., Peqlizza, L., & Marchesi, C. (2001). The Parma high school epidemiological survey: Obsessive compulsive symptoms. *Acta Psychiatrica Scandinavia, 103*, 441–446.

Malcarne, V. L., & Hansdottir, I. (2001). Vulnerability to anxiety disorders in childhood and adolescence. In R. E. Ingram & J. M. Price (Eds.), *Vulnerability to psychopathology: Risk across the lifespan* (pp. 271–303). New York: Guilford.

Malecki, C. K., & Elliott, S. N. (2002). Children's social behaviors as predictors of academic achievement: A longitudinal analysis. *School Psychology Quarterly, 17*, 1–23.

March, J. S. (1997). *Multidimensional anxiety scale for children*. San Antonio, TX: Pearson Education.

March, J. S., Biederman, J., Wolkow, R., Safferman, A., Mardekian, J., Cook, E. H., et al. (1998). Sertraline in children and adolescents with obsessive-compulsive disorder: A multicenter randomized controlled trial. *Journal of the American Medical Association, 280*, 1752–1756.

March, J. S., & Mulle, K. (1998). *OCD in children and adolescents*. New York: Guilford.

Mars Area School District v. Laurie L., 827 A. 2d 1249 (Pa. Cmwlth, 2003).

Martell, C. R., Addis, M. E., & Jacobson, N. S. (2001). *Depression in context: Strategies for guided action*. New York: W. W. Norton.

Mash, E. J., & Dozois, D. J. A. (2003). In E. J. Mash & R. A. Barkley (Eds.), *Child psychopathology* (2nd ed.), (pp. 3–71). New York: Guilford.

Masi, G., Favilla, L., Mucci, M., & Millepiedi, S. (2000). Depressive comorbidity in children and adolescents with generalized anxiety disorder. *Child Psychiatry and Human Development, 30*, 305–315.

Mataix-Coles, D., Rauch, S. L., Manzo, P. A., Jenike, M. A., & Baer, L. (1999). Use of factor analyzed symptom dimensions to predict outcome with serotonin reuptake inhibitors and placebo in the treatment of obsessive-compulsive disorders. *American Journal of Psychiatry, 156*, 1409–1416.

Maughan, A., & Cichetti, D. (2002). Impact of child maltreatment and interadult violence on children's emotion regulation abilities and socioemotional adjustment. *Child Development, 73*, 1525–1542.

Mayo Clinic. (2008). *Anxiety treatment and drugs*. Available at http://www.mayoclinic.com/health/anxiety/DS01187/DSECTION=treatments-and-drugs.

McClure, E. B., & Pine, D. S. (2006). Social anxiety and emotion regulation: A model for developmental psychopathology perspectives on anxiety disorders. In D. Cichetti & D. J. Cohen (Eds.), *Developmental psychopathology (2nd ed.), Vol. 3: Risk, disorder, and adaptation* (pp. 470–502). New York: Wiley.

McConaughey, S. H., & Achenbach, T. M. (2001). *Structured clinical interview for children and adolescents. (SCICA)*. Burlington, VT: University of Vermont, Research Center for Children, Youth, & Families.

McGee, R., Feehan, M., Williams, S., & Anderson, J. (1992). DSM-III disorders from age 11 to age 15 years. *Journal of the American Academy of Child and Adolescent Psychiatry, 29*, 611–619.

Meichenbaum, D. (1977). *Cognitive-behavior modification: An integrative approach*. New York: Plenum.

Mellings, T. M. B., & Alden, L. E. (2000). Cognitive processes in social anxiety: The effects of self-focus, rumination, and anticipatory processing. *Behaviour Research and Therapy, 38*, 243–257.

Mendelson, T., Rehkopf, D. H., & Kuzbansky, L. D. (2008). Depression among Latinos in the United States: A meta-analytic review. *Journal of Consulting and Clinical Psychology, 76*, 355–366.

Mendenhall, A. N., Fristad, M. A., & Early, T. J. (2009). Factors influencing service utilization and mood symptom severity in children with mood disorders: Effects of Multi-Family Psychoeducation Groups (MFPG). *Journal of Consulting and Clinical Psychology, 77*, 463–473.

Menutti, R. B., Christner, R. W., & Freeman, A. (2006). An introduction to a school-based cognitive-behavioral framework. In R. B. Menutti, A. Freeman, & R. W. Christner (Eds.), *Cognitive-behavioral interventions in educational settings: A handbook for practice* (pp. 3–19). New York: Routledge.

Merrell, K. W. (2003). *Behavioral, social, and emotional assessment of children and adolescents* (2nd ed.). Mahwah, NJ: Erlbaum.

Merrell, K. W., Carrizales, D., Feuerborn, L., Gueldner, B. A., & Tran, O. K. (2007). *Strong kids: A social and emotional learning curriculum.* Baltimore: Brookes.

Merrell, K. W., & Gueldner, B. A. (2010). Preventive interventions for students with internalizing disorders: Effective strategies for promoting mental health in schools. In H. M. Walker & M. R. Shinn (Eds.), *Interventions for achievement and behavior problems in a three-tier model including RTI* (pp. 799–823). Bethesda, MD: National Association of School Psychologists.

Merrell, K. W., & Walters, A. S. (1998). *Internalizing symptoms scale for children.* Austin, TX: PRO-ED.

Merry, S., McDowell, H., Hetrick, S., Bir, J., & Muller, N. (2004) Psychological and/or educational interventions for the prevention of depression in children and adolescents. (Cochrane Review). *The cochrane library* (Issue 2). Chichester, UK: Wiley.

Mesquita, B., & Albert, D. (2007). The cultural regulation of emotion. In J. J. Gross (Ed.), *Handbook of emotion regulation* (pp. 486–503). New York: Guilford.

Messick, S. (1983). Assessment of children. In P. H. Mussen (Series Ed.) & W. Kessen (Vol. Ed), *Handbook of child psychology: Vol. 1. History, theory, and methods* (4th ed.), (pp. 477–425). New York: Wiley.

Meyer, S. E., Chrousos, G. P., & Gold, P. W. (2001). Major depression and the stress system: A life span perspective. *Development and Psychopathology, 13,* 565–580.

Miklowitz, D. J., & Scott, J. (2009). Psychosocial treatments for bipolar disorder: Cost-effectiveness, mediating mechanisms, and future directions. *Bipolar Disorders, 11*(Suppl 2), 110–122.

Mineka, S., Watson, D. W., & Clark, L. A. (1998). Psychopathology: Comorbidity of anxiety and unipolar mood disorders. *Annual Review of Psychology, 49,* 377–412.

Moreau, D. L., & Follet, C. (1993). Panic disorders in children and adolescents. *Child and Adolescent Clinics of North America, 2,* 581–602.

Moskos, M., Olson, L., Halbern, S., Keller, T., & Gray, D. (2005). Utah youth suicide survey: Psychological autopsy. *Suicide and Life-Threatening Behavior, 35,* 536–546.

Mr. I. v. Maine School Administrative Dist. No. 55, 480 F.3d 1 (1st Cir. 2007).

Mufson, L., Dorta, K. P., Moreau, D., & Weissman, M. M. (2004). *Interpersonal psychotherapy for depressed adolescents* (2nd ed.). New York: Guilford.

Mufson, L., Dorta, K. P., Wickramartne, P., Nomura, Y., Olfson, M., & Weissman, M. M. (2004). A randomized effectiveness trial of interpersonal psychotherapy for depressed adolescents. *Archives of General Psychiatry, 63,* 577–584.

Mufson, L., Gallagher, T., Dorta, K. P., & Young, J. F. (2004). Interpersonal psychotherapy for adolescent depression: Adaptation for group therapy. *American Journal of Psychotherapy, 58,* 220–237.

Mufson, L., Moreau, D., Weissman, M. M., Wickramartne, P., Martin, J., & Samoilov, A. (1994). The modification of interpersonal psychotherapy with depressed adolescents ITP-A: Phase I and phase II studies. *Journal of the American Academy of Child and Adolescent Psychiatry, 33,* 695–705.

Mufson, L., Weissman, M. M., Moreau, D., & Garfinkel, R. (1999). Efficacy of interpersonal psychotherapy for depressed adolescents. *Archives of General Psychiatry, 56,* 573–579.

Muirs, P., Meesters, C., Merckelbach, H., Sermon, A., & Zwakhalen, S. (1998). Worry in normal children. *Journal of the American Academy of Child and Adolescent Psychiatry, 37,* 703–710.

Muris, P., Merkelbach, H., Gadet, B., & Moulaert, V. (2000). Fear, worries, and scary dreams in 4- to 12-year old children: Their content, developmental pattern, and origins. *Journal of Clinical Child Psychology, 29,* 43–52.

Nation, M., Crusto, C., Wandersman, A., Kumpfer, K. L., Seybolt, D., Morrissey-Kane, E., & Davino, K. (2003). What works in prevention: Principles of effective intervention programs. *American Psychologist, 58*, 449–456.

National Institute of Mental Health (NIMH). (n. d.) *Anxiety disorders*. Bethesda, MD: National Institute of Mental Health. (Available online at http://www.nimh.nih.gov/health/publications/anxiety-disorders/nimhanxiety.pdf)

National Institute of Mental Health (NIMH). (1998). *Priorities for prevention research at NIMH: A report by the National Advocacy Mental Health Council Workgroup on Mental Disorders Prevention Research*. Bethesda, MD: National Institute of Mental Health.

National Institute of Mental Health (NIMH). (2001). *National advisory mental health council workshop on mental disorders prevention research: Priorities for prevention research at NIMH*. Available at http://www.journals.apa.org/prevention/volume4/pre040017a.html.

Nelson, E. C., Grant, J. D., Bucholz, K. K., Glowinski, A., Madden, P. A. F., Reich, W., & Heath, A. C. (2000). Social phobia in a population-based female adolescent twin sample: Comorbidity and associated suicide-related symptoms. *Psychological Medicine, 30*, 797–804.

Newman, D. L., Moffit, T. E., Caspi, A., & Magdol, L. (1996). Psychiatric disorder in a birth cohort of young adults: Prevalence, comorbidity, clinical significance, and new case incidence from ages 11-21. *Journal of Consulting and Clinical Psychology, 64*, 552–562.

Nielson, T. A., Laberge, L., Paquet, J., Tremblay, R. E., Vitaro, F., & Montplasir, J. (2000). Development of disturbing dreams during adolescence and their relation to anxiety symptoms. *Sleep, 23*, 727–736.

Nolen-Hoeksema, S. (2000). The role of rumination in depressive disorders and mixed anxiety/depressive symptoms. *Journal of Abnormal Psychology, 109*, 504–511.

Nolen-Hoeksema, S., Girgus, J. S., & Seligman, M. E. P. (1992). Predictors and consequences of childhood depressive symptoms: A 5-year longitudinal study. *Journal of Abnormal Psychology, 101*, 405–422.

Ochsner, K. N., Bunge, S. A., Gross, J. J., & Gabrieli, J. D. E. (2002). Rethinking feelings: An fMRI study of the cognitive regulation of emotion. *Journal of Cognitive Neuroscience, 14*, 1215–1229.

Office of Special Education Programs. (2010). *What is school-wide positive behavioral interventions and supports?* Washington, DC: Technical Assistance Center on Positive Behavioral Interventions and Supports. (http://www.pbis.org/school/what_is_swpbs.aspx).

Offord, D. R., Boyle, M. H., Racine, Y. A., Fleming, J. E., Cadman, D. T., Blum, H. M., Bryne, C., Links, P. S., Lipman, E. L., MacMillan, H. L., Grant, N. I. R., Sanford, M. N., Szatmari, P., Thomas, H., & Woodward, C. A. (1992). Outcome, prognosis, and risk in a longitudinal follow-up study. *Journal of the American Academy of Child and Adolescent Psychiatry, 31*, 916–923.

Ollendick, T. H. (1983). Reliability and validity of the fear survey schedule for children-revised (FSSC-R). *Behaivour Research and Therapy, 32*, 635–638.

Ollendick, T. H. (1995). Cognitive behavioral treatments of panic disorder with agoraphobia in adolescents: A multiple baseline design analysis. *Behavior Therapy, 26*, 517–532.

Ollendick, T. H., & King, N. J. (2000). Empirically supported treatments for children and adolescents. In P. C. Kendall (Ed.), *Child and adolescent therapy* (pp. 386–425). New York: Guilford.

Ollendick, T. H., King, N. J., & Chorpita, B. F. (2006). Empirically supported treatments for children and adolescents: The movement to evidence-based practice. In P. C. Kendall (Ed.), *Child and adolescent therapy: Cognitive-behavioral procedures* (3rd ed., pp. 492–520). New York: Guilford.

Ollendick, T. H., Mattis, S. G., & King, N. J. (1994). Panic disorder in children and adolescents: A review. *Journal of Child Psychology and Psychiatry, 35*, 113–134.

Ollendick, T. H., Yang, R., King, N. J., Dong, Q., & Akande, A. (1996). Fears in American, Australian, Chinese, and Nigerian children and adolescents: A cross-cultural study. *Journal of Child Psychology and Psychiatry, 37*, 213–220.

Patterson, G. R., & Stoolmiller, M. (1991). Replications of a dual failure model for boys' depressed mood. *Journal of Consulting and Clinical Psychology, 59*, 491–498.

Pawlak, C., Pascual-Sanchez, T., Rae, P., Fischer, W., & Ladame, F. (1999). Anxiety disorders, comorbidity, and suicide attempts in adolescence: A preliminary investigation. *European Psychiatry, 14*, 132–136.

Payne, A. P., & Eckert, R. (2010). The importance of provider, program, school, and community predictors of the implementation quality of school-based prevention programs. *Prevention Science, 11*, 126–141.

Pennington, B. F. (2002). *The development of psychopathology.* New York: Guilford.

Perrin, S., & Last, C. G. (1997). Worrisome thoughts in children referred for anxiety disorder. *Journal of Clinical Child Psychology, 26*, 181–189.

Pfeffer, C. R., Klerman, G. L., Hurt, S. W., Kakuma, T., Peskin, J. R., & Siefker, C. A. (1993). Suicidal children grow up: Rates and psychosocial risk factors for suicide attempts during follow-up. *Journal of the American Academy of Child and Adolescent Psychiatry, 38*, 106–113.

Phillips, L., Bull, R., Adams, F., & Fraser, L. (2002). Positive mood and executive function: Evidence from Stroop and fluency tasks. *Emotion, 2*, 12–22.

Pianta, R., Steinberg, M., & Rollins, K. (1995). The first two years of school: Teacher-child relationships and deflections in children's classroom adjustment. *Development and Psychopathology, 7*, 295–212.

Piers, E. V., Harris, D. B., & Herzberg, D. S. (2002). *Piers-Harris self-concept scale for children* (2nd ed.). Los Angeles, CA: Western Psychological Services.

Pincus, D. B., & Friedman, A. G. (2004). Improving children's coping with everyday stress: Transporting treatment interventions to the school setting. *Clinical Child and Family Psychology Review, 7*, 223–240.

Pine, D. S., Cohen, E., Cohen, P., & Brook, J. S. (2000). Social phobia and the persistence of conduct problems. *Journal of Child Psychology and Psychiatry, 41*, 657–665.

Pine, D. S., Cohen, P., Gurley, D., Brook, J., & Ma, Y. (1998). The risk for early-adulthood anxiety and depressive disorders in adolescents with anxiety and depressive disorders. *Archives of General Psychiatry, 55*, 56–64.

Pine, D. S., & Grun, J. S. (1999). Childhood anxiety: Integrating developmental psychopathology and affective neuroscience. *Journal of Child and Adolescent Psychopharmacology, 9*, 1–11.

Plutchik, R. (1980). *Emotion: A psychoevolutionary synthesis.* New York: Harper & Row.

Pössel, P., Horn, A. B., Green, G., & Hautzinger, M. (2004). School-based prevention of depression symptoms in adolescents: A 6-month follow-up. *Journal of the American Academy of Child and Adolescent Psychiatry, 43*, 1003–1010.

Poznanski, E. O., & Mokros, H. B. (1996). *Children's depression rating scale-revised.* Los Angeles, CA: Western Psychological Services.

Prinstein, M. J., Boergers, J., & Vernberg, E. M. (2001). Overt and relational aggression in adolescents: Social-psychological adjustment of aggressors and victims. *Journal of Clinical Child Psychology, 30*, 479–491.

Puig-Antich, J., & Chambers, W. (1978). *The schedule for affective disorders and schizophrenia for school-age children.* New York: New York State Psychiatric Association.

Rapee, R. M. (2002). The development and modification of temperamental risk for anxiety disorders: Prevention of a lifetime of anxiety. *Biological Psychiatry, 52*, 947–957.

Rashid, T., & Anjum, A. (2008). Positive psychotherapy for young adults and children. In J. R. Z. Abela & L. Hankin (Eds.), *Handbook of depression in children and adolescents* (pp. 250–287). New York: Guilford.

Rathus, J. H., & Miller, A. I. (2002). Dialectical behavior therapy adapted for suicidal adolescents. *Suicide and Life-Threatening Behavior, 32*, 146–157.

Reddy, L. A., Newman, E., De Thomas, C. A., & Chun, V. (2009). Effectiveness of school-based prevention and intervention programs for children and adolescents with emotional disturbance: A meta-analysis. *Journal of School Psychology, 47*, 77–99.

Reich, W., Welner, A., & Herjanic, B. (1997). *Diagnostic interview for children and adolescents-IV.* North Tonawanda, NY: Multi-Health Systems.

Reinecke, M. A., Datillio, F. M., & Freeman, A. (2006). *Cognitive therapy with children and adolescents* (2nd ed.). New York: Guilford.

Research Units of Pediatric Psychopharmacology (RUPP) Anxiety Group. (2001). Fluvoxamine for the treatment of anxiety disorders in children and adolescents. *New England Journal of Medicine, 344*, 1279–1285.

Research Units of Pediatric Psychopharmacology (RUPP) Anxiety Group. (2003). Searching for moderators and mediators of pharmacological treatment effects in children and adolescents with anxiety disorders. *Journal of the American Academy of Child and Adolescent Psychiatry, 42*, 13–21.

Reynolds, W. M. (1987). *Suicidal ideation questionnaire-junior*. Odessa, FL: Psychological Assessment Resources.

Reynolds, W. M. (1988). *Suicidal ideation questionnaire*. Odessa, FL: Psychological Assessment Resources.

Reynolds, W. M. (1989). *Reynolds adolescent depression scale: Professional manual*. Odessa, FL: Psychological Assessment Resources.

Reynolds, W. M. (1998). *Adolescent psychopathology scale*. Lutz, FL: Psychological Assessment Resources.

Reynolds, W. M. (2000). *Adolescent psychopathology scale-short form*. Lutz, FL: Psychological Assessment Resources.

Reynolds, W. M. (2002). *Reynolds adolescent depression scale-2*. Lutz, FL: Psychological Assessment Resources.

Reynolds, W. M. (2010). *Reynolds child depression scale-2*. Lutz, FL: Psychological Assessment Resources.

Reynolds, C. R., & Kamphaus, R. W. (2004). *Behavior assessment system for children-2*. Bloomington, MN: Pearson Assessments.

Reynolds, W. M., & Mazza, J. M. (1999). Assessment of suicidal ideation among inner-city children and young adolescents: Reliability and validity of the suicidal ideation questionnaire-JR. *School Psychology Review, 28*, 17–30.

Reynolds, C. R., & Richmond, B. O. (1985). *Revised children's manifest anxiety scale*. Los Angeles, CA: Western Psychological Services.

Reynolds, C. R., & Richmond, B. O. (2008). *Revised children's manifest anxiety scale-2*. Los Angeles, CA: Western Psychological Services.

Rhoades, M. M., & Kratochwill, T. R. (1992). Teacher reactions to behavioral consultation: An analysis of language and involvement. *School Psychology Quarterly, 7*, 47–59.

Rice, F., Harold, G. T., & Thapar, A. (2002). Assessing the effects of age, sex and shared environment on the genetic etiology of depression in childhood and adolescence. *Journal of Child Psychology and Psychiatry and Allied Disciplines, 43*, 1039–1051.

Richters, J. E., & Cichetti, D. (1993). Mark Twain meets DSM-III-R: Conduct disorder, development, and the concept of harmful dysfunction. *Development and Psychopathology, 5*, 5–29.

Riddle, M., Reeve, E., Varyura-Tobias, J., Yang, H. M., Claghorn, J. L., Gaffney, G., et al. (2001). Fluvoxamine for children and adolescents with obsessive-compulsive disorder: A randomized controlled multicenter trial. *Journal of the American Academy of Child and Adolescent Psychiatry, 40*, 222–229.

Roberts, C., Kane, R., Bishop, B., Matthews, H., & Thompson, H. (2004). The prevention of depressive symptoms in rural children: A follow-up study. *International Journal of Mental Health Prevention, 6*, 4–16.

Roberts, J., & Monroe, S. M. (1994). A multidimensional model of self-esteem in depression. *Clinical Psychology Review, 14*, 161–181.

Roberts, R. E., Roberts, C. R., & Chen, Y. R. (1997). Ethnocultural differences in prevalence of adolescent depression. *Journal of Community Psychology, 25*, 95–110.

Robinson, J. L., Kagan, J., Reznick, J. S., & Corley, R. (1992). The heritability of inhibited and uninhibited behavior: A twin study. *Developmental Psychology, 28*, 1030–1037.

Rohde, P., Lewinshohn, P. M., & Seely, J. R. (1994). Are adolescents changed by an episode of major depression? *Journal of the American Academy of Child and Adolescent Psychiatry, 33*, 1289–1298.

Rose, D. T., & Abramson, L. Y. (1992). Developmental predictors of depressive cognitive style: Research and theory. In D. Cichetti & S. L. Toth (Eds.), *Rochester symposium on developmental psychopathology* (Vol. 4, pp. 323–349). Rochester, NY: University of Rochester Press.

Rosselló, J., & Bernal, G. (1999). The efficacy of cognitive-behavioral and interpersonal treatments for depression in Puerto Rican adolescents. *Journal of Consulting and Clinical Psychology, 67*, 734–745.

Roth, J. L., & Brooks-Gunn, J. (2003). Youth development programs: Risk, development, and policy. *Journal of Research on Adolescence, 8*, 423–459.

Roth, J. L., Brooks-Gunn, J., Murray, I., & Foster, W. (1998). Promoting healthy adolescents: Synthesis of youth development program evaluations. *Journal of Adolescent Health, 32*, 170–182.

Rothbart, M. K., & Bates, J. E. (2006). Temperament. In N. Eisenberg & W. Damon (Eds.), *Handbook of child psychology, Vol. 3, Social, emotional, and personality development* (6th ed.), (pp. 99–166). New York: Wiley.

Rothbart, M. K., Posner, M. I., & Hershey, K. (1995). Temperament, attention, and developmental psychopathology. In D. Cichetti & J. D. Cohen (Eds.), *Handbook of developmental psychopathology* (Vol. 1), (pp. 315–340). New York: Wiley.

Rudolph, K. D. (2002). Gender differences in emotional responses to interpersonal stress during adolescence. *Journal of Adolescent Health, 30*, 3–13.

Rudolph, K. D., & Clark, A. G. (2001). Conceptions of relationships in children with depressive and aggressive symptoms: Social-cognitive distortion or reality? *Journal of Abnormal Child Psychology, 29*, 41–56.

Rudolph, K. D., & Hammen, C. (1999). Age and gender as determinants of stress exposure, generation, and reactions in youngsters; A transactional perspective. *Child Development, 70*, 660–677.

Rudolph, K. D., Hammen, C., & Burge, D. (1994). Interpersonal functioning and depressive symptoms in childhood: Addressing the issues of specificity and comorbidity. *Journal of Abnormal Child Psychology, 22*, 355–371.

Rudolph, K. D., Kurlakowsky, K. D., & Conley, C. S. (2001). Developmental and social-emotional origins of depressive control-related beliefs and behavior. *Cognitive Therapy and Research, 25*, 447–475.

Rutter, M. (1989). Psychosocial risk trajectories and beneficial starting points. In S. Doxiadis & S. Stewart (Eds.), *Early influences shaping the individual* (pp. 220–239). New York: Plenum Press.

Rutter, M. (1990). Psychosocial resilience and protective mechanisms. In J. E. Rolf, A. S. Masten, D. Cichetti, K. H. Nuechterlein, & S. Weintraub (Eds.), *Risk and protective factors in the development of psychopathology* (pp. 181–214). New York: Cambridge University Press.

Rutter, M., MacDonald, H., LeCouteur, A., Harrington, R., Bolton, P., & Bailey, A. (1990). Genetic factors in child psychiatric disorders-II. Empirical findings. *Journal of Child Psychology and Psychiatry, 31*, 39–83.

Ryan, N. D. (2003). Medication treatment. *CNS Spectrums, 8*, 283–287.

Ryff, C. D., & Keyes, C. I. M. (1995). The structure of psychological well-being revisited. *Journal of Personality and Social Psychology, 69*, 719–727.

Ryff, C. D., & Singer, B. (2002). From social structure to biology: Integrative science to pursuit of human health and well-being. In C. R. Snyder & S. J. Lopez (Eds.), *Handbook of positive psychology* (pp. 541–555). New York: Oxford University Press.

Rynn, M. A., Siqueland, L., & Rickels, K. (2001). Placebo-controlled trail of sertraline in the treatment of children with generalized anxiety disorder. *American Journal of Psychiatry, 158*, 2008–2014.

Sattler, J. M., & Hoge, R. D. (2008). *Assessment of children: Behavioral, social, and clinical foundations* (5th ed.). San Diego, CA: Sattler Publishing.

Schmidt, N. B., & Lerew, D. R. (2002). Prospective evaluation of perceived control, predictability, and anxiety sensitivity in the pathogenesis of panic. *Journal of Psychopathology and Behavioral Assessment, 24*, 207–214.

Schmidt, N. B., Lerew, D. R., & Jackson, R. J. (1997). The role of anxiety sensitivity in the pathogenesis of panic: Prospective evaluation of spontaneous panic attacks during acute stress. *Journal of Abnormal Psychology, 106*, 355–364.

Schulte, A. C., & Osborne, S. S. (2003). When assumptive worlds collide: A review of definitions of collaboration in consultation. *Journal of Educational and Psychological Consultation, 14*, 109–138.

Schwartz, D., Gorman, A. H., Duong, M. T., & Nakamoto, J. (2008). Peer relationships and academic achievement as interacting predictors of depressive symptoms during middle childhood. *Journal of Abnormal Psychology, 117*, 289–299.

Schwartz, C. E., Wright, C. I., Shin, L. M., Kagan, J., & Rauch, S. L. (2003). Inhibited and uninhibited infants grown up: Adult amygdalar response to novelty. *Science, 300*, 1952–1953.

Section 504 of the Rehabilitation Act of 1973, 29 U.S.C. § 794.

Seely, J. R., Rohde, P., & Jones, L. B. (2010). School-based prevention and intervention for depression and suicidal behavior. In M. R. Shinn & H. M. Walker (Eds.), *Interventions for achievement and behavior problems in a three-tier model including RTI* (pp. 363–396). Bethesda, MD: National Association of School Psychologists.

Seligman, M. E. P. (1975). *Helplessness: On depression, development, and death*. San Francisco: Freeman.

Seligman, M. E. P. (1998). The American way of blame. *APA Monitor, 29(7)*, 3. Washington, DC: American Psychological Association.

Seligman, M. E. P. (2002). *Authentic happiness: Using the new positive psychology to realize your potential for lasting fulfillment*. New York: Free Press.

Seligman, M. E. P., Berkowitz, M. W., Catalano, R. F., Damon, W., Eccles, J. S., Gillham, J. E., et al. (2005). The positive perspective on youth development. In D. L. Evans, E. B. Foa, R. E. Gur, H. Hendin, C. P. O'Brien, M. E. P. Seligman, et al. (Eds.), *Treating and preventing adolescent mental health disorders: What we know and what we don't know* (pp. 498–527). Oxford, UK: Oxford University Press.

Shaffer, D., Fisher, P., Lucas, C. P., Dulcan, M. K., & Schwab-Stone, M. E. (2000). NIMH diagnostic interview schedule for children version IV (NIMH DISC-IV): Description, differences from previous versions, and reliability of some common diagnoses. *Journal of the American Academy of Child and Adolescent Psychiatry, 39*, 28–38.

Shaffer, D., Garland, A., Vieland, V., Underwood, M., & Busner, C. (1991). The impact of curriculum-based suicide prevention programs for teenagers. *Journal of the American Academy of Child and Adolescent Psychiatry, 30*, 588–596.

Shaffer, D., Gould, M. S., Fisher, P., Trautman, P., Moreau, D., Kleinman, M., et al. (1996). Psychiatric diagnosis in child and adolescent suicide. *Archives of General Psychiatry, 53*, 339–348.

Shaffer, D., Lucas, C. P., & Richters, J. E. (Eds.). (1999). *Diagnostic assessment in child and adolescent psychopathology*. New York: Guilford.

Shaffer, D., & Pfeffer, C. R. (2001). Practice parameters for the assessment and treatment of children and adolescents with suicidal behavior. *Journal of the American Academy of Child and Adolescent Psychiatry, 40*(Suppl), 45S–23S.

Shaffer, D., Vieland, V., Garland, A., Rojas, M., Underwood, M., & Busner, C. (1990). Adolescent suicide attempters: Response to suicide prevention programs. *Journal of the American Medical Association, 264*, 3151–3155.

Shankman, S. A., Klein, D. N., Torpey, D. C., Olino, T. M., Dyson, M. W., Kim, J., et al. (2011). Do positive and negative temperament traits interact in predicting risk for depression? A resting EEG study of 329 preschoolers. *Development and Psychopathology, 23*, 551–562.

Shannon, K. E., Beauchaine, T. P., Brenner, S. L., Neuhaus, E., & Gatzke-Kopp, L. (2007). Familial and temperamental predictors of resilience in children at risk for conduct disorder and depression. *Development and Psychopathology, 19*, 701–727.

Sheeber, L., Hops, H., Alpert, A., Davis, B., & Andrews, J. A. (1997). Family support and conflict: Prospective relations in adolescent depression. *Journal of Abnormal Child Psychology, 25,* 333–344.

Sheffield, J., Spence, S. H., Rapee, R. M., Kowalenko, N., Wginall, A., Davis, A., et al. (2006). Comparison of universal, indicated, and combined universal plus indicated approaches to the prevention of depression among adolescents. *Journal of Consulting and Clinical Psychology, 74,* 66–79.

Shochet, I. M., & Ham, D. (2004). Universal school-based approaches to preventing adolescent depression: Past findings and future directions of the resourceful adolescent program. *International Journal of Mental Health Promotion, 6,* 17–25.

Silberg, J., Pickles, A., Rutter, M., Hewitt, J., Simonoff, E., Maes, H., Carbonneau, R., Murrelle, L., Foley, D., & Eaves, L. (1999). The influence of genetic factors and life stress on depression among adolescent girls. *Archives of General Psychiatry, 56,* 225–232.

Silk, J. S., Nath, S. R., Siegel, I. R., & Kendall, P. C. (2000). Conceptualizing mental disorders in children: Where have we been and where are we going? *Development and Psychopathology, 12,* 712–735.

Silverman, W. K., & Albano, A. M. (1996a). *Anxiety disorders interview schedule for DSM-IV—child version: Parent interview schedule.* New York: Oxford University Press.

Silverman, W. K., & Albano, A. M. (1996b). *Anxiety disorders interview schedule for DSM-IV—child version: Child interview schedule.* New York: Oxford University Press.

Silverman, W. K., Flesig, W., Rabian, B., & Peterson, R. A. (1991). Childhood anxiety sensitivity index. *Journal of Clinical Child Psychology, 20,* 162–168.

Silverman, W. K., & Ginsburg, G. S. (1995). Specific phobias and generalized anxiety disorder. In J. S. March (Ed.), *Anxiety disorders in children and adolescents* (pp. 151–180). New York: Guilford.

Simons, A. D., Rohde, P., Kennard, B. D., & Robins, M. (2005). Relapse and recurrence prevention in the treatment for adolescents with depression study. *Cognitive and Behavioral Practice, 12,* 240–251.

Slenkovich, J. (1992a). Can the language "social maladjustment" in the SED definition be ignored? *School Psychology Review, 21,* 21–22.

Slenkovich, J. (1992b). Can the language "social maladjustment" in the SED definition be ignored? The final words. *School Psychology Review, 21,* 43–44.

Smith, P., Perrin, S., Yule, W., & Rabe-Hesketh, S. (2001). War exposure and maternal reactions in the psychological adjustment of children from Bosnia-Herzegovina. *Journal of Child Psychology and Psychiatry, 42,* 395–404.

Sommers-Flanagan, J., & Campbell, D. G. (2009). Psychotherapy and (or) medications for depression in youth? An evidence-based review with recommendations for treatment. *Journal of Contemporary Psychotherapy, 39,* 111–120.

Sonntag, H., Wittchen, H. U., Hofler, M., Kessler, R. C., & Stein, M. B. (2000). Are social fears and DSM-IV social anxiety disorder associated with smoking and nicotine dependence in adolescents in adolescents and young adults? *European Psychiatry, 15,* 67–74.

Sonuga-Barke, E. J. S. (1998). Categorical models of childhood disorder: A conceptual and empirical analysis. *Journal of Clinical Child and Adolescent Psychology, 39,* 115–133.

Southam-Gerow, M. A., Kendall, P. C., & Weersing, V. R. (2001). Examining outcome variability: Correlates of treatment response in a child and adolescent anxiety clinic. *Journal of Clinical Child Psychology, 30,* 422–436.

Spell, A. W., Kelley, M. L., Wang, J., Self-Brown, S., Davidson, K. L., et al. (2008). The moderating effects of maternal psychopathology on children's adjustment post-Hurricane Katrina. *Journal of Clinical Child and Adolescent Psychology, 37,* 553–563.

Spence, S. H. (1998). A measure of anxiety symptoms among children. *Behavior Research and Therapy, 36,* 545–566.

Spence, S. H., Burns, J., Boucher, S., Glover, S., Graetz, B., Kay, D., et al. (2005). The *beyondblue* schools research initiative: Conceptual framework and intervention. *Australasian Psychiatry, 13,* 159–164.

Spence, S. H., Rapee, R., McDonald, C., & Ingram, M. (2001). The structure of anxiety symptoms among preschoolers. *Behavior Research and Therapy, 39*, 1293–1316.

Spence, S. H., Sheffield, J., & Donovan, C. L. (2003). Preventing adolescent depression: An evaluation of the problem solving for life program. *Journal of Consulting and Clinical Psychology, 71*, 3–13.

Spence, S. H., Sheffield, J., & Donovan, C. L. (2005). Long-term outcome of a school-based universal approach to prevention of depression in adolescents. *Journal of Consulting and Clinical Psychology, 73*, 160–167.

Spence, S. H., & Shortt, A. L. (2007). Can we justify the widespread dissemination of universal, school-based interventions for the prevention of depression among children and adolescents? *Journal of Child Psychology and Psychiatry, 48*, 526–542.

Spielberger, C. (1973). *State-trait anxiety inventory for children.* Palo Alto, CA: Consulting Psychologists Press.

Sroufe, L. A. (1997). Psychopathology as an outcome of development. *Development and Psychopathology, 9*, 251–268.

Sroufe, L. A., Carlson, E. A., Levy, A. K., & Egeland, B. (1999). Implications of attachment theory for developmental psychopathology. *Development and Psychopathology, 11*, 1–13.

Stark, K. D., & Kendall, P. C. (1996). *Taking action workbook.* Ardmore, PA: Workbook Publishing.

Stein, M. B., Fuetsch, M., Muller, N., Hofler, M., Lieb, R., & Wittchen, H. U. (2001). Social anxiety disorder and the risk of depression: A prospective community study of adolescents and young adults. *Archives of General Psychiatry, 59*, 251–256.

Stein, J. A., Newcomb, M. D., & Bentler, P. M. (1986). Stability and change in personality: A longitudinal study from early adolescence to young adulthood. *Journal of Research in Personality, 20*, 276–291.

Steketee, G., Chambless, D. L., & Tran, G. Q. (2001). Effects of axis I and axis II comorbidity on behavior therapy outcomes for obsessive compulsive disorder and agoraphobia. *Comprehensive Psychiatry, 42*, 76–86.

Stice, E., Rohde, P., Gau, J. M., & Wade, E. (2010). Efficacy trial of a brief cognitive-behavioral depression prevention program for high risk adolescents: Effects at 1- and 2-year follow-up. *Journal of Consulting and Clinical Psychology, 78*, 856–867.

Stice, E., Shaw, H., Bohon, C., Marti, C., & Rohde, P. (2009). A meta-analytic review of depression prevention programs for children and adolescents: Factors that predict magnitude of intervention effects. *Journal of Consulting and Clinical Psychology, 77*, 486–503.

Strack, F., Schwarz, N., Bless, H., & Kuebler, A. (1993). Awareness of the influence of culture as a determinant of assimilation versus contrast. *European Journal of Social Psychology, 23*, 55–62.

Strauss, C. C., & Last, C. G. (1993). Social and simple phobias in children. *Journal of Anxiety Disorders, 7*, 141–152.

Strauss, C. C., Lease, C. A., Last, C. G., & Francis, G. (1988). Overanxious disorder: An examination of developmental differences. *Journal of Abnormal Child Psychology, 16*, 433–443.

Street, H., Nathan, P., Durkin, K., Morling, J., Dhazari, M. A., Carson, J., & Durkin, E. (2004). Understanding the relationships between well-being, goal-setting, and depression in children. *Australian Journal of Psychiatry, 38*, 155–161.

Sugai, G., & Horner, R. H. (2006). A promising approach for expanding and sustaining school-wide positive behavior support. *School Psychology Review, 33*, 245–259.

Sullivan, P. F., Neal, M. C., & Kendler, K. S. (2000). Genetic epidemiology of major depression: Review and meta-analysis. *American Journal of Psychiatry, 157*, 1552–1562.

Summerfelt, L. J., Richter, M. A., Antony, M. M., & Swinsion, R. P. (1999). Symptom structure in obsessive-compulsive disorder: A confirmatory factor analytic study. *Behaviour Research and Therapy, 37*, 297–311.

Swedo, S. E. (1994). Sydenham's chorea: A model for childhood neuropsychiatric disorders. *Journal of the American Medical Association, 272*, 1788–1791.

Swedo, S. E., Leonard, H. L., Garvey, M., Mittleman, B., Allen, A. J., Perlmtter, S., et al. (1998). Pediatric autoimmune neuropsychiatric disorders associated with streptococcal infections: Clinical description of the first 50 cases. *American Journal of Psychiatry, 155*, 264–271.

Swedo, S. E., Rapoport, J. L., Leonard, H., Lenane, M., & Cheslow, D. (1989). Obsessive-compulsive disorder in children and adolescents: Clinical phenomenology of 70 consecutive cases. *Archives of General Psychiatry, 46*, 335–341.

Tackett, J. L., & Kruger, R. F. (2005). Interpreting personality as a vulnerability for psychopathology. In B. L. Hankin & J. R. Z. Abela (Eds.), *Development of psychopathology: A vulnerability-stress perspective* (pp. 199–214). Thousand Oaks, CA: Sage.

Teplin, L. A., Abram, K. M., McClelland, G. M., Dulcan, M. K., & Mericle, A. A. (2002). Psychiatric disorders in youth in juvenile detention. *Archives of General Psychiatry, 59*, 1133–1143.

Terr, L. C. (1979). Children of Chowchilla: A study of psychic trauma. *Psychoanalytic Study of the Child, 34*, 552–623.

Terr, L. C. (1983). Chowchilla revisited: The effects of psychic trauma four years after a school-bus kidnapping. *Journal of Psychiatry, 140*, 1543–1550.

Thapar, A., & McGuffin, P. (1995). Are anxiety symptoms in children heritable? *Journal of Child Psychology and Psychiatry, 36*, 439–447.

Thomas, K. M., Drevets, W. C., Dahl, R. E., Ryan, N. D., Birmaher, B., Eccard, C. H., et al. (2001). Amygdala response to fearful faces in anxious and depressed children. *Archives of General Psychiatry, 58*, 1057–1063.

Thompson, R. A. (1994). Emotion regulation: In search of definition. In N. A. Fox (Ed.), The development of emotion regulation: Biological and behavioral considerations. *Monographs of the Society for Research in Child Development, 59*(2–3, Serial No. 240), 25–52.

Thompson, M., Kaslow, N. J., Weiss, B., & Nolen-Hoeksema, S. (1998). Children's attributional style questionnaire-revised: Psychometric examination. *Psychological Assessment, 10*, 166–170.

Thompson, R. A., & Meyer, S. (2007). Socialization of emotion regulation in the family. In J. J. Gross (Ed.), *Handbook of emotion regulation* (pp. 249–268). New York: Guilford.

Tillman, R., & Geller, B. (2003). Definitions of rapid, ultra-rapid, and ultradian cycling and of episode duration in pediatric and adult bipolar disorders: A proposal to distinguish episodes from cycles. *Journal of Child and Adolescent Psychopharmacology, 13*, 267–271.

Tomarken, A. J., & Keener, A. D. (1998). Frontal brain asymmetry and depression: A self-regulatory perspective. *Cognition and Emotion, 12*, 387–420.

Topolski, T. D., Hewitt, J. K., Eaves, L., Meyer, J. M., Silberg, J. L., Simonoff, E., et al. (1999). Genetic and environmental influences on ratings of manifest anxiety by parents and children. *Journal of Anxiety Disorders, 13*, 371–397.

Topolski, T. D., Hewitt, J. K., Eaves, L., Silberg, J. L., Meyer, J. M., Rutter, M., Pickles, A., & Simonoff, E. (1997). Genetic and environmental influences on child reports of manifest anxiety and symptoms of separation anxiety and overanxious disorders: A community-based twin study. *Behavior Genetics, 27*, 15–28.

Toth, S. L., & Cichetti, D. (1996). Patterns of relatedness and depressive symptomatology in maltreated children. *Journal of Consulting and Clinical Psychology, 64*, 32–41.

Toth, S. L., Manly, J. T., & Cichetti, D. (1992). Child maltreatment and vulnerability to depression. *Development and Psychopathology, 4*, 97–112.

Toth, S. L., Maughan, A., Manly, J. T., Spagnola, M., & Cichetti, D. (2002). The relative efficacy of two interventions in altering maltreated children's representational models: Implications for attachment theory. *Development and Psychopathology, 14*, 777–808.

Treadwell, K. H., & Kendall, P. C. (1996). Self-talk in anxiety-disordered youth: States of mind, content specificity, and treatment outcome. *Journal of Consulting and Clinical Psychology, 64*, 841–950.

Treatment for Adolescents with Depression Team. (2004). Fluoxetine, cognitive-behavioral therapy, and their combination for adolescents with depression. *Journal of the American Medical Association, 292*, 807–820.

Tucker, D. M., Derryberry, D., & Luu, P. (2000). Anatomy and physiology of human emotion: Vertical integration of brainstem, limbic, and cortical systems. In J. C. Borod (Ed.), *The neuropsychology of emotion* (pp. 56–79). London: Oxford University Press.

Turner, S. M., Beidel, C., & Cooley-Quille, M. R. (1995). Two year follow-up of social phobics treated with social effectiveness therapy. *Behaviour Research and Therapy, 33*, 553–556.

Turner, S. M., Beidel, C., & Costello, A. (1987). Psychopathology in the offspring of anxiety disorder patients. *Journal of Consulting and Clinical Psychology, 55*, 229–235.

U.S. Department of Health and Human Services (1999). *Mental health: A report of the surgeon general*. Rockville, MD: U.S. Department of Health and Human Services, Substance Abuse and Mental Health Services Administration, Center for Mental Health Services, National Institutes of Health, National Institute of Mental Health.

Umbreit, J., Ferro, J. B., Liaupsin, C. J., & Lane, K. L. (2007). *Functional behavioral assessment and function-based intervention: An effective, practical approach*. Upper Saddle River, NJ: Pearson Education.

Valleni-Basile, L. A., Garrison, C. Z., Jackosn, K. L., Waller, J. L., McKeown, R. E., Addy, C. L., & Cuffe, S. P. (1994). Frequency of obsessive-compulsive disorder in a community sample of young adolescents. *Journal of the American Academy of Child and Adolescent Psychiatry, 33*, 782–791.

Vasey, M. W., Crnic, K. A., & Carter, W. G. (1994). Worry in childhood: A developmental perspective. *Cognitive Therapy and Research, 18*, 529–549.

Vasey, M. W., & Dadds, M. R. (2001). An introduction to the developmental psychopathology of anxiety. In M. W. Vasey & M. R. Dadds (Eds.), *The developmental psychopathology of anxiety* (pp. 3–26). New York: Oxford University.

Vermetten, E., Vythilingam, M., Southwick, S. M., Charney, D. S., Bremmer, J. D., et al. (2003). Long-term treatment with paroxetine increases verbal declarative memory and hippocampal volume in post-traumatic stress disorder. *Biological Psychiatry, 54*, 693–702.

Viken, R. J., Rose, R. J., Kaprio, J., & Koskenvuo, M. (1994). A developmental genetic analysis of adult personality: Extraversion and neuroticism from 18 to 59 years of age. *Journal of Personality and Social Psychology, 66*, 722–730.

Vittengl, J. R., Clark, L. A., Dunn, T. W., & Jarrett, R. B. (2007). Reducing relapse and recurrence in unipolar depression: A comparative meta-analysis of cognitive-behavioral therapy's effects. *Journal of Consulting and Clinical Psychology, 75*, 475–488.

Vuilleumier, P. (2003). How brains behave: Neural mechanisms of emotional attention. *Trends in Cognitive Science, 9*, 585–594.

Wagner, K. D., Ambrosini, P., Rynn, M., Wohlberg, C., Yang, B., Greenbaum, M. S., et al. (2003). Efficacy of sertraline in the treatment of children and adolescents with major depressive disorder: Two randomized controlled trials. *Journal of the American Medical Association, 290*, 1033–1041.

Walker, H. M., & Severson, H. H. (1992). *Systematic screening for behavior disorders (SSBD)* (2nd ed.). Longmont, CO: Sopris West.

Walker, H. M., & Shinn, M. R. (2010). Systemic, evidence-based approaches for promoting positive outcomes within a multitier framework: Moving from efficacy to effectiveness. In M. R. Shinn & H. M. Walker (Eds.), *Interventions for achievement and behavior problems in a three-tier model including RTI* (pp. 1–26). Bethesda, MD: National Association of School Psychologists.

Walsh, T. M., Stewart, S. H., McLaughlin, E., & Comeau, N. (2004). Gender differences in childhood anxiety sensitivity index (CASI) dimensions. *Journal of Anxiety Disorders, 18*, 696–706.

Watson, D. (2000). *Mood and temperament*. New York: Guilford.

Watson, D., Clark, L. A., & Harkness, A. R. (1994). Structures of personality and their relevance to psychopathology. *Journal of Abnormal Psychology, 103*, 346–353.

Watson, J. B., & Raynor, P. (1920). Conditioned emotional reactions. *Journal of Experimental Psychology, 3*, 1–4.

Wechsler, D. (1991). *Wechsler intelligence scale for children-third edition (WISC-III)*. San Antonio, TX: Psychological Corporation.

Weems, C. E., Silverman, W. K., & LaGreca, A. M. (2000). What do youth referred for anxiety problems worry about? Worry and its relation to anxiety and anxiety disorders in children and adolescents. *Journal of Abnormal Child Psychology, 28,* 63–72.

Weems, C. E., & Watts, S. E. (2005). Cognitive models of childhood anxiety. In C. M. Velotis (Ed.), *Anxiety disorder research* (pp. 205–232). Hauppauge, NY: Nova Science.

Weissman, M. M., Gammon, G. D., John, K., Merikangas, K. R., Warner, V., Prusoff, B. A., & Sholomskas, D. (1987). Children of depressed parents: Increased psychopathology and early onset of major depression. *Archives of General Psychiatry, 43,* 847–853.

Weissman, M. M., Leckman, J. R., Merikangas, K. R., Gammon, G. D., & Prusoff, B. A. (1984). Depression and anxiety disorders in parents and children: Results from the Yale Family Study. *Archives of General Psychiatry, 41,* 845–852.

Weissman, M. M., Markowitz, J. C., & Klerman, G. L. (2000). *Comprehensive guide to interpersonal psychotherapy*. New York: Basic Books.

Weissman, M. M., Wolk, S., Goldstein, R. B., Moreau, D., Adams, P., Greenwald, S., Klier, C. M., Ryan, N. D., Dahl, R. E., & Wickramaratne, P. (1999). Depressed adolescents grown up. *Journal of the American Medical Association, 281,* 1707–1713.

Weisz, J. R., McCarty, C. A., & Valeri, S. M. (2006). Effects of psychotherapy for depression in children and adolescents: A meta-analysis. *Psychological Bulletin, 132,* 132–149.

Weisz, J. R., Suwanlert, W., Chaiyasit, W., Weiss, B., Achenbach, T. M., & Walker, B. R. (1987). Epidemiology of behavioral and emotional problems among Thai and American children. *Journal of the American Academy of Child and Adolescent Psychiatry, 26,* 890–897.

Welsh, M., Parke, R. D., Widaman, K., & O'Neil, R. (2001). Linkages between children's social and academic competence: A longitudinal analysis. *Journal of School Psychology, 39,* 463–481.

Werner, E. E. (1995). Resilience in development. *Current Directions in Psychological Science, 4,* 81–85.

Werry, J. S. (2001). Pharmacological treatments of autism, attention deficit hyperactivity disorder, oppositional defiant disorder, and depression in children and youth: Commentary. *Journal of Clinical Child Psychology, 30,* 110–113.

West, P., & Sweeting, H. (2003). Fifteen, female, and stressed: Changing patterns of psychological distress over time. *Journal of Child Psychology and Psychiatry, 44,* 399–411.

Wewetzer, C., Jans, T., Muller, B., Neudorfl, A., Bucherl, U., Remschmidt, H., Warnke, A., & Herptetz-Dahlman, B. (2001). Long-term outcome and prognosis of obsessive-compulsive disorder with onset in childhood or adolescence. *European Child and Adolescent Psychiatry, 10,* 37–46.

Whitaker, A., Johnson, J., Shaffer, D., Rapoport, J. L., Kalikow, K., Walsh, B. T., et al. (1990). Uncommon troubles in young people: Prevalence estimates of selected psychiatric disorders in a nonreferred adolescent population. *Archives of General Psychiatry, 47,* 487–496.

Williams, N. L., Reardon, J. M., Murray, K. T., & Cole, T. M. (2005). Anxiety disorders: A developmental vulnerability-stress perspective. In B. L. Hankin & J. R. Z. Abela (Eds.), *Development of psychopathology: A vulnerability-stress perspective* (pp. 289–327). Thousand Oaks, CA: Sage.

Witt, J. C., Erchul, W. P., McKee, W. T., Pardue, M. M., & Wickstrom, K. F. (1991). Conversational control in school-based consultation: The relationship between consultant and consultee topic determination and consultation outcome. *Journal of Educational and Psychological Consultation, 2,* 101–116.

Wittchen, H., Stein, M., & Kessler, R. (1999). Social fears and social phobia in a community sample of adolescents and young adults. *Psychological Medicine, 29,* 309–323.

Wittchen, H. U., Zhao, S., Kessler, R. C., & Eaton, W. W. (1994). DSM-III-R generalized anxiety disorder in the National Comorbidity Survey. *Archives of General Psychiatry, 51,* 355–364.

Wood, J. J., McLeod, B. D., Sigman, M., Hwang, W., & Chu, B. C. (2003). Parenting and childhood anxiety: Theory, empirical findings, and future directions. *Journal of Child Psychology and Psychiatry, 44,* 134–151.

Woodward, L. J., & Ferguson, D. M. (2001). Life course outcomes of young people with anxiety disorders in adolescence. *Journal of the American Academy of Child and Adolescent Psychiatry, 40,* 1086–1093.

World Health Organization. (1993). *The ICD-10 classification of mental and behavioural disorders: Diagnostic criteria for research.* Geneva: World Health Organization.

Yonkers, K. A., Warshaw, M. R., Maisson, A. O., & Keller, M. B. (1996). Phenomenology and course of generalized anxiety disorder. *British Journal of Psychiatry, 168,* 308–313.

Yonkers, K. A., Zlotnick, C., Allsworth, J., Warsahw, M., Shea, T., & Keller, M. B. (1998). Is the course of panic disorder the same in men and women? *American Journal of Psychiatry, 155,* 596–602.

Young, J. E. (1999). *Cognitive therapy for personality disorders: A schema-focused approach* (3rd ed.). Sarasota, FL: Professional Resource Press.

Young Mun, E., Fitzgerald, H. E., Von Eye, A., Puttler, L. I., & Zucker, R. A. (2001). Temperamental characteristics as predictors of externalizing and internalizing child behavior problems in the contexts of high and low parental psychopathology. *Infant Mental Health Journal, 22,* 393–415.

Young, J. F., & Mufson, L. (2008). Interpersonal psychotherapy for treatment and prevention of adolescent depression. In J. R. Z. Abela & B. L. Hankin (Eds.), *Handbook of depression in children and adolescents* (pp. 288–306). New York: Guilford.

Youngstrom, E. A. (2009). Definitional issues in bipolar disorder over the life cycle. *Clinical Psychology: Science and Practice, 16,* 140–160.

Youngstrom, E. A. (2010). *Bipolar disorder in children and adolescents.* Workshop presented at the Annual Convention of the National Association of School Psychologists, Chicago, IL.

Zirkel, P. (2003). Top five Section 504 errors. *ELA Notes, 38(3),* 5. Dayton, OH: Education Law Association

About the Author

Thomas J. Huberty is Professor of School Psychology at Indiana University. He received his Ph.D. in Educational (School) Psychology from the University of Missouri in 1980. His teaching and research interests are in anxiety and depression, developmental psychopathology, personality assessment, cognitive–behavioral interventions, mental health of children and youth, and special education and mental health law. Professional experiences include working as a psychologist in community mental health, developmental disabilities, pediatric psychology, public schools, and Head Start. He is a licensed psychologist in Indiana, is board certified in School Psychology by the American Board of Professional Psychology, and is a Fellow of the American Academy of School Psychology. In addition, he has been an administrative law judge/independent hearing officer for more than 20 years for due process hearings under the auspices of the Individuals with Disabilities Education Act (IDEA) and Section 504 of the Rehabilitation Act of 1973. In that role, he has presided over numerous due process hearings and has issued many legally binding decisions regarding students with special needs.

Index

T.J. Huberty, *Anxiety and Depression in Children and Adolescents:
Assessment, Intervention, and Prevention*, DOI 10.1007/978-1-4614-3110-7,
© Springer Science+Business Media, LLC 2012

CPSIA information can be obtained at www.ICGtesting.com
Printed in the USA
LVOW100500230313

325696LV00008B/147/P